Guide to Internal Medicine

Guide to Internal Medicine

● *Editors*

Douglas S. Paauw, MD

Associate Professor of Medicine,
Coordinator for Student Teaching,
Division of General Internal Medicine,
Department of Medicine,
University of Washington School of Medicine,
Seattle, Washington

Lisanne R. Burkholder, MD, MPH

Acting Instructor of Medicine,
Division of General Internal Medicine,
Department of Medicine,
University of Washington School of Medicine,
Seattle, Washington

Mary B. Migeon, MD

Acting Instructor of Medicine,
Division of General Internal Medicine,
Department of Medicine,
University of Washington School of Medicine,
Seattle, Washington

with 59 illustrations

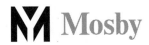

St. Louis Baltimore Boston Carlsbad Chicago Minneapolis New York Philadelphia Portland
London Milan Sydney Tokyo Toronto

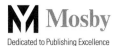

Mosby
Dedicated to Publishing Excellence

Acquiring Editor: Beverly J. Copland
Associate Developmental Editor: Shelby McCoy
Project Manager: Carol Sullivan Weis
Senior Production Editor: Rick Dudley
Designer: Jennifer Marmarinos

Composition by Top Graphics
Printing/binding by Quebecor, Kingsport, Tennessee

Mosby, Inc.
11830 Westline Industrial Drive
St. Louis, Missouri 63146

Library of Congress Cataloging in Publication Data
Guide to internal medicine / editors, Douglas S. Paauw, Lisanne R.
   Burkholder, Mary B. Migeon.—1st ed.
      p.   cm.
   Includes index.
   ISBN 0-323-00921-2
   1. Internal medicine.   I. Paauw, Douglas S. (Douglas Stephen),
1958- . II. Burkholder, Lisanne R.   III. Migeon, Mary B.
   [DNLM: 1. Internal Medicine. 2. Internal Medicine Examination
Questions.   WB 115 G946 1999]
RC46.G896   1999
616—dc21
DNLM/DLC
for Library of Congress   99-14131
                                                               CIP

99 00 01 02 03 / 9 8 7 6 5 4 3 2 1

Contributors

Amy Baernstein, MD
Acting Instructor,
Division of General Internal Medicine,
Department of Medicine,
University of Washington School of Medicine,
Seattle, Washington

Ernie-Paul Barrette, MD
Assistant Professor of Medicine,
Division of General Internal Medicine,
Department of Medicine,
University of Washington School of Medicine,
Seattle, Washington

Clarence H. Braddock III, MD, MPH
Assistant Professor of Medicine,
Adjunct Assistant Professor of Medical History and Ethics,
Adjunct Assistant Professor of Health Services,
Director, Center for Education and Development,
Veterans Administration—Puget Sound,
Department of Medicine,
University of Washington School of Medicine,
Seattle, Washington

Janis D. Bridge, MD, MPH
Acting Instructor of Medicine,
Division of General Internal Medicine,
Department of Medicine,
University of Washington School of Medicine,
Seattle, Washington

Lisanne R. Burkholder, MD, MPH
Acting Instructor of Medicine,
Division of General Internal Medicine,
Department of Medicine,
University of Washington School of Medicine,
Seattle, Washington

Sarah L. Clever, MD
Resident Physician,
Division of General Internal Medicine,
Department of Medicine,
University of Washington School of Medicine,
Seattle, Washington

Debra D. Dahlen, MD
Senior Fellow,
Division of Hematology,
Department of Medicine,
University of Washington School of Medicine,
Seattle, Washington

Dawn E. DeWitt, MD, MSc, FACP
Assistant Professor of Medicine,
Division of General Internal Medicine,
Department of Medicine,
University of Washington School of Medicine,
Seattle, Washington

Kelly Edwards, MA
Project Manager, Bioethics Education Project,
Department of Medical History and Ethics,
University of Washington School of Medicine,
Seattle, Washington

Gregory C. Gardner, MD
Associate Professor,
Division of Rheumatology,
Department of Medicine,
University of Washington School of Medicine,
Seattle, Washington

Barak Gaster, MD
Acting Assistant Professor of Medicine,
Division of General Internal Medicine,
Department of Medicine,
University of Washington School of Medicine,
Seattle, Washington

Michael J. Geist, MD
Madrona Medical Group,
Bellingham, Washington

Karna Gendo, MD
Chief Resident, Ambulatory Care,
Harborview Medical Center,
Department of Medicine,
University of Washington School of Medicine,
Seattle, Washington

Bruce Gilliland, MD, FACP
Professor of Medicine,
Professor of Laboratory Medicine,
Department of Medicine,
University of Washington School of Medicine,
Seattle, Washington

Deborah L. Greenberg, MD
Assistant Professor of Medicine,
Division of General Internal Medicine,
Department of Medicine,
University of Washington School of Medicine,
Seattle, Washington

Noreen R. Henig, MD
Senior Fellow, Pulmonary and Critical Care Medicine,
Department of Medicine,
University of Washington School of Medicine,
Seattle, Washington

John B. Holroyd, MD
Chief Resident, Ambulatory Care,
University of Washington Medical Center,
Department of Medicine,
University of Washington School of Medicine,
Seattle, Washington

Serena P. Koenig, MD
Instructor of Medicine,
Department of Internal Medicine,
Harvard Medical School,
Boston, Massachusetts

Mary B. Laya, MD, MPH
Assistant Professor of Medicine,
Division of General Internal Medicine,
Department of Medicine,
University of Washington School of Medicine,
Seattle, Washington

Terry J. Mengert, MD
Associate Professor of Medicine,
Division of Emergency Medicine,
Department of Medicine,
University of Washington School of Medicine,
Seattle, Washington

Mary B. Migeon, MD
Acting Instructor of Medicine,
Division of General Internal Medicine,
Department of Medicine,
University of Washington School of Medicine,
Seattle, Washington

George Novan, MD
Clinical Associate Professor of Medicine,
Department of Medicine,
University of Washington School of Medicine,
Seattle, Washington;
Director, Internal Medicine Spokane,
Spokane, Washington

Douglas S. Paauw, MD, FACP
Associate Professor of Medicine,
Coordinator for Student Teaching,
Division of General Internal Medicine,
Department of Medicine,
University of Washington School of Medicine,
Seattle, Washington

Linda Pinsky, MD
Assistant Professor of Medicine,
Adjunct Assistant Professor of Medical Education,
Division of General Internal Medicine,
Department of Medicine,
University of Washington School of Medicine,
Seattle, Washington

Heidi S. Powell, MD
Acting Assistant Professor of Medicine,
Division of General Internal Medicine,
Department of Medicine,
University of Washington School of Medicine,
Seattle, Washington

Alexander D. Schafir, MD
Assistant Professor of Medicine,
Medical Director, Internal Medicine Clinic,
Oregon Health Sciences University,
Portland, Oregon

John V.L. Sheffield, MD
Assistant Professor of Medicine,
Division of General Internal Medicine,
Department of Medicine,
University of Washington School of Medicine,
Seattle, Washington

C. Scott Smith, MD, FACP
Associate Professor of Medicine,
Adjunct Associate Professor of Medical Education,
Division of General Internal Medicine,
Department of Medicine,
University of Washington School of Medicine,
Seattle, Washington

James P. Souza, MD
Staff Physician,
Veterans Administration Medical Center,
Boise, Idaho

Thomas O. Staiger, MD
Assistant Professor of Medicine,
Division of General Internal Medicine,
Department of Medicine,
University of Washington School of Medicine,
Seattle, Washington

John Daryl Thornton, MD
Chief Resident,
Seattle VA Medical Center,
Department of Medicine,
University of Washington School of Medicine,
Seattle, Washington

Jeffrey I. Wallace, MD, MPH
Assistant Professor of Medicine,
Division of Gerontology and Geriatric Medicine,
Department of Medicine,
University of Washington School of Medicine,
Seattle, Washington

James P. Willems, MD
Chief Medicine Resident,
University of Washington Medical Center,
Department of Medicine,
University of Washington School of Medicine,
Seattle, Washington

Emily Y. Wong, MD
Assistant Professor of Medicine,
Division of General Internal Medicine,
Department of Medicine,
University of Washington School of Medicine,
Seattle, Washington

To
Kathy and Carly
Blaine and Kristen
Jacques, Sophie, and Jonathan
In memory of George Aagaard

Preface

Here at last is all you need to know to enjoy and succeed in the internal medicine clerkship. This guide blends the best of the how-to manuals with essential concepts from traditional medicine texts and also covers outpatient medicine. Using this guide, you can master key skills and knowledge useful to you throughout your medical training.

The guide is divided into three sections covering basic skills, common symptoms, and common conditions. These topics are easily read cover-to-cover during a medicine clerkship. Throughout the text you will find questions frequently asked during rotations. *Key points* in each chapter help you focus your learning. *Practice cases* apply your learning to real clinical scenarios. *Learning objectives* accompany answers to each case-based problem, reiterating key information to be gleaned from the chapter. A *multiple-choice exam* at the end of the guide tests your mastery of the material and prepares you for your clinical exams.

Although the guide specifically targets medical students, it is a valuable resource for learners and educators in a wide variety of medical settings, including internal medicine, family practice, physician assistant, and nurse practitioner programs.

Acknowledgments

We would like to thank: Jackie Swihart, Kellie Engle, Marsha Donaldson, and Karen McMasters for invaluable administrative assistance in preparing the manuscript; Daniel Bor for legal advice; D.C. Dugdale and Dawn DeWitt for sage advice about the world of publishing; Michael Richardson for enthusiastic and generous sharing of his extensive radiologic website resources; and to our students, who inspire us with their enthusiasm and whose thoughtful feedback helped shape this book.

Contents

SECTION 3   Patients Presenting With a Known Condition

Guide to Internal Medicine

Introduction to the Medicine Clerkship

1

Secrets to Being a Successful Medical Student

Medicine is not a trade to be learned but a profession to be entered. It is an ever widening field that requires continued study and prolonged experience in close contact with the sick. All that the medical school can hope to do is to supply the foundations on which to build.

Francis W. Peabody, 1927

What can I do to be successful in the Internal Medicine clerkship?

Within the confines of the lecture hall, success is often defined by grades. In the clerkships, performance evaluations remain very important, but as you enter the clinical years, you must seek to define personal goals and definitions of success that are broader than pass/fail. For the purpose of the medicine clerkship, you may hope to learn how to provide excellent patient care, develop your history-taking and physical examination skills, improve your presentations, acquire time-management skills, become a careful diagnostician, or simply survive the experience. Whatever your initial goals, one important measure of success is the degree to which a student acquires knowledge, clinical skills, work habits, values, and behavioral attributes that can serve as a foundation for subsequent training and career. In these introductory pages, the suggestions made are based on years of experience working with students and will hopefully help you excel in the clerkship and enjoy the experience.

Be enthusiastic

Your energy level, desire to learn, and spirit will motivate your residents and attendings to teach and involve you in patient care. With enthusiasm, a student with an average knowledge base can provide fantastic care and be a vital team member. Without enthusiasm, a brilliant student may appear disinterested and be a less effective team member and physician.

Know your patients

An excellent student has complete command of a patient's history, physical examination, and laboratory test results, strives to understand basic pathophysiologic principles underlying patient conditions, is aware of diagnostic and therapeutic options available, and seeks to understand the personal and social factors that may influence the patient's response to therapy.

Care about your patients

Assume personal responsibility for the quality of care your patients receive. Monitor their progress closely, and spend time at the bedside to discuss matters other than symptoms. Although team hierarchy gives residents and attendings precedence, your patients will view you as their primary physician if you establish a caring rapport.

Communicate with precision

Your chart notes and oral presentations are your opportunity to demonstrate your fund of knowledge, problem-solving skill, and ability to think clearly. Legible and precise order writing is essential to good patient care. Careful explanation of the treatment plan to nursing staff will ensure that your intended plan is followed.

Distinguish between major and minor problems

As important as being able to identify all of your patient's problems is the ability to put major and minor problems in perspective. At first, it is natural to consider all problems important, but time constraints make it essential that you prioritize when presenting cases and planning your workday. Attend to all of your patient's issues, but keep a steady focus on the big picture. This will allow you to budget time more efficiently and manage patients more effectively.

Acknowledge your knowledge deficits and seek guidance whenever necessary

At the beginning of the clerkship, you are not expected to know much about taking care of patients. When you encounter uncertainty, take note of it and do not try to hide it from others. Seek guidance from house staff, nurses, attendings, patients, therapists, and the literature. Do not judge yourself harshly. Instead, get excited to learn something new. Your patients will be better off.

Develop sound reading habits to use throughout your career

It is impossible to know everything, but it is a good idea to avoid being ignorant about the same thing twice. Each day, keep a list of things you do not understand and read about them later. You may be amazed by how much you retain when the material you read is relevant to your patients.

Behave professionally

It is expected that you will approach patients with empathy and respect their individual dignity and confidentiality. Strive to be cooperative, patient, and attentive at all times, even with difficult persons. It is a privilege to care for fellow human beings. When in doubt, follow the Golden Rule.

Be a team player

Medical care is provided by professionals from multiple disciplines who share the common goal of serving the patient. To contribute, you must understand the special role of nurses, therapists, and pharmacists and use them appropriately. Strong team spirit can motivate you to provide excellent care despite fatigue and stress. Earn respect by being respectful.

Work well with nurses

Nurses spend their entire day at your patient's bedside and can provide valuable insight into patient progress. Experienced nurses know a lot about patient assessment and ways to provide comfort. Some students find this intimidating and end up treating nurses unpleasantly. It is far preferable to acknowledge nursing expertise openly and try to learn from the suggestions made.

Strike a healthy balance between medicine and personal life

Sleep, exercise, good food, and leisure activities with family and friends are vital to your soul. To sustain your energy and focus at the hospital, you must attend to your personal happiness. A healthy balance in your life can help you cope with the anxiety of adapting to your new role and responsibilities and to accept this challenge eagerly. If all goes well on the rotation, you will glimpse the profound satisfaction available to those who care for the sick and gain insight into the kind of doctor you want to become.

2

Day-to-Day Inpatient Skills

What are a student's responsibilities on a ward team?

On the inpatient wards, you are expected to be your team's "expert" on all patients you admit and to participate actively in all aspects of their care. In addition to knowing everything about your patients (and always having patient data readily available), you should write all but emergent orders (cosigned by house staff or attending), represent and speak for your team wherever your patients are discussed, complete chart notes in a timely manner, perform procedures with appropriate supervision, and contribute to all diagnostic and treatment planning. You may also be asked to research interesting aspects of your patients' cases and teach the team during rounds. In addition, you should pay attention on rounds to learn from all patients on the team, and you should be ready and willing to help care for any patient as necessary. Finally, students can be a very important source of energy, enthusiasm, curiosity, and fresh humanitarian spirit for their teams. This energy is often crucial to team morale.

Do I need to preround?

Yes! The work day officially begins with work rounds, at which time the team sets a plan for the day for each patient. Before work rounds, you should preround, which consists of reviewing chart notes, checking vital signs, doing a directed physical examination, and checking laboratory test values. Allow 10 to 15 minutes per patient and be ready to start work rounds on time.

How much information should I gather in the H&P?

Your history and physical (H&P) should be complete on every patient you admit. Outstanding physicians take excellent histories and possess superior physical examination skills. The history provides information to make most diagnoses, and optimal patient care depends on the accuracy of this information and the strength of the doctor-patient relationship created in the process. With practice and repetition, you will gain confidence in your ability to identify your patients' problems and become more efficient, but the medicine clerkship is not a place to cut corners.

What is a good presentation?

Many students approach case presentations as if their primary purpose was student evaluation. In fact, the main object of the presentation is to convey the essentials of the patient's illness to team members so that all can learn and participate in subsequent discussions of management. This requires more than a simple recitation of what a patient told you; it should be an organization of the problems, your assessment, and your plan. At the end of a good presentation, your team should understand a patient's most pressing issues and your plan to address them. Be prepared to discuss these. Attributes of good work rounds presentations include:

- **Brevity:** The goal is 3 to 5 minutes for a new patient (less for daily progress reports). At first, you will need to learn from your resident what information is appropriate; you only have time for crucial details. Expect questions and leave time for them.
- **Organization:** Practice on your on-call day. Do not improvise. People expect to hear information presented in a certain order. Disorganization creates confusion.
- **Eye contact:** Engage your team and they will listen. Presenting from memory greatly enhances your ability to achieve this goal. Never ever read from your H&P.

What should I include in my write-ups?

Of all the notes in your patient's chart, yours should be the most complete. Initial write-ups generally average 3 to 6 pages and should succinctly review the history, examination, laboratory test values, diagnostic reasoning, and plan. The following are a few suggestions of ways to avoid common pitfalls:

- **Chronology:** Use day of admission as a consistent point of reference ("3 days prior to admission [PTA], she noticed chest pain. 1 day PTA, she noted shortness of breath.").
- **Pertinent negatives:** Include these at the end of the history of present illness (HPI) to reflect the differential diagnosis.

- **Abbreviations:** Use only familiar abbreviations; write everything else out.
- **Organization:** Use an outline for past medical history (PMH), examination, and plan so details can be found at a glance.
- **Completeness:** Describe physical findings completely; be attentive to detail.

How do I write a good Assessment and Plan?

The Assessment & Plan section is probably the source of greatest confusion for most students. It is actually quite simple. First, state the problem (diagnosis, symptom, sign, or laboratory result). Second, give a realistic differential diagnosis for that problem. Third, state which diagnosis is most likely and why others are not, incorporating data from your H&P. Finally, for each problem, list the diagnostic and therapeutic plan so that readers can rapidly find and review your plan. By following this formula, you will avoid the two most common mistakes:

- **Don't ramble:** Rambling assessments that regurgitate textbook differentials and pathophysiology reflect poor synthesis of information and are not relevant to the case.
- **Don't be too brief:** Very brief assessments reflect poor understanding of the differential diagnosis and rationale for evaluation and treatment.

What should I try to learn when reading about my patients?

To monitor your patients effectively and contribute to diagnostic and therapeutic decision-making, begin by reviewing the following information:

- **Pathophysiology:** Disease processes of the major diagnoses in your patients
- **Typical signs and symptoms:** For the major conditions in the differential diagnosis
- **Diagnostic algorithm:** Rationale for tests, sequence of testing, cost, and potential ramifications of test results on therapeutic options
- **Treatment algorithm:** Rationale for choosing treatment options, including efficacy and cost
- **Drug side effects:** Side effects/toxicities, drug interactions, and convenience

Which reading sources are most useful?

Anything you read in the attempt to provide excellent patient care will be better retained than information reviewed out of context, but different sources have different attributes. *Syllabi/spiral-bound manuals* provide concise reviews with practical management advice. *Texts* are strong on pathophysiology and typical disease signs and symptoms but can be out of date regarding workup and therapy. Texts tend to pack details densely, so some students have difficulty distinguishing and remembering key information. *MEDLINE* is a comprehensive on-line guide to the medical literature. Being able to construct a literature search to answer a clinical question is an essential skill, but be sure you have a firm grasp of the basics first and that the articles you pull are relevant to your patient.

3

Day-to-Day Outpatient Skills

How do I prioritize the outpatient visit?

Whereas inpatients often have a single problem leading to hospitalization, outpatients usually present several issues for you to address in a brief period of time. Often you will not have time to deal with every issue and must determine which to address in a single visit. Each visit should begin with an attempt to set an agenda for that visit. Before entering the room, review the problem list and set some goals. When you see the patient, ask what goals they have: "What are your concerns today?" After you have heard the patient's list, try to cover key management goals and special patient concerns, and avoid overlooking potentially serious new problems. You may respond: "Those are a lot of important issues. Let's cover your blood pressure and sore leg today. We probably won't have time to discuss the chronic shoulder pain, but let's do that carefully next time, okay?"

What is an appropriate examination?

Your examination should address the problems of the day. For a patient with a sore throat, vital signs and a good HEENT (head, eyes, ears, nose, and throat), neck, and lung examination should suffice. A complete examination is generally done only with new patients or those with vague or troubling symptoms, and when patients request it specifically.

What should I present to my attending?

In clinic, your presentations should clarify the issues you discussed and your plan for each. Be sure to let your attendings know when you are running behind and how they might help you most. One popular and effective format is as follows:

Frame the patient and identify a question that you want the attending to address

Mr. K is a 45-year-old man with diabetes, hypertension, and depression. He is here for a new lesion on his leg and for a blood pressure check. I'd like you to look at his leg with me, and I need your thoughts on his blood pressure (BP).

Give an efficient, problem-based history, examination, and plan

Leg lesion. He noticed this lesion a few months ago, and it's gradually grown. He doesn't recall injuring himself, and it's nontender. He has not had fever or chills. On examination, the temperature is 37°; and on his right anterior shin he has a smooth, shiny, well-demarcated plaque with central atrophy and telangiectasia. The surrounding leg and skin are normal in appearance and sensation is intact. Because he's diabetic, I was originally concerned about infection, but there are no signs or symptoms of that. Could you look at it with me?

Blood pressure. He's had hypertension for 5 years, and it had been well controlled until recently when his medication doses have had to be increased. He's currently taking atenolol 50 mg, hydrochlorothiazide 25 mg, and lisinopril 20 mg. He does not drink and has always been compliant with his medications. Now his pressures at home range from 140s to 150s over 90s. In clinic today, his pressure is 152/92 and pulse is 54. There is no edema. I hear a bruit over the right femoral artery. I am concerned that he might be developing renovascular disease, and I'd like to order a renal artery duplex.

Other issues. We didn't talk about his diabetes today. I'd like to schedule an appointment for follow-up in 2 weeks to go over that and his test results.

Get feedback
Any suggestions for me?

What should I include in my notes?

When reviewing your clinic notes, a reader should be able to rapidly identify your patient's problems, medications, and management plan. With the exception of the Assessment & Plan section, clinic notes are generally much more concise than ward notes. Basic elements include:

- **Initial diagnosis/chief complaint (ID/CC):** Briefly frame the patient and purpose of the visit
- **Problem list**

- **Medications**
- **Current concerns:** Concise histories of problems addressed
- **Examination:** Detailed descriptions of examination performed that day
- **Laboratory test values:** Summarize key findings only
- **Assessment & Plan:** For each problem, discuss your rationale and plan

What is my responsibility for follow-up?

It is your responsibility to follow up on your patient's test results and determine appropriate timing for a return visit. Before a patient leaves clinic, review how they will learn of test results. You may need to devise a system to remind you to look up results. When tests are back, you should either send a letter or make a phone call to the patient. In some clinics, patients can call in for results, but this may not be adequate for abnormal results. You should also discuss when the patient should return to clinic. There are no clear guidelines to follow, so this can be deceptively difficult. Ask your attending if you are unclear. From the standpoint of your education, scheduling return visits before you leave the rotation will enhance your experience significantly.

When should I read?

Although clinic rotations generally include more free time than exists on ward rotations, some find it difficult to incorporate reading into diagnostic and therapeutic decision-making in clinic. Several little breaks in the clinic routine exist, however, and you can use each to advantage. Read *before the visit,* especially when you know the chief complaint and are unsure what an appropriate history and examination would entail. Ask your attending for guidance on what to read. A few minutes of advance preparation can save time in the room. Read *before the examination* to look up something during the minute a patient takes to disrobe, but be quick! Read *before your presentation* to clarify questions about diagnosis, elements of the story, examination, or laboratory test results before you present to the attending. Read *between visits* to take advantage of any gaps in your student schedule.

4

Communicating With Patients

What barriers to communicating with patients will I encounter?

Most physicians begin their careers hoping to convey caring, respect, and compassion. This becomes a challenge in a busy day filled with multiple distractions and patient-care demands. Through training, physicians are taught to elicit specific pertinent positive and negative findings on history and physical to fit patient symptoms and examination findings into defined sets of diagnostic criteria. This clashes with patients' needs to feel heard, respected, and understood as individuals. The busy physician's desire for concise data organized in diagnostic packages can be frustrated by human storytelling, which often unfolds in circuitous, unpredictable, and revealing ways. Cross-cultural differences between physicians and patients often widen this gap. A power imbalance is also inherent in the physician-patient interaction and may impede good communication. Finding ways to appreciate the breadth of human expression while you are in the midst of gathering data is key to fostering long-term job satisfaction.

How can my nonverbal cues help communicate caring and respect to patients?

Nonverbal cues can reduce the inherent power imbalance, can improve your ability to convey respect and caring, and may be more important than what you say. Sit across from the patient at eye level to avoid the power difference implied by looming above a patient. Maintain good eye contact. Practice respectful listening, an exercise in sharing rather than taking control of the conversation. Furtive glances at a watch signal that you have other more important things to do. Instead, it is better to openly acknowledge time limits and plan with the patient for the best use of time. Stay on schedule, especially in clinic, respecting patients' busy lives. The examination is another powerful venue for nonverbal cues. Do not poke and prod to extract information with your hands. Instead, listen gently, respectfully, and deliberately with your hands. Your patients will feel the difference.

What can I say during a visit with a patient to improve communication?

Physicians interrupt patients on average within the first 7 to 11 seconds of history. To avoid this annoying pattern, initially say very little. Say hello using the patient's name. Introduce yourself. Ask what he or she wants to accomplish in the visit and allow the patient to respond without interruption. After several minutes, if you feel it is necessary, you can gently redirect patients with rambling stories: "Now let's get back to your chest pain," or "We need to stay focused or I won't be very helpful to you," or "I'm afraid we won't accomplish your goals for this visit if we stray too far from your chest pain." Some specifics about how you ask questions may be helpful. Begin with open-ended questions. Try not to assume the answer in how you ask the question. During the examination, keep the patient involved as a partner in the experience by explaining what you are doing as you go. Reassure patients as you perform the examination that things are normal. Briefly review your findings at the end of the examination. Give patients permission to stop you if the examination is too uncomfortable, especially for pelvic examinations.

What do I accomplish with a good history?

You accomplish many things during the history. Incidentally, it may be wise to think of "hearing" a history rather than "taking" one. Use verbal and nonverbal cues to establish a partnership of trust and mutual understanding. Set boundaries and expectations. Elicit patient perceptions about illness (i.e., "What does this illness mean to you?") and about the role they expect their physician to play in their health care (i.e., "What do you hope I can do to help you?"). And, of course, ask about all those pertinent positive and negative clues to diagnose illness.

How do I communicate test results?

Set patient expectations when you order the test about when and how you will communicate results. Also, explain what you are hoping to learn from the test. In the inpatient setting, laboratory and test results that provide significant new information should be shared with patients daily, ideally as soon as they are available. Be brief. Use language the patient can understand to explain the meaning of the test. You may start by asking the patient if he or she remembers your earlier conversation about why the test was obtained. This helps you assess if they have understood prior discussions. Follow-up of test results is trickier in the outpatient setting. You may send a letter if things are normal (warn patients that this takes several weeks), or call if things are abnormal.

How do I give bad news?

Often, it is effective to start with a screening question to assess the patient's understanding of why the test was obtained, what they think is likely to be found, and what they are ready to hear. This may make it easier to confirm their suspicions with the bad result (e.g., "Do you understand why we got that CT scan of your abdomen?"). Keep it simple, short, and direct (e.g., "I have bad news. The CT scan shows cancer"). Give the patient time to absorb bad news; a pause is useful for this. Offer to answer questions at the time and again later once the patient has had time to deal with the news. If you do not know the answer to a question, say so and offer to find out. It is often reassuring for patients to hear that you are going to be there to see them through whatever happens next.

How do I do a successful bedside presentation?

Bedside presentation is a tradition that has unfortunately fallen out of favor with residents. Bedside presentations work well as the format for daily morning work rounds. With the entire team and patient present, the intern or student succinctly presents pertinent information regarding a patient's admission or hospital care and discusses the plan for the day. Generally, patients prefer hearing bedside presentations on work rounds rather than hearing pieces of conversations about them (or other patients) from the hallway. Bedside presentations provide an efficient way of updating the patient and team simultaneously, including the patient as a partner in plans, making rounds professional and succinct, and allowing quick confirmation of findings. Specific approaches to bedside rounds may vary by team and teaching institution. It is useful to orient the patient to the goals of this daily routine on their first day ("I'm going to tell the team why you came to the hospital and share the information we've gathered about you overnight"). Most patients respond appropriately when encouraged to participate ("Please correct my mistakes, and ask questions if anything isn't clear"). Some teams feel most comfortable speaking directly to the patient and using lay terms while remaining succinct in the presentation and discussion. Many residents object to bedside rounds for fear unanswerable questions may arise, or the patient may see that there are different opinions about how to proceed. However, this can also be seen as a strength of bedside rounds. Unanswerable questions or ambiguities about medical decisions can be openly acknowledged, with a plan of how to find the answer and when to get back to the patient with more information. Most patients appreciate being involved in this way and benefit greatly from seeing the complex and inexact nature of the decision-making process of medicine.

5

Ethics in Medicine

CONFIDENTIALITY

What does the duty of confidentiality require?

Confidentiality is one of the core tenets of medical practice. The obligation of confidentiality prohibits the physician from disclosing information about the patient's case to other parties without permission and encourages the physician to take precautions to ensure that only authorized access to information occurs. Discussions about patients with other physicians are often critical for patient care and are an integral part of the learning experience in a teaching hospital. These discussions are justifiable, so long as precautions are taken to limit the ability of others to hear or see confidential information.

What kinds of disclosure are inappropriate?

The realities of communication in medical practice make it difficult to protect patient confidentiality. Inappropriate disclosure of information occurs when cases are discussed in the elevator or hallway, when extra copies of handouts with patient information on them are left out, or when patient family members are informed, even about minor care issues, against the patient's wishes. The patient's right to privacy is not being respected in these situations.

When should confidentiality be breached?

Confidentiality is not an absolute obligation and may be broken if there is concern for the safety of specific persons or for public welfare. Clinicians have a duty to protect identifiable individuals from any serious threat of harm if they have information that could prevent the harm. In the most clear-cut cases of limited confidentiality, physicians are required by state law to report certain communicable or infectious diseases to public health authorities, such as acquired immunodeficiency syndrome (AIDS), gonorrhea, syphilis, hepatitis A and B, measles, and tuberculosis. Suspected cases of child, dependent adult, and elder abuse are reportable, as are gunshot wounds. Local municipal code and institutional policies can vary regarding what is reportable and standards of evidence required. It is best to ask about your institution's policy.

INFORMED CONSENT

What is informed consent?

The most important goal of informed consent is to allow the patient to be an informed participant in health care decisions. It originates from the legal and ethical right the patient has to direct what happens to his or her body and from the ethical duty of the physician to involve the patient in his or her health care. The term *basic consent* entails letting the patient know what you would like to do and asking him or her if that will be all right; it is appropriate for simple procedures, such as drawing blood. Decisions that merit this streamlined approach have a high level of community consensus and a low level of risk. A more formal process of informed consent should occur for more invasive procedures, such as lumbar puncture or thoracentesis. The more formal process includes a discussion of several aspects of the procedure (Box 5-1) and a consent form signed by the patient and filed in the chart.

BOX 5-1   Elements to Discuss When Obtaining Formal Patient Consent

- Nature of the decision/procedure
- Reasonable alternatives to the proposed intervention
- Relevant risks, benefits, and uncertainties related to each alternative
- Assessment of patient understanding
- Acceptance of the intervention by the patient

What are my responsibilities during the informed consent discussion?

Consent is only valid if given voluntarily by a patient competent to make the decision. Patients often feel powerless and vulnerable, and it is easy for coercive situations to arise in this setting. To encourage voluntariness, the physician must make clear to the patient that he or she is participating in a decision and not merely signing a form. With this understanding, the informed consent process should be seen as an invitation to the patient to participate in decisions. The physician is also generally obligated to share the reasoning process and provide a recommendation to the patient. Comprehension on the part of the patient is equally as important as the information provided. Consequently, the discussion should be carried on in lay terms and the patient's understanding should be assessed along the way.

What sorts of interventions require informed consent?

For a wide range of decisions, written consent is not required, but some meaningful discussion is needed. For instance, a man contemplating having a prostate-specific antigen (PSA) screen for prostate cancer should know the relevant arguments for and against this screening test, discussed in lay terms. Most health care institutions have policies that state which health interventions require a signed consent form. For example, surgery, anesthesia, and other invasive procedures are usually in this category.

Is there such a thing as implied consent?

Consent can be implied, rather than obtained, in emergency situations when the patient is unconscious or incompetent and no surrogate decision-maker is available. This is based on the principle of beneficence, which requires a physician to act on the patient's behalf when the patient's life is at stake. The patient's presence in the hospital ward, intensive care unit (ICU), or clinic does not imply consent to undergo treatment or procedures.

DO-NOT-RESUSCITATE ORDERS

What is a do-not-resuscitate order?

A do-not-resuscitate (DNR) order means that the patient will not receive cardiopulmonary resuscitation (CPR) if he or she is found with no pulse or respirations. In some cases, your patient will have a DNR order on the chart. In many cases, the question has never been addressed, and you will need to discuss preferences with your patient regarding CPR. Deciding whether to forgo future resuscitation involves careful consideration of potential clinical benefit and the patient's preferences.

Real or perceived differences in these two considerations make decisions to forgo CPR difficult.

When can CPR be withheld?

If your patient stops breathing or his or her heart stops beating in the hospital, the standard of care is to perform CPR in the absence of a valid physician's order to withhold it. CPR can be withheld when the patient, or the legal surrogate if the patient is not competent, clearly indicates that he or she does not want CPR should the need arise. It can also be withheld when CPR is deemed futile (judged to be of no medical benefit).

When is CPR "futile"?

CPR is futile when it offers the patient no clinical benefit; in such cases, you are ethically justified in withholding it. CPR has been prospectively evaluated in a wide variety of clinical situations. Knowing the probability of success with CPR can help determine futility. For instance, CPR has virtually 0% probability of success in the following clinical circumstances: septic shock, acute stroke, metastatic cancer, and severe pneumonia. Even in other clinical situations, survival after CPR is extremely limited.

How should the patient's quality of life be considered in decisions about CPR?

CPR might also be judged futile when the patient's quality of life is so poor that no meaningful survival is expected even if CPR were successful at restoring circulatory stability. Judging quality of life tempts prejudicial statements about patients with chronic illness or disability. There is substantial evidence that patients with chronic conditions often rate their quality of life much higher than healthy people would. Nevertheless, many would agree that patients in a permanent unconscious state possess a quality of life that virtually no one would accept. Therefore CPR is usually considered futile for patients in a persistent vegetative state.

Are "slow codes" ever justified?

"Slow codes" are those in which a half-hearted effort at resuscitation is made. Physicians may be tempted to resort to using a slow code when there is disagreement between the patient and the physician about the utility of CPR. Slow codes are not ethically justified.

What if the patient is unable to say what his or her wishes are?

In some cases, the decision about CPR must be made when the patient is unable to participate. There are two general approaches to this dilemma. One is to use an ex-

---

BOX 5-2 Hierarchy for Choosing a Surrogate Decision-Maker

1. Legal guardian with health care decision-making authority
2. Individual given durable power of attorney for health care decisions
3. Spouse
4. Adult children of patient (all in agreement)
5. Parents of patient
6. Adult siblings of patient (all in agreement)

BOX 5-3 Criteria Indicating Patient Competence to Make Treatment Decisions

- Understands the clinical information presented
- Appreciates the situation, including the consequences of refusing treatment
- Is able to display reason in deliberating about his or her choices
- Clearly communicates choice

---

isting *advance directive,* a document that indicates with some specificity the decisions the patient would like made should he or she be unable to participate. The other solution involves identifying a surrogate decision-maker. The law recognizes a hierarchy of family relationships in determining which family member should be the official "spokesperson" (Box 5-2), although ideally all close family members and significant others should be involved in the discussion and reach some consensus.

TERMINATION OF LIFE-SUSTAINING TREATMENTS

When is it justifiable to discontinue life-sustaining treatments?

Occasionally, you will have patients who are receiving treatments or interventions that keep them alive, and you will face the decision of whether to discontinue these treatments. Examples include dialysis for acute or chronic renal failure and mechanical ventilation for respiratory failure. In some circumstances, these treatments are no longer of benefit, whereas in others the patient or family no longer wants the treatment. If the patient has the ability to make decisions, fully understands the consequences of the decision, and states he or she no longer wants a treatment, it is justifiable to withdraw the treatment. Treatment withdrawal is also justifiable if the treatment no longer offers benefit to the patient.

Do different standards apply to withholding and withdrawing care?

Many clinicians feel that it is easier to not start (withhold) a treatment, such as mechanical ventilation, than to stop (withdraw) it. Although there is a natural tendency to believe this, there is no ethical or legal distinction between withholding and withdrawing treatment.

What if you are not sure if the patient is competent?

Patients must be "competent" to make treatment decisions. A better term is "decision-making capacity" to avoid confusion with legal determinations of competence. For example, an elderly grandfather may be found incompetent to manage a large estate but may still have intact capacity to make treatment decisions. The capacity to make treatment decisions, including withholding or withdrawing treatment, is considered intact if the patient satisfies all four basic criteria (Box 5-3). If the patient does not meet these criteria, then his or her decision-making capacity should be questioned and the surrogate decision-maker should be consulted. Sometimes the patient is awake, alert, and conversant, but his or her decisions seem questionable or irrational. It is important to distinguish an irrational decision from simple disagreement. In these situations, talk with the patient to clarify the reasoning.

What about the patient whose decision-making capacity varies from day to day?

Patients can move in and out of a coherent state from medication effects or their underlying disease. You should do what you can to catch a patient in a lucid state, lightening up on the medications if necessary, to include him or her in the decision-making process.

Does depression or other mental illness impair a patient's decision-making capacity?

Patients with active mental illness, including depression, should have their decision-making capacity evaluated carefully, usually by a psychiatrist. Patients should not be presumed to be unable to make treatment decisions. In several studies, patients voice similar preferences for life-sustaining treatments when depressed as they do after treatment of depression.

Key Points

- With a few exceptions, patient information should be kept in confidence.
- The ethical principle of respect for persons creates an obligation for physicians to foster patient participation in health care decisions.
- DNR orders should be written when the patient (or surrogate) states such a preference.
- Competent, fully informed patients have the right to refuse life-sustaining treatments.

CASE 5-2

A 64-year-old woman with multiple sclerosis is hospitalized. The team thinks that she may need to be placed on a feeding tube soon to ensure adequate nourishment. They ask the patient about this in the morning, and she agrees. However, in the evening (before the tube has been placed), the patient becomes disoriented and seems confused about her decision to have the feeding tube placed. She tells the team she does not want it in. They revisit the question in the morning, when the patient is again lucid. Unable to recall her state of mind from the previous evening, the patient again agrees to the procedure.

A. Is this patient competent to decide?

B. Which preference should be honored?

CASE 5-1

A 60-year-old man has a heart attack and is admitted to the medical floor with a very poor prognosis. He asks that you not share any of his medical information with his wife because he does not think she will be able to take it. His wife catches you in the hall and asks about her husband's prognosis.

A. Will you tell his wife?

B. What are you required to do legally?

CASE 5-3

Mr. H is a 24-year-old man who resides in a skilled nursing facility, where he is undergoing rehabilitation from a cervical spine injury. The injury left him quadriplegic. He has normal cognitive function and no problems with respiration. He is admitted to your service for treatment of pneumonia. The resident suggests antibiotics, chest physiotherapy, and hydration. One day while signing out Mr. H to the cross-covering intern, the intern says, "He should be a DNR, based on medical futility."

A. Is his case medically futile?

B. If so, why?

Practical Skills for the Medical Student

HOW TO READ ELECTROCARDIOGRAMS

How do I report ECG findings in my note?

A normal report covers the six key features of an electrocardiogram (ECG): "Normal sinus rhythm, rate of 70, normal axis, intervals, chamber sizes, and no ischemic changes."

How do I recognize normal sinus rhythm?

Normal sinus rhythm (Figure 6-1) occurs when orderly depolarization begins in the sinus node, progresses through the atria (P wave), traverses the atrioventricular (AV) node (PR interval), then passes through the ventricles (QRS complex), causing a ventricular contraction. After depolarization is finished, there is a brief pause (ST segment), and then the ventricles repolarize (T wave). Thus, in normal sinus rhythm, every QRS complex is preceded by a P wave and every P is followed by a QRS, with a constant PR interval for every beat.

How do I calculate the rate?

The heart rate is the number of ventricular contractions per minute. On a standard ECG, a little box passes by in 0.04 seconds, a big box in 0.2 seconds. Estimate the rate by counting the big boxes between each QRS complex and memorizing the corresponding rate (Table 6-1). Alternatively, use rate = 300/B, where B is the number of large boxes between each QRS complex.

Why is it useful to understand vectors?

Understanding vectors in the limb and precordial leads allows you to localize heart muscle injury (Table 6-2). Also, with vectors, you can calculate axis, which helps identify ventricular hypertrophy. You will need to read an ECG text for details about vectors. Normal axis of the QRS reflects the left ventricle's great muscle bulk, which points down and to the left between leads aV_F and I. Thus, if QRS is upward in both I and aV_F, the axis is normal. Left ventricular hypertrophy shifts the axis to the left and creates a negative QRS in lead aV_F. Right ventricular hypertrophy shifts the axis down and to the right, with a resultant negative QRS in lead I.

What specific changes will my patient with myocardial damage show on ECG?

In general, ST segment changes and flipped T waves occur with early myocardial damage; significant Q waves appear 24 to 48 hours later. The spectrum of injury ranges from reversible ischemia to irreversible infarction (Figure 6-2). T wave inversions are a nonspecific sign of myocardial ischemia or early infarction. Normal T waves follow the direction of the QRS complex but flip to the opposite direction with myocardial injury.

What are intervals all about?

Prolonged intervals represent delays in conduction. A PR interval greater than 1 big box indicates AV nodal block and can be caused by myocardial infarction (MI) or medications such as digoxin or diltiazem. QRS widening to beyond 3 small boxes (or 0.12 seconds) is caused by interventricular conduction delay, such as a bundle branch block. Detect left bundle branch block by the "rabbit ears" (RR′) in leads V_5-V_6. Right bundle branch block causes "rabbit ears" (RR′) in leads V_1-V_2. QT prolongation is important because it can lead to torsades de pointes, a deadly ventricular arrhythmia. The QT interval depends on the heart rate and is normal if it is less than half the RR interval. QT prolongation occurs with tricyclic antidepressant overdose, hypomag-

TABLE 6-1
Calculating Rate by the Number of Large Boxes Between QRS Complexes

Boxes between QRS complexes	1	2	3	4	5
Rate (beats per minute)	300	150	100	75	60

TABLE 6-2
Contiguous Leads That Localize Acute Myocardial Infarction

LOCATION	LEADS AFFECTED (ST, T, Q CHANGES)
Anterior wall of LV	V_1-V_4
Inferior wall of LV	II, III, aV_F
Lateral wall of LV	I, aV_L, V_5, V_6
Posterior wall of LV	V_1-V_2 (large R waves)
Septal wall	V_1-V_2
RV	Right-sided precordial leads

LV, Left ventricle; *RV*, right ventricle.

TABLE 6-3
Criteria for LV Hypertrophy Using Wave Amplitudes

R wave in aV_L	>11 mm high
(S in V_1 or V_2) + (R in V_5 or V_6)	>35 mm high

Waves: P, Q, R, S, T

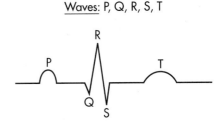

Intervals: PR, QRS, ST, QT

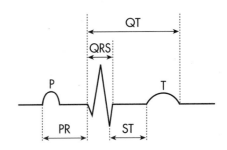

Figure 6-1 Components of a normal ECG tracing.

nesemia, hypocalcemia, some antiarrhythmic drugs, and interactions of some medications (e.g., cisapride with erythromycin).

How do I detect chamber wall hypertrophy or enlargement?

Left ventricular hypertrophy creates a leftward axis, large S waves in leads V_1-V_2, and large R waves in aV_L, V_5, and V_6 (Table 6-3). Right ventricular hypertrophy creates large R waves in leads V_1-V_2. Left atrial enlargement is best seen in V_1 as a late negative deflection in a biphasic P wave. The negative portion of the P wave must be greater than 1 mm deep and 1 box wide. Right atrial enlargement creates a large peaked P wave greater than 2.5 mm high, best seen in lead II.

HOW TO READ AN ABDOMINAL FILM

When should I obtain abdominal films?

Not all patients with abdominal pain require x-rays, which are often nonspecific. Obtain films to rule out perforation, obstruction, or chronic pancreatitis (Figure 6-3).

How do I order abdominal films?

Order an abdominal series: chest x-ray, supine and upright abdominal films. The chest x-ray shows the lung fields and diaphragms. This screens for pulmonary pathology (pneumonia) presenting with abdominal symptoms and for free air in the abdomen.

What key findings should I look for in an abdominal series?

Free air, a surgical emergency until proven otherwise, is best seen on chest x-ray as a dark crescent under the right diaphragm in contrast to the radiodense liver. If the patient cannot stand, a cross-table lateral with the patient's left side down will show free air. Common causes are bowel wall perforation from duodenal ulcer, diverticula, or cancer. Another critical finding is dilated colon from obstruction or ileus. If markedly dilated,

A   Reversible ischemia

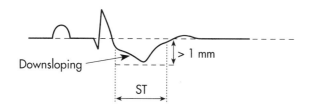

- Downsloping ST segment depression > 1 mm below baseline

B   Irreversible infarction
Early (minutes/hours)

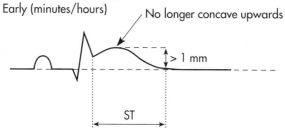

- ST segment elevation > 1 mm above baseline
- In 2 or more contiguous leads

C   Irreversible infarction
Late (hours/days)

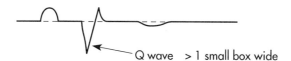

- T wave inversion
- Q waves > 1 box wide and deep
- In 2 or more contiguous leads

D   Pericarditis

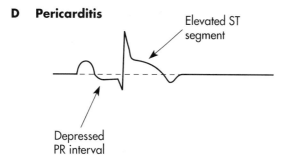

- Diffuse ST segment elevation
- Diffuse PR segment depression

Figure 6-2 ST segment and Q waves changes with myocardial damage **(A-C)** or pericardial inflammation **(D).**

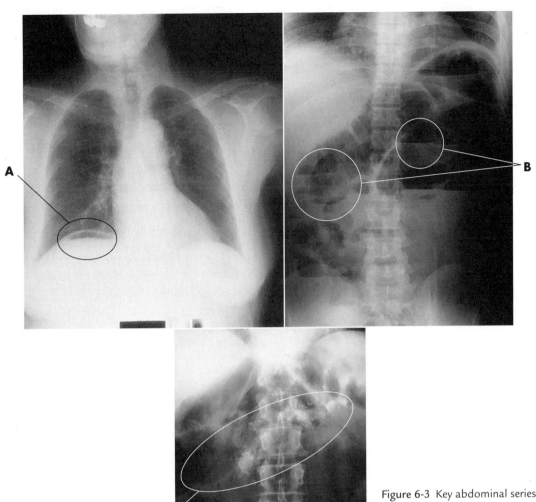

Figure 6-3 Key abdominal series findings. **A,** *Free air* indicates perforation. **B,** *Air fluid levels* of bowel obstruction. **C,** *Pancreatic calcifications* are pathognomonic for chronic pancreatitis.

toxic megacolon secondary to *Clostridium difficile* should be considered—also a risk for perforation.

What constitutes dilation for large and small bowel?

Roughly 3 cm for small intestine, 6 cm for large intestine, and 9 cm for the cecum. To discern between large and small bowel, use anatomy: small bowel valvulae are circumferential; in the large bowel, haustrations only partially embrace the circumference and give a scalloped border.

How can I tell the difference between ileus and bowel obstruction?

In both conditions, air-fluid levels and dilation are seen. Air in the rectum suggests ileus. In true obstruction, no air passes, so the rectum collapses within 24 hours.

Also, air-fluid levels the same height throughout the gut suggest obstruction, rather than the varying levels seen in ileus.

What other findings can be helpful?

Extensive stool suggests constipation. Arterial calcification raises concern for mesenteric ischemia. Gallstones or kidney stones may be seen. Pneumatosis, or air in the bowel wall, is a grim indicator of mesenteric necrosis. Hepatomegaly, splenomegaly, or enlarged kidneys may be suggested. Finally, bowel wall thickening from edema can be seen.

HOW TO READ CHEST FILMS

What should I look for on a chest film?

The key to chest x-ray reading is to proceed systematically through six major steps (Box 6-1). This ensures that nothing will be overlooked. Remember that the hardest lesion to see on x-ray is the second one.

Why is technique important?

Technique will vary from film to film and must be taken into account. Anterior-posterior (AP) films are shot with the film behind the patient's back. The divergence of x-ray beams exaggerates heart size. Posterior-anterior (PA) and lateral films are better but require the patient to stand. Appropriate exposure barely reveals the vertebrae behind the heart. With overpenetration, darkened normal lungs may be mistaken for emphysema. Underpenetration or poor inspiration will increase interstitial markings. Adequate inspiration is determined by counting at least 10 posterior ribs (appear horizontal) in the lung field. Patient rotation artificially widens the mediastinal profile; normally the vertebrae line up between the clavicular heads (Figure 6-4).

What can be seen in bones and soft tissue?

Bony fractures, dislocations, and lytic lesions from cancer should be sought. Examine soft tissue for swelling or subcutaneous air suggestive of pneumothorax. Severe osteoporosis can be seen as transparent bone or vertebral compression fractures, best seen on the lateral view.

BOX 6-1   Key Elements of Reading a Chest X-ray

A = Airways and lung fields
B = Bones and soft tissue
C = Cardiac contour and mediastinum
D = Diaphragms and costophrenic angles
E = Examine technique
F = Foreign bodies, tubes, and wires

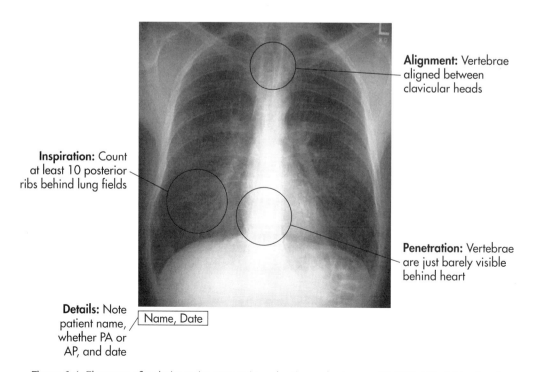

Alignment: Vertebrae aligned between clavicular heads

Inspiration: Count at least 10 posterior ribs behind lung fields

Penetration: Vertebrae are just barely visible behind heart

Details: Note patient name, whether PA or AP, and date

Name, Date

Figure 6-4 Elements of techniques important in evaluating a chest x-ray. (© 1997, Mike Richardson.)

What causes a widened mediastinum?

Aside from patient rotation, thoracic aortic aneurysm, tumor, or lymphadenopathy can widen the mediastinum.

Why should I look at the diaphragms and costophrenic angles?

Free air under the diaphragm occurs with bowel perforation. A blunted costophrenic angle may be the only sign of pleural effusion and should prompt obtaining decubitus films (patient lying on the side) to evaluate the amount of pleural fluid and if it is free flowing or loculated.

What is a silhouette sign?

The silhouette sign occurs when fluid or infection in the lung is adjacent to and therefore obliterates the border of the hemidiaphragm or heart. For example, if the right heart border is poorly seen, this is a right middle lobe silhouette sign, indicating a right middle lobe infiltrate (Figure 6-5). Similarly, a right lower lobe pneumonia will obliterate the right hemidiaphragm.

What does pneumonia look like?

Pneumonia may have many appearances, including a silhouette sign, diffuse interstitial infiltrates, or unexplained pleural effusions. In a volume-depleted patient, an infiltrate may be very subtle. Apical infiltrates can occur with any form of pneumonia but are classic for tuberculosis (TB).

What acute catastrophes should I not miss on chest x-ray?

Certain conditions should never be missed (Table 6-4).

What causes nodules in the lung parenchyma?

Cancer, either primary or metastatic, arteriovenous malformations, focal infection or abscess, hamartomas, and granulomas can all appear as nodules.

TABLE 6-4
Castastrophes Not to Miss on Chest X-ray

FINDING	CONDITION
Subdiaphragmatic "free" air	Intestinal perforation
Widened mediastinum	Aortic aneurysm or dissection
Mediastinal air	Esophageal rupture
Mediastinal shift, air in the pleural space	Pneumothorax

What are clues to volume overload or congestive heart failure?

Look for an enlarged cardiac silhouette greater than half the width of the thorax on PA view, interstitial prominence, Kerley B lines, and cephalization. *Kerley B lines* are thin horizontal lines at the periphery of the lung field. *Cephalization* is the engorgement of vessels in the upper lung fields. Under normal conditions, gravity makes vessels more prominent at the bottom of the lung field. *Blunting of the costophrenic angles* suggests pleural effusion.

HOW TO PERFORM BASIC PROCEDURES AND BODY FLUID ANALYSIS

What is the first step for any procedure?

Any invasive procedure requires informed consent. To obtain consent, explain the indication for the procedure, what the procedure involves, the risks (i.e., what a reasonable person would want to know), the alternatives to the procedure, and the consequences of not having the procedure. Patient competence is essential in this process. Patients under 18 years of age and those with altered mental status are not considered competent. In these cases, a surrogate decision-maker is sought. In an emergency, informed consent is not necessary if the procedure can be life-saving. The signed consent should be properly documented in the medical record.

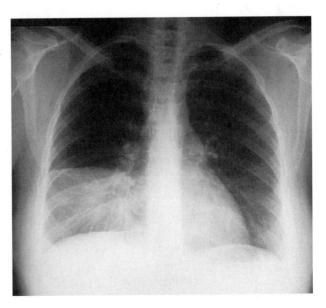

Figure 6-5 Loss of the right heart silhouette with right middle lobe pneumonia. NOTE: Right diaphragm is still clearly seen. (© 1997, Mike Richardson.)

What habits facilitate a successful procedure?

Take time at the outset to collect and arrange supplies, place a waste receptacle within easy reach, review technique, and position the patient. Wash hands before each procedure, and always use sterile technique. Out of respect for the hospital staff, clean up after the procedure and dispose of all sharp implements appropriately.

How do I document a procedure?

There is a standard format for procedure notes (Box 6-2).

LUMBAR PUNCTURE

What are the indications for lumbar puncture?

Any patient with unexplained fever and mental status changes should undergo lumbar puncture (LP) to rule out central nervous system (CNS) infection. Patients with new-onset "worst headache of their life" require LP in the face of a negative computed tomography (CT) scan to rule out subarachnoid hemorrhage and rare conditions, such as carcinomatous meningitis and Guillain-Barré syndrome. LP can be used to treat normal pressure hydrocephalus and to administer intrathecal chemotherapy or epidural anesthesia.

When is LP contraindicated?

Increased intracranial pressure is an absolute contraindication to LP because of the risk of causing uncal herniation. It should be suspected when patients have papilledema or risk factors for space-occupying lesions (i.e., HIV, CNS tumor, trauma, focal neurologic examination, and new seizure). Under these circumstances, a CT scan is mandatory. In other cases, CT scan is standard but likely unnecessary. Coagulopathy is a relative contraindication to LP.

BOX 6-2   Standard Procedure Note

Date and time _____
Procedure _____
Indication _____
Operators _____

Consent was obtained after explanation of risks and benefits. Area prepped and draped in sterile fashion. ____ ml of 1% lidocaine injected. ____ ml fluid withdrawn without complication and sent for _____. Wound cleansed and dressed.

Signature _____

What are the key steps in performing an LP?

Lie the patient on his or her side at the edge of the bed nearest you at a comfortable height. The patient's hip bones should be perpendicular to the bed with knees to chest for best access to the intervertebral space. Mark the L4 space at the level of the iliac crests. Prepare and drape the low back in sterile fashion, and apply anesthesia to the skin as a wheal, then to the deep tissues, making sure you are not injecting a vessel by pulling back on the plunger each time. Insert the spinal needle, aiming for the umbilicus. Obtain an opening pressure and collect several milliliters of cerebrospinal fluid (CSF) in each of four vials. Replace stylet before removing spinal needle.

What are the complications of LP?

The complications are post-LP headache, infection, hemorrhage, or uncal or tonsillar herniation.

What CSF tests should I order, and how do I interpret them?

Order cell count and differential, glucose, protein and bacterial cultures, and Gram stain. Glucose should be 50% to 60% of the simultaneous blood glucose. If it is lower, consider bacterial (including tuberculous) meningitis and parameningeal infection. Normal CSF white blood cell (WBC) count is 0 to 5 cells per mm^3. The differential is crucial because predominance of neutrophils suggests bacterial infection. Mononuclear cells are more common with viral, fungal, and tuberculous meningitis. However, neutrophils may predominate in early viral infection. Protein is usually less than 60 mg/dl. High protein is seen in all CNS infections, although it is highest with bacterial processes. An isolated increase in protein may be seen in patients with diabetes. Other tests to order can include cytology (if malignancy is suspected) or cryptococcal antigen, fungal stain, and culture in the immunocompromised patient. Specific viral testing is also available.

THORACENTESIS

What are the indications for thoracentesis?

Patients with new or unexplained pleural effusion require thoracentesis for diagnosis. Effusions often accompany pneumonia and should be tapped to rule out pleural space infection requiring drainage. Thoracentesis can also be used therapeutically for large, symptomatic effusions.

When is thoracentesis contraindicated?

Relative contraindications to thoracentesis include coagulopathy, cutaneous infections at the puncture site, and uncooperative patients. Small effusions may be more safely tapped with ultrasound guidance.

What are the key steps to thoracentesis?

Position the patient sitting on the edge of the bed, leaning over a tray table. Raise the bed to a comfortable height for you. Locate and mark your puncture site by percussing the chest. Be certain your mark is at the upper border of a rib to avoid the vascular bundle. Prepare and drape in sterile fashion. Apply anesthesia generously, especially at the parietal pleura. Advance the needle over the top of a rib while pulling back on the plunger until fluid is reached. A diagnostic tap requires about 30 ml of fluid. Therapeutic taps should not exceed 1.5 L to avoid reexpansion pulmonary edema. Fluid collection devices vary. With every device, it is crucial to avoid introducing air into the pleural space. Combat negative intrapleural pressure by having the patient exhale any time you must open the system to change devices. Obtain and review a postprocedure x-ray to rule out pneumothorax.

What are the complications of thoracentesis?

Pneumothorax, hepatic or splenic puncture, infection, hemothorax, and reexpansion pulmonary edema are the complications.

What pleural fluid tests should I order, and how do I interpret the results?

Order cell count and differential, protein, serum lactate dehydrogenase (LDH), glucose, bacterial cultures, and cytology. Simultaneous serum LDH, protein, and glucose are helpful. Other tests to order as circumstances warrant include amylase and lipids. Cultures for TB, even in the presence of disease, are low yield. pH has fallen out of favor because of the difficulty with accuracy but can be helpful in determining if chest-tube drainage is needed. Based on these results, your next task is to discern exudates from transudates (Table 6-5).

Differential diagnosis of exudates includes uninfected parapneumonic effusion, empyema, neoplasm, subdiaphragmatic abscess, pulmonary embolism, pancreatitis, rheumatoid and lupus arthritis, sarcoidosis, and Dressler's syndrome (after pericardiotomy or myocardial infarction). Causes of transudates include congestive heart failure, cirrhosis, and nephrotic syndrome.

PARACENTESIS

What are the indications for paracentesis?

New-onset ascites requires paracentesis for diagnosis. Patients with chronic ascites and new abdominal pain, fever, or unexplained increase in ascites should be tapped to evaluate for spontaneous bacterial peritonitis (SBP). In ascites compromising respiratory status or patient comfort, larger volumes of 2 to 5 L can be tapped therapeutically.

When is paracentesis contraindicated?

Paracentesis is hardly ever contraindicated. Most patients with ascites have coagulopathy; this is not a contraindication because the risk of serious bleeding is low (2%) even with coagulopathy.

What are the key steps to paracentesis?

Identify the puncture site. The left lower quadrant in the midclavicular line avoids the bladder, liver, and all but the largest spleens. The patient can be supine or slightly rotated to the left side. Prepare and drape as for other procedures. Apply anesthesia generously, especially to the parietal peritoneum. To avoid fluid leakage, advance the needle through a zigzag path in the subcutaneous tissue (Figure 6-6). Pull back on the plunger as you advance. As with thoracentesis, collection devices

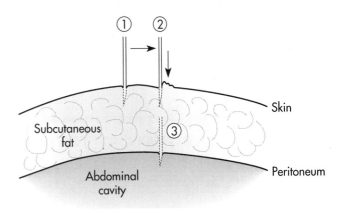

Figure 6-6 Zigzag path through the subcutaneous fat to prevent leakage after paracentesis. *1,* Enter skin; *2,* pull skin 1 to 2 cm away from original entry site with needle perpendicular to skin surface; *3,* advance needle through peritoneum.

TABLE 6-5		
Interpreting Pleural Fluid		
TEST	**EXUDATE**	**TRANSUDATE**
LDH	>200	<200
Pleural LDH/serum LDH	>0.6	<0.6
Protein	>3 g/dl	<3 g/dl
Pleural protein/serum protein	>0.5	<0.5
Pleural glucose/serum glucose	<0.5	>0.5
Cell count (per mm³)	>1000	<1000

will vary. After collection, withdraw the needle and place a pressure dressing over the site.

What are the complications of paracentesis?

The complications are bowel perforation, bladder perforation, abdominal wall hematoma, and infection.

What peritoneal fluid tests should I order, and how do I interpret the results?

Order cell count and differential, protein, bacterial cultures, and cytology. Cell count is the single most important test for deciding presence of infection. Diagnostic criteria for spontaneous bacterial peritonitis are WBC greater than 500 per mm³ or neutrophils greater than 250 per mm³. WBC greater than 10,000 indicates peritonitis, such as from perforated duodenal ulcer, and is an indication for an immediate CT scan. Calculate the serum-ascites albumin gradient (SAAG) as indicated by the name: serum albumin minus the ascites albumin. A SAAG greater than 1.1 is consistent with low-protein ascitic fluid resulting from portal hypertension. A SAAG less than 1.1 is consistent with high-protein peritoneal fluid as a result of TB or peritoneal carcinomatosis. Also, a total ascitic protein greater than 3 gm/dl suggests malignancy or TB. Bacterial cultures are best obtained by inoculating blood culture bottles at the bedside with 10 ml or more per bottle. Cultures for TB in peritoneal fluid are low yield. Yields from cytology examination are better if several liters are sent.

> ## Key Points
> - Proper patient and operator position is key to a comfortable and safe procedure.
> - Peritoneal fluid analysis is different than LP and thoracentesis fluid in that bacterial infection is *more* likely if the peritoneal fluid protein level is low.
> - Generous anesthesia, especially at parietal surfaces, is important for patient comfort and cooperation.
> - Use your knowledge of risks, complications, and indications in obtaining patient consent.

ABNORMAL LABORATORY TESTS

My clinic patient has an abnormal laboratory test. What should I do next?

Not long into your outpatient rotation, you will probably be faced with an abnormal blood test result. Clinic test results are often available only after the patient has left, unlike on the hospital ward. In the outpatient set-

ting, you have several options for follow-up: have the patient return for more history or examination, order more blood tests, refer for a diagnostic study, refer for consultation, or simply observe over time. Many sections of this book will provide specific guidance in interpreting test results. Included below are some tests not discussed in other chapters.

What is the role of screening laboratory tests?

Some physicians routinely obtain screening panels of laboratory tests; patients may also request these. However, there is no evidence that these "routine" screening tests are helpful in healthy patients. They generate false-positive results and unexpected abnormalities that worry patients and perplex providers. Because the abnormal range for each test includes normal outliers at the high and low ends, a random set of 20 laboratory tests will have, on average, one abnormal result just by chance. To avoid this trap, order tests only to pursue your evaluation of symptoms and signs of disease.

Are there any laboratory tests that I should order routinely?

In a well adult with no symptoms and a normal examination, the only reasonable screening tests are total cholesterol and high-density lipoprotein (HDL). Some also check glucose, PSA in men over age 50 years, hematocrit in menstruating women, and thyroid-stimulating hormone (TSH) in older women, to screen for diabetes, prostate cancer, iron deficiency, and thyroid disease, respectively. These screening tests are not uniformly agreed upon (see Chapter 18).

WHITE BLOOD CELL COUNT

What does an elevated WBC count (leukocytosis) mean?

The most common causes of leukocytosis are infection and steroids. Bacterial infections usually cause elevation of the neutrophil count with "left shift," meaning an increase in immature forms of neutrophils called *bands*. Toxic granulation may also be present with infection, a sign that neutrophils are actively producing digestive enzymes to fight intruding bacteria. Viral infection can cause elevated lymphocytes or atypical lymphocytes. In hospitalized patients, it is not uncommon to see a mild stress-related leukocytosis. The pearl to differentiating this from other causes is that it usually rapidly resolves when the patient's condition is more stable, often within 24 hours. Leukemia is an infrequent but significant cause of leukocytosis, usually with immature blast forms in the peripheral circulation.

My patient has elevated eosinophils. What could be causing this?

Eosinophilia may be due to neoplasm, allergy (including drug reactions), Addison's disease, collagen vascular disease, or parasitic infection (mnemonic NAACP).

ERYTHROCYTE SEDIMENTATION RATE

When should I be concerned about an elevated erythrocyte sedimentation rate?

The erythrocyte sedimentation rate (ESR) increases with age. A useful clinical pearl is that an ESR greater than half the age of the patient is almost always pathologic and warrants evaluation. More specifically, normal values for men are less than (age)/2, and for women are less than (age + 10)/2. For example, an 80-year-old woman should have an ESR less than (80 + 10)/2, or 45. With an ESR greater than 100, the diagnosis is usually obvious during initial evaluation. An elevated ESR is the only hint of disease in 0.06% of cases, that is, extremely rarely.

Is the ESR helpful for those with vague symptoms or positive review of systems?

A normal ESR will only reasonably exclude the diagnosis of temporal arteritis (TA) and polymyalgia rheumatica (PMR) but no other disorder. A normal ESR is not strong enough evidence to exclude a serious illness. In fact, it is routinely normal in infectious mononucleosis and typhoid fever and in 10% of patients with active TB.

What causes an ESR greater than 100?

Infection is the most common cause, followed by malignancy and collagen vascular disease. Infections raising the ESR include TB, pulmonary infections, syphilis, chronic bacterial infections (e.g., osteomyelitis, endocarditis, septic arthritis, liver/spleen/perinephric abscess), urinary tract infections, and AIDS. Malignancy accounts for 15% of ESRs greater than 100 and is almost always metastatic when the ESR is that high. Most likely cancers include multiple myeloma, lymphoma, and breast, lung, and colon cancers. Rheumatologic diseases can have a striking elevation in the ESR, especially TA, PMR, rheumatoid arthritis, and lupus erythematosus.

What evaluation should I pursue when the ESR is greater than 100?

Perform careful history and physical examination, including pelvic examination and stool hemoccult. This should suggest a diagnosis. Blood tests and imaging studies do not substitute for a detailed history and physical. Pursue the laboratory tests and studies most likely to confirm the diagnosis. Consider complete blood count with differential and urinalysis to look for infection; electrolytes, blood urea nitrogen (BUN), and creatinine to check kidney function and acid-base status; and liver function tests (albumin, alanine aminotransferase [ALT], aspartate aminotransferase [AST], alkaline phosphatase [alk phos], lactate dehydrogenase, and bilirubin) to look for hepatic injury. Because myeloma is more common with these extreme elevations in ESR, consider serum and urine protein electrophoresis (SPEP, UPEP). Obtain chest radiograph to look for lung infection, vasculitis, or tumor. In 5% to 10% of cases with an ESR of greater than 100, no cause will be found.

What about less extreme values, that is, ESR 35 to 75?

Many of these will be normal when rechecked in several weeks. This should be the extent of the workup in an asymptomatic patient. For persistently elevated values, a careful history and examination and careful use of the above tests will lead to the answer. In the asymptomatic patient with a benign examination, almost all elevated ESR results will go unexplained.

ALKALINE PHOSPHATASE

How should I evaluate an elevated alk phos?

Biliary obstruction and bone diseases are the main causes of an elevated alk phos. To sort out which is present, obtain a γ-glutamyltransferase (GGT) or 5'-nucleotidase; either of which will be elevated with biliary tree pathology but not with bone disease. Alk phos isoenzymes also determine the source but take several weeks. If biliary pathology is suggested, look for gallstones or tumor compressing the biliary tree (pancreatic, cholangiocarcinoma) by abdominal CT scan. Also consider autoimmune disease, such as primary biliary cirrhosis, which is diagnosed by a positive antimitochondrial antibody test in greater than 90% of cases. Alk phos can also be elevated in hepatitis or cirrhosis, although it is rarely more than 1 to 2 times the upper limits of normal and not usually greater than the ALT. When bone disease is likely, consider fractures, Paget's disease, bone metastases, or infection.

TUMOR MARKERS

What are tumor markers?

Tumor markers are substances produced in excess by particular tumors and found in the blood (Table 6-6). Tumor markers are too nonspecific to use for diagnosis or general screening. They can be used to assess

TABLE 6-6
Common Tumor Markers and Their Clinical Use

TUMOR MARKER	ASSOCIATED TUMOR	CLINICAL USE
α-fetoprotein	Germ cell cancer, liver cancer	Classify tumor type, follow for recurrence; suggest source of liver mass; screen high-risk cirrhosis patients
β-HCG	Germ cell tumor	Classify tumor type
CEA	Colon cancer	Follow for recurrence; suggest source of liver mass
CA-125	Ovarian cancer	Follow for recurrence

completeness of resection, or follow for recurrence after treatment. Occasionally, they can suggest a diagnosis when findings are nonspecific. For example, in the case of a liver mass, elevated α-fetoprotein suggests primary liver tumor, whereas an elevated carcinoembryonic antigen (CEA) suggests colon cancer metastatic to the liver. Patients with cirrhosis at high risk for hepatocellular carcinoma (i.e., resulting from hepatitis B or C or hemachromatosis) may undergo annual α-fetoprotein screening. Germ cell tumors are classified based on whether they make β-human chorionic gonadotrophin (β-HCG) or α-fetoprotein.

TABLE 6-7
Calculating Sensitivity and Specificity

TEST	DISEASE	
	Present	*Absent*
Positive	A (true positive)	B (false positive)
Negative	C (false negative)	D (true negative)

Sensitivity: $\dfrac{A}{(A + C)}$ *or* $\dfrac{\text{(true positive test results)}}{\text{(all patients with disease)}}$

Specificity: $\dfrac{D}{(D + B)}$ *or* $\dfrac{\text{(true negative test results)}}{\text{(all patients without disease)}}$

HOW TO INTERPRET SENSITIVITY AND SPECIFICITY

What are sensitivity and specificity?

When diagnosing or treating a condition, we need to know how accurate the test is. For example, in a screening test such as PSA, we want a balance between a big net that catches all prostate cancers (sensitivity) and yet still omits those cases that are not cancer (specificity). Unfortunately, PSA does not meet either of these goals. Put another way, sensitivity is the proportion of people with the condition who test positive; specificity is the proportion of persons without the condition who test negative. A test's sensitivity and specificity can be calculated by using a 2 × 2 table (Table 6-7).

How do levels of sensitivity and specificity affect how I interpret a test?

Some people find the mnemonics *SpPIN* and *SnNOUT* helpful. If a test has high *Sp*ecificity, a *P*ositive test rules the condition *IN*. If a test has high *Sn*sitivity, a *N*egative result rules *OUT* the condition. For example, a peritoneal fluid wave on physical examination is 92% specific for ascites. Therefore, if a fluid wave is present, you can rule ascites in (a highly *sp*ecific test, *p*ositive finding, rule it *in*). On the other hand, in a study of patients at a veteran's hospital, a history of ankle edema was 93% sensitive for the presence of ascites. Therefore, if the pa-

tient has no history of ankle edema, you can rule ascites out (*s*ensitive test, *n*egative finding, rule it *out*).

If my patient has a positive test, what is the likelihood that he or she actually has the condition?

Sensitivity and specificity relate to characteristics of the test itself. The question of likelihood turns the focus to the characteristics of the patient being tested. We ask, "Given a positive test, what is the probability that this patient actually has the condition?" or, "Given a negative test, what is the probability that the patient does not have this condition?" The statistical terms for these concepts are positive and negative predictive value (PPV and NPV), respectively. The predictive value is dependent on the estimated prevalence of a disease, or *pretest probability*. To determine how likely it is that a positive test indicates disease, you must have this estimate of the patient's risk, as well as the sensitivity and specificity of the test being applied.

What are the steps to calculating the predictive values?

Calculate predictive values using the same 2 × 2 table (Table 6-8). Pick an arbitrary number of patients, such as 1000, and multiply by the pretest probability to get the "disease present" and "disease absent" totals. Then

TABLE 6-8
Calculating Predictive Value*

TEST	DISEASE	
	Present	*Absent*
Positive	A (true positive)	B (false positive)
Negative	C (false negative)	D (true negative)

Positive Predictive Value:

$$\frac{A}{(A + B)} \ or \ \frac{\text{(true positive test results)}}{\text{(all positive test results)}}$$

Negative Predictive Value:

$$\frac{D}{(D + C)} \ or \ \frac{\text{(true negative test results)}}{\text{(all negative test results)}}$$

*Requires prior knowledge of sensitivity, specificity, and pretest probability, i.e., prevalence of disease.

TABLE 6-9
Predictive Values of Renal Artery Duplex in Renal Artery Stenosis*

DUPLEX	RENAL ARTERY STENOSIS	
	Present in 20	*Absent in 980*
Positive	A = 18†	B = 60
Negative	C = 2	D = 920‡

$$\text{PPV:} \ \frac{18}{(18 + 60)} = 23\% \qquad \text{NPV:} \ \frac{920}{(2 + 920)} = 99.8\%$$

*Pretest probability = **2%** prevalence of renal artery stenosis in general population. Assume 1000 patients, therefore 20 have disease, 980 do not have disease.
Sensitivity = **92%**, specificity = **94%** for renal artery duplex.
†Calculated from known sensitivity of 92%; 92% of 20 = 18 true positives.
‡Calculated from known specificity of 94%; 94% of 980 = 920 true negatives.

multiply the total "disease present" by the sensitivity to get A = true positives. For D = true negatives, multiply the "disease absent" by the specificity. To get C and B, subtract A from total "disease present" and D from the total "disease absent," respectively. Finally, for PPV, divide the true positives, A, by the total positive tests, A plus B. For NPV, divide D by total negative tests, D + C.

How are predictive values and these calculations applied to a real clinical scenario?

For example, the renal artery duplex is a highly sensitive (92%) and specific (94%) test for renal artery stenosis as a cause of hypertension. However, because the incidence of the disease is so low (2%) in the general population, the PPV is 23% while the NPV is 99.8% (Table 6-9). So back to the question, "My patient has a positive renal artery duplex. Does she really have renal artery stenosis?" The answer is, "This patient, despite the positive test result, only has a 1 in 4 chance (23%) of truly having renal artery stenosis."

CASE 6-1

A 24-year-old woman desires an HIV test. She is an intravenous (IV) drug user and obtains drugs through prostitution. Assume a pretest probability of 25%. Sensitivity and specificity are 98%.
A. Using a 2 × 2 table, calculate the predictive value of a positive test.
B. Now calculate the PPV in a monogamous woman with no risk factors who has a pretest probability of 1/1000.

HOW TO USE ANTIBIOTICS

How do I approach the task of choosing and dosing antibiotics?

Learning about all antibiotics is almost impossible, given the large number of choices available. To complicate matters, many antibiotics sound alike, especially cephalosporins. Your decision to use an individual antibiotic will be based on several factors: coverage of the likely or cultured organisms, drug allergy history, formulary availability, and cost. Once you decide which drug to use, consult a pocket pharmacopeia for dosing and remember to adjust for renal function.

What is empiric therapy?

Empiric therapy is best-guess therapy when a specific pathogen is not yet known. Patients have signs of infection, but definitive culture of blood, urine, or body fluid takes several days. In the interim before the pathogen is known, antibiotics are frequently begun. In many cases, especially with pneumonia or skin infections, a specific pathogen may never be isolated, and the whole treatment course is based on the most likely pathogen in a given setting.

What is a good starting point for picking antibiotic therapy?

Learn a few antibiotics appropriate for use with common bacterial pathogens: *Staphylococcus aureus;* gram-negative rods; anaerobes; *Enterococcus;* and atypical organisms, such as *Chlamydia, Legionella,* and *Mycoplasma* (Table 6-10).

When do I worry about *S. aureus* infections?

S. aureus is a very common pathogen, and its drug resistance makes it particularly troublesome. Typical situations for *S. aureus* infections include endocarditis in IV drug users, skin and wound infection, and nosocomial pneumonia.

What are good drugs for treating *S. aureus* infections?

S. aureus infections are divided into methicillin-sensitive and methicillin-resistant (MRSA) infections. In otherwise healthy patients when MRSA is unlikely, the best initial IV drugs for *S. aureus* infections are nafcillin or first-generation cephalosporins, such as cefazolin (Box 6-3). Oral options are dicloxacillin and cephalexin. If the patient has a life-threatening penicillin allergy, vancomycin is the best option. When MRSA is likely, as in frequently hospitalized or institutionalized patients, vancomycin is used for empiric coverage until sensitivities are available. Oral vancomycin is not absorbed and should only be used for topical therapy of *Clostridium difficile* colitis. Other drugs with good *S. aureus* activity

include clindamycin; quinolones; second- and third-generation cephalosporins; or combination penicillin products with β-lactamase inhibitors, such as ampicillin/clavulanate, piperacillin/tazobactam, or ticarcillin/clavulanate.

How does anyone keep the cephalosporins straight?

The cephalosporins are confusing because they have similar names. Classify them by generation, with first-generation drugs having better gram-positive coverage and third-generation drugs having better gram-negative coverage.

> Gram positives: 1st > 2nd > 3rd generation
> Gram negatives: 3rd > 2nd > 1st generation

Other special features of cephalosporins include the following: (1) cefotetan and cefoxitin are the only ceph-

---

BOX 6-3   Best Drugs for Methicillin-Sensitive *S. aureus*

- Nafcillin
- First-generation cephalosporin
- Vancomycin (for penicillin allergic)

TABLE 6-10
Antibacterial Spectrum of Commonly Used Antibiotics

ANTIBIOTIC	EXCELLENT ACTIVITY (>90% ISOLATES SENSITIVE)	FAIR ACTIVITY (70% TO 90% ISOLATES SENSITIVE)	POOR ACTIVITY
Penicillin	*Streptococcus* species except *Enterococcus* Oral anaerobes	*Enterococcus*	Aerobic gram-negative rods *Staphylococcus aureus* Atypical organisms
Ampicillin	*Streptococcus* species Oral anaerobes	*Haemophilus influenzae*	Most aerobic gram-negative rods *S. aureus* Atypical organisms
Trimethoprim/Sulfamethoxazole	*Streptococcus* species except *Enterococcus* *E. coli*	*S. aureus*	Anaerobes Hospital-acquired gram-negative rods
Clindamycin	*Streptococcus* species except *Enterococcus* Anaerobes *S. aureus*		Aerobic gram-negative rods Atypical organisms
Ciprofloxacin Ofloxacin	Aerobic gram-negative rods *S. aureus*	*Streptococcus* species	Anaerobes *Enterococcus*
Levofloxacin Grepafloxacin Trovafloxacin	Aerobic gram-negative rods *S. aureus*/*Streptococcus*	Anaerobes (trovafloxacin only)	*Enterococcus*

alosporins with good anaerobe activity (both are second generation); (2) ceftazidime and cefoperazone are the only third-generation cephalosporins with activity against *Pseudomonas aeruginosa*; cefepime is a "fourth"-generation cephalosporin that has antipseudomonal activity; (3) ceftriaxone is a third-generation cephalosporin that can be given once a day; and (4) no cephalosporin covers *Enterococcus* (group D streptococcus).

When do I worry about gram-negative or anaerobic infections?

Gram-negative bacteria are generally seen with genitourinary tract infections (e.g., pyelonephritis, urinary tract infection or infection from a bowel source (e.g., biliary tract disease or peritonitis from bowel wall perforation). In addition to gram-negative rods, the bowels can also be the source of anaerobes and/or gram-positive cocci, such as *Enterococcus*. The oral gingiva is another common source of anaerobic infections (e.g., tooth abscess, aspiration pneumonia). A subcategory of less common gram-negative rods includes nosocomial, or hospital-acquired, gram-negative rods, such as *Klebsiella* or *Pseudomonas*.

What are the best antibiotics for treating gram-negative infections?

Aminoglycosides and the monobactam aztreonam provide narrow coverage of aerobic gram-negative rods only. They are useful for almost all gram-negative infections, although they are usually not used alone as empiric therapy because of their narrow spectrum. For situations in which multiple types of organisms are possible, choose broader-spectrum empiric therapy, such as quinolones (which provide superb gram-negative coverage), extended-spectrum penicillins (e.g., mezlocillin, piperacillin, or ticarcillin), third- or fourth-generation cephalosporins, imipenem or meropenem. Of this group, imipenem and meropenem have the broadest spectrum of activity, including gram-positive organisms, as well as aerobic and anaerobic gram-negative rods. Although it is tempting to always use the broadest antibiotics, this in fact wipes out normal colonizing gut and vaginal flora. Choose the narrowest spectrum possible, and narrow therapy promptly when culture results are available.

What antibiotics provide excellent coverage for anaerobic infections?

Anaerobes can be either gram-negative or gram-positive and are distinguished by their inability to grow well in the presence of oxygen. Their response to antibiotics is unique. Anaerobic infections of the mouth are generally sensitive to penicillin or ampicillin. By contrast, anaerobes of the gastrointestinal tract (especially *Bacteroides fragilis*) manufacture β-lactamase; therefore these "below the diaphragm" anaerobes are frequently resistant to penicillin. The best anaerobe drugs in this situation are clindamycin, metronidazole, a penicillin derivative/β-lactamase inhibitor combination, cefotetan, cefoxitin, imipenem, or meropenem. Trovafloxacin is the only member of the quinolone class with anaerobe activity (Box 6-4).

How do you treat enterococcal infections?

These are difficult to treat. Ampicillin has the most activity, but resistance is growing. Penicillin and vancomycin are other options. For enterococcal bacteremia, aminoglycosides are frequently combined with ampicillin or vancomycin for synergy. Only about one third of enterococcal strains have sensitivity to aminoglycosides.

What drugs are best for the atypical organisms *Legionella, Chlamydia, Mycoplasma*?

Erythromycin and fluoroquinolone are the traditional drugs for these infections. Azithromycin and clarithromycin are newer medications in the same class as erythromycin and are just as effective against atypical organisms with the benefit of less frequent dosing but with the drawback of higher cost.

How do I know the cost of antibiotics?

In general, the drug cost of new antibiotics is greater than older antibiotics. For IV antibiotics the number of doses is the biggest determining factor in cost. The administration cost of an IV antibiotic is $18 to $24 per dose. As a result, an expensive once-daily IV antibiotic will have a lower daily cost than a cheaper IV antibiotic, which needs to be given several times a day. For example, ceftriaxone 2 g IV q24h = $50 (cost of 2 g ceftriaxone) + $20 for 1 IV administration = $70 per day is cheaper than ampicillin 1 g IV q6h = $6 (cost of 4 doses of 1 g ampicillin) + $80 for 4 IV administrations = $86.

BOX 6-4 Best Drugs for Anaerobes

- Clindamycin
- Metronidazole
- Penicillin derivative with β-lactamase inhibitor
- Cefotetan/cefoxitin
- Meropenem/imipenem

Key Points ··

- Nafcillin and first-generation cephalosporins are the most potent antibiotics for methicillin-sensitive *S. aureus*.
- In general, for gram-positive coverage by the cephalosporins, 1st > 2nd > 3rd generation. Gram-negative coverage is 3rd > 2nd > 1st generation.
- The best antibiotics for anaerobe coverage are clindamycin, metronidazole, β-lactam + β-lactamase inhibitor combinations and cefotetan/cefoxitin.

BOX 6-5   Common Indications for Intubation

Apnea
Poor airway protection
PaO_2 <55 mm Hg despite FiO_2 of >60%
Respiratory rate >30-40 or <10
Increased intracranial pressure

HOW TO APPROACH THE ACUTELY ILL PATIENT

How do I recognize an acutely ill patient?

Acutely ill patients require rapid assessment and simultaneous intervention to stabilize their situation. Observe immediate obvious worrisome clues, such as respiratory distress, pallor, cyanosis, unusual behavior, altered consciousness, or diaphoresis. Trust your instincts. A patient is considered unstable if vital signs are markedly abnormal; check for hypotension or severe hypertension, altered respiratory rate, and marked tachycardia or bradycardia. Mental status is sometimes considered a fifth vital sign that, if acutely altered, also makes a patient unstable. Some chief complaints are so worrisome that patients are considered unstable until proven otherwise (e.g., chest pain, severe dyspnea or headache, or sudden neurologic abnormality).

When do I call a code?

Call a code when a patient is found without respirations or pulse or in a situation in which immediate help is required to avert a cardiopulmonary arrest. If you find a patient in this condition, tell the nearest staff person to "call a code," then stay by the patient and support their ABCs (airway, breathing, and circulation), including CPR if indicated, until help arrives. Calling a code triggers a rapid response by a team of physicians, respiratory therapists, and nurses and includes a code cart containing emergency medications and a cardioverter/defibrillator.

What do I do first?

Call for help and immediately notify your supervising physician. Then perform a primary survey to address the ABCs. If you encounter a life-threatening problem in the primary survey, deal with it right away. Establish and protect the *airway* and consider intubation if the gag reflex is absent. Provide *breathing* support and oxygen and follow pulse oxymetry. Use oxygen cautiously (at low flow rates) in patients with chronic obstructive pulmonary disease. Consider intubating patients with severe respiratory distress (Box 6-5). Address *circulatory* issues (cardiac arrest, hemorrhage, hypotension, and IV access), and begin continuous cardiac and blood pressure monitoring. For hypotension, order fluid in rapid boluses (i.e., 0.5-1 L normal saline) and reassess after each bolus: look for improvements in blood pressure and pulse rate, and for fluid overload by listening for rales in the lungs. This avoids unmonitored high flow rates that may cause volume overload. Some add a "D" to the primary survey to address *deficit in mental status* and treat with naloxone (0.4-2 mg IV), glucose (1 amp D50W IV) and thiamine (100 mg IM or IV), as indicated by the clinical picture.

In a patient in distress, what other key information might be helpful?

In addition to current vitals signs and screening exam, an arterial blood gas, complete blood count, electrolytes, bicarbonate, glucose, and renal function may be useful. ECG and portable chest x-ray may also be appropriate. A quick assessment of recent medical events and medications from the chart notes, laboratory test values, and discussion with other care providers may provide useful clues to what is going on.

2

Patients Presenting With a Symptom, Sign, or Abnormal Lab Value

7

Abdominal Pain

ETIOLOGY

There are so many causes of abdominal pain. How do I begin to categorize them?

It is useful to differentiate chronic (>1 month) from acute pain. Common causes of chronic and acute abdominal pain are listed along with risk factors (Tables 7-1 and 7-2). In elderly patients, beware that chronic pain may actually be a subtle presentation of an acute process. Reasons for this include milder or more diffuse symptoms resulting from impaired immunity, impaired mentation, effects of medications, or concurrent illness. With focal pain, location is also helpful in narrowing the differential (Figure 7-1). Diffuse pain is most commonly caused by early appendicitis (first few hours), ischemic bowel disease, and bowel obstruction.

What are some abdominal catastrophes I shouldn't miss?

Abdominal aortic aneurysm rupture, bowel perforation, ischemic bowel, and ectopic pregnancy can cause rapid clinical decline and death, especially if diagnosis is delayed. Aortic aneurysm rupture usually causes sudden, diffuse pain radiating to the back and may interfere with blood flow to the lower extremities or spine. Bowel perforation causes diffuse pain with evolving peritoneal signs and sepsis. Ischemic bowel causes diffuse pain with a remarkably soft abdominal examination and usually occurs in patients with risk factors for atherosclerosis. Ectopic pregnancy should be suspected in all sexually active women with lower abdominal pain.

What important extraabdominal problems masquerade as abdominal pain?

Atypical angina may present as epigastric pain but is usually associated with exercise and relieved by resting and may have associated dyspnea or nausea. Also, be-ware of the lower-lobe pneumonia or pulmonary embolus (PE) that irritates the diaphragm and masquerades as upper quadrant pain. Occasionally, lower abdominal pain is caused by a hip problem. Abdominal wall pain from muscle strain, hernia, nerve entrapment, rectus sheath hematoma, or herpes zoster (i.e., shingles) may mimic an intraabdominal process. Abdominal wall pain is usually worse on palpation in a half–sit-up position (Carnett's sign), whereas intraabdominal processes are less painful in this position.

What diagnoses should I think of when patients give a history of pain worsened by eating?

Pancreatitis, gallstones, mesenteric ischemia, reflux esophagitis, small bowel obstruction, irritable bowel syndrome, and, occasionally, atypical angina can all cause postprandial pain.

EVALUATION

How do I approach history taking when there are so many questions I could ask?

Ask an open-ended question to get a brief description of onset and location of the pain (e.g., "Tell me more about your pain"). From there, second-year students are taught to obtain a history by asking all patients all questions about every aspect of their pain (Box 7-1). It takes significant stamina to get detailed answers to all the questions. This technique can also swamp students with information without distinguishing important from irrelevant data. Hypothesis testing is an alternative approach used intuitively by masters of the trade. In this streamlined approach the physician first generates a mental list of common causes of pain in the location, or of the character, described spontaneously by the patient. The physician then asks the patient key questions to see which entity on the list of possibilities is the closest fit. Hypothesis testing builds a good knowledge base and requires thinking on one's feet during the interview.

TABLE 7-1

Causes of Chronic Abdominal Pain, Associated Risk Factors, and Key Presenting Features

COMMON CAUSES	RISK FACTORS	KEY PRESENTING FEATURES
Peptic ulcer disease	NSAIDs, prednisone, alcohol, caffeine	Improved with antacids Worse with hunger or spicy food, NSAIDs Melena
Reflux disease	Obesity	Acid or food regurgitation Symptoms worse supine
Gallstone disease	"Fat, 40, female"	Right upper quadrant pain Pain radiates to right shoulder Postprandial pain, especially after fatty food
Irritable bowel syndrome	Anxious, female Young to middle-aged	No nocturnal symptoms Improved with defecation
Obstipation	Elderly, narcotics, calcium channel blockers	Inability to pass stool Hard stool
Atypical angina	Hypertension, family history of MI, hyperlipidemia, smoking, diabetes	Worse with exercise, eating Associated dyspnea, diaphoresis, nausea

TABLE 7-2

Risk Factors Associated With Common Causes of Acute Abdominal Pain

CAUSES	RISK FACTOR
COMMON	
Appendicitis	Generally young but not always
Gallstone disease	"Fat, 40, female"
Ischemic bowel	Elderly, atherosclerotic risk factors
LESS COMMON	
Ectopic pregnancy	Sexually active women, prior PID, IUD
PID	Sexually active women, prior STD, IUD, douching
Pancreatitis	Gallstone disease, alcohol use, high triglycerides, medications
Obstipation	Elderly, narcotic use, calcium channel blockers
Bowel obstruction	Prior abdominal surgery, hernia

PID, Pelvic inflammatory disease; *IUD,* intrauterine device; *STD,* sexually transmitted disease.

Beware that this technique can backfire if used before the patient is allowed to tell a full story because key pieces of information may be missed. If the cause of pain is still unclear after several iterations of hypothesis testing, the traditional, exhaustive approach of questioning may be necessary. The student write-up should reflect the hypothesis-testing approach by pointing out the suspected diagnosis and pertinent negatives to exclude other contenders in the differential.

BOX 7-1   Questions to Ask Patients About Abdominal Pain

Onset and duration
Character and severity of pain
Location and radiation
Progression of symptoms over time
Associated symptoms
Relation to meals, exercise, defecation
Change in stool or flatus
Exacerbating and relieving factors
History of recent travel, infectious exposure, alcohol use
Medications

What specific questions should I ask when patients have focal pain?

Here is an example of how to use hypothesis testing for a patient with focal epigastric pain. First, think of the common causes of epigastric pain: gastroesophageal reflux disease (GERD), peptic ulcer disease (PUD), gallstones, and atypical cardiac ischemia (although not as common, it should not be missed). To distinguish between these possibilities, ask patients about the key features of each (see Table 7-1). In this way, a few questions can quickly prioritize the differential diagnosis for pain in any location.

What specific questions should I ask when patients have diffuse abdominal pain?

Potential causes of poorly localized pain include ischemic bowel, abdominal aortic aneurysm rupture, bowel obstruction, obstipation, pancreatitis, and spontaneous

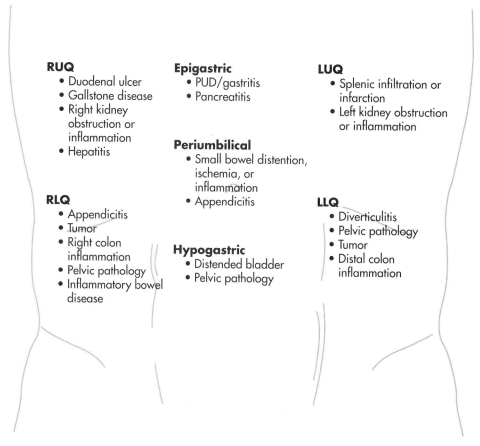

RUQ
- Duodenal ulcer
- Gallstone disease
- Right kidney obstruction or inflammation
- Hepatitis

RLQ
- Appendicitis
- Tumor
- Right colon inflammation
- Pelvic pathology
- Inflammatory bowel disease

Epigastric
- PUD/gastritis
- Pancreatitis

Periumbilical
- Small bowel distention, ischemia, or inflammation
- Appendicitis

Hypogastric
- Distended bladder
- Pelvic pathology

LUQ
- Splenic infiltration or infarction
- Left kidney obstruction or inflammation

LLQ
- Diverticulitis
- Pelvic pathology
- Tumor
- Distal colon inflammation

Figure 7-1 Common causes of abdominal pain by location in the abdomen.

bacterial peritonitis. Ask about atherosclerotic risk factors to assess for ischemic bowel and aortic aneurysm. Ask about postprandial symptoms and weight loss because these often accompany ischemic bowel. Inability to pass stool suggests obstipation or obstruction, and feculent emesis suggests obstruction. Radiation to the back makes aortic dissection or pancreatitis more likely. Liver disease or ascites with fever is concerning for spontaneous bacterial peritonitis. Postprandial nausea or vomiting with prior gallstone disease, alcohol use, or hypertriglyceridemia is suspicious for pancreatitis.

What clues are helpful in the social history?

Age, gender, and presence of specific risk factors are important clues. Older patients may suffer from ischemic bowel, complications of gallstone disease, diverticulitis, or obstipation. Older men with benign prostatic hypertrophy may have painful bladder distension as a result of outlet obstruction. Sexually active women may have pelvic inflammatory disease (PID) or ectopic pregnancy. Women with chronic pelvic pain of unclear cause even after extensive workup may have depression or prior sex-

ual abuse contributing to a somatoform disorder. Infectious exposures, such as IV drug use or unprotected intercourse, place patients at risk for hepatitis. Sick contacts or travel to areas with poor sanitation are risk factors for hepatitis A, viral gastroenteritis, or infectious diarrhea. Nonsteroidal antiinflammatory drugs (NSAIDs), steroids, caffeine, or alcohol are risks for PUD. Alcohol overuse is also a risk factor for pancreatitis or chronic liver disease.

What are some "red flags" in history or physical that I shouldn't miss?

Before you launch into the internist's usual reverie of an exhaustive history and physical, remember that a prolonged history-taking could delay urgent intervention in a very ill patient. It is wise to do a quick initial evaluation for abnormal vital signs and peritoneal signs to get a sense of the urgency of intervention. Red flags (concerning signs) for malignancy include weight loss, sweats, fevers, and early satiety. Melena may signal a malignancy or other source of gastrointestinal (GI) bleed that requires intervention. Dyspnea may signal acidemia or a cardiac or pulmonary problem masquerading as abdominal pain. A mass on examination may simply be due to obstipation but could be a tumor or distended bladder. Peritoneal signs warrant urgent evaluation and intervention. Fever suggests infection or some tumors, although it is not always present with either of these conditions. Fever with jaundice and right upper quadrant pain is likely ascending cholangitis, requiring urgent GI referral for possible endoscopy. Patients on steroids may have a blunted response to acute processes, so they should be assumed to have an acute process until proven otherwise.

What are helpful findings on physical examination in patients with abdominal pain?

Tachycardia or hypotension suggests a serious illness, requiring rapid assessment. Peritoneal signs (involuntary guarding and rebound tenderness) occur when the peritoneal lining is irritated, usually by infection or blood. Patients with peritoneal signs are usually lying very still to avoid movement. Turner's and Cullen's signs are ecchymoses seen on the flank and around the umbilicus, respectively, in patients with retroperitoneal hemorrhage. A Sister Joseph's nodule is an indurated nodule of metastatic cancer in the umbilicus seen in patients with GI malignancy. The pelvic examination is very important in women with abdominal pain. Cervical motion tenderness and purulent cervical discharge suggest PID. Adnexal fullness or tenderness may accompany ectopic pregnancy or tuboovarian abscess. Hernia may be the cause of a bowel obstruction. Shifting dullness or a fluid wave may suggest ascites and some coincident complication of liver disease.

What studies are warranted in patients with mild or chronic abdominal pain?

Generally, patients with chronic or mild pain do not require urgent evaluation. In fact, most patients with chronic pain have already undergone prior evaluation without revealing a diagnosis, and further investigation is not simple or revealing. A history of physical or sexual abuse is more likely in such patients. In those who have not had testing or who have other focal symptoms, tailor workup to confirm diagnostic suspicions from history and examination. You have time to try empiric antacids, review prior test results, and pursue workup in a serial fashion, one test at a time. Obtain ultrasound if you suspect gallstones. Lower abdominal pain suggesting irritable bowel syndrome without bloody stool or weight loss requires no tests. Order colonoscopy when weight loss, stool habit changes, or bloody stool suggest inflammatory bowel disease or colon cancer.

What workup should I order in acutely ill patients with abdominal pain?

In patients with severe or poorly localized pain, inadequate history, or vital signs or peritoneal signs worrisome for severe illness, standard laboratory workup includes urinalysis and "belly labs" (i.e., complete blood count, arterial blood gas, electrolytes, liver function tests, and an amylase or lipase). Obtain a pregnancy test in all sexually active women with severe lower abdominal pain. Abdominal x-ray series may detect obstruction, perforation, or obstipation. Blood cultures are warranted in febrile patients. Do not forget the bladder or kidney as a potential source of pain. Bladder catheterization or ultrasound may reveal a bladder outlet obstruction. Obtain abdominal imaging if you suspect cholecystitis, cholangitis, appendicitis, abdominal aortic aneurysm, or ectopic pregnancy. In patients whose cause of abdominal pain remains cryptic after initial evaluation, ask about abuse or depression. If you have reason to suspect extraabdominal source of pain, get a chest x-ray and ECG.

TREATMENT

The underlying cause should be treated. Patients with an unclear source of acute abdominal pain accompanied by peritoneal signs may need urgent exploratory surgery. Please also see relevant sections on dyspepsia (Chapter 13), liver disease (Chapter 26), GI bleeding (Chapter 16), and solid tumors (Chapter 28) for more details about treatment of specific conditions.

When should I hospitalize patients with abdominal pain?

Reasons for admitting a patient with abdominal pain include peritoneal signs, unstable vital signs, suspected cholangitis, cholecystitis, appendicitis, bowel obstruction or perforation, tuboovarian abscess, and patients with pyelonephritis or PID who need IV antibiotics because of nausea and vomiting.

Key Points

- Narrow the differential diagnosis of abdominal pain by location and how long the pain has been present.
- Get a pregnancy test and perform a pelvic examination in all young women with lower abdominal pain.
- A painful but soft abdomen in an elderly person is ischemic bowel disease until proven otherwise.
- Myocardial infarction and pulmonary pathology can masquerade as abdominal pain.

CASE 7-1

A 25-year-old woman has crampy right lower quadrant abdominal pain. She takes oral contraceptives and is monogamous with her current partner. She recently finished a course of antibiotics for sinusitis but otherwise has been healthy without prior surgeries or hospitalizations. Her pulse is 90, blood pressure is 110/75, and temperature is 99.6° F. Her examination reveals a soft abdomen with focal tenderness in the right lower quadrant.

A. What clues do you have in her history to help you make a differential diagnosis?

B. What other questions do you want to ask to narrow your differential diagnosis?

C. You obtain the additional history that she has had this pain in the right lower quadrant for about 3 days and that there have been three prior episodes of similar symptoms in the last year, all of which resolved after a week or so. Prior episodes have been associated with some diarrhea, and this time she noticed blood-streaked stool. Her periods have been regular and her last one began 3 weeks ago. What would you order now?

CASE 7-2

An 80-year-old man is brought to the emergency room with severe, acute, diffuse abdominal pain associated with a single, large, loose stool. He has a history of congestive heart failure (CHF) and recently increased his diuretic dose. He has also lost 10 pounds over the last 2 months. When you ask why, he reports he no longer enjoys eating because he experiences diffuse abdominal pain every time he eats. On examination, heart rate is 112, blood pressure is 120/80, respiratory rate is 28, and abdomen is soft but diffusely tender without organomegaly or guarding. Rectal examination reveals a diffusely large prostate and guaiac-positive stool.

A. What is your differential diagnosis?

B. How will you evaluate him?

chapter

8

Anemia

ETIOLOGY

What is anemia?

Anemia is a decrease in red cell mass. Because red cell mass is difficult to measure directly, hemoglobin and hematocrit (Hct) are used as surrogate measures. Hemoglobin of less than 12 in women and 13 in men defines anemia. Hematocrit is roughly 3 times the hemoglobin. Hemoglobin and hematocrit measures are plasma volume–dependent. They are falsely elevated in dehydration and falsely decreased in volume overload (e.g., cirrhosis or CHF).

How does anemia occur?

Blood loss is the most common cause of anemia, usually from gastrointestinal bleeding or menses. Any other disruption in the red cell life cycle will cause anemia, including inadequate production or excessive destruction. Any of these causes may coexist. Red cell *production* is abnormal if the bone marrow does not have necessary building blocks, such as iron or vitamin B_{12}, or if the marrow is damaged as a result of drugs, fibrosis, or cancer infiltration. *Destruction* occurs by hemolysis, either within blood vessels (intravascular) or in the spleen (extravascular).

How do the reticulocyte count and MCV help determine etiology?

The normal bone marrow responds to anemia by releasing more reticulocytes (immature red cells). With hemolysis or acute blood loss, the reticulocyte count increases. A normal marrow response is reflected in a corrected reticulocyte index of greater than 2 to 3. Lower values, no matter what the cause of anemia, suggest that the bone marrow is not functioning normally, that is, there is a production problem. In this case the mean corpuscular volume (MCV) will help distinguish causes (Table 8-1).

What causes the changes in red cell size reflected in an abnormal MCV?

Enlarged red cells often develop when abnormal deoxyribonucleic acid (DNA) synthesis delays nuclear maturation of erythrocyte precursors, as in vitamin B_{12} or folate deficiency. Alcohol may be the most common cause of macrocytic anemia. Between 40% and 90% of alcoholic patients have an MCV greater than 100, mostly resulting from a direct effect of alcohol on the bone marrow, although occasionally caused by folate deficiency. Small red cells occur with problems in hemoglobin synthesis, as with iron deficiency or thalassemia.

How do people get deficient of folate or vitamin B_{12}?

Folate deficiency generally results from inadequate nutritional intake of leafy green vegetables and citrus fruits and is especially seen in severely disabled patients. Deficiency also results from problems with absorption (as with small bowel disease or the use of phenytoin or phenobarbital) or increased demand (as in pregnancy, psoriasis, chemotherapy, or hemolytic anemia). The body stores only a 3-month supply of folate, so deficiency can develop after a short period of time. In contrast, the liver stores 3 to 5 years of B_{12}, so a nutritional deficiency alone almost never occurs. Vitamin B_{12} requires binding to intrinsic factor from the stomach to be absorbed in the terminal ileum. B_{12} deficiency is usually caused by pernicious anemia, a destruction of the parietal cells that make intrinsic factor in the stomach. Achlorhydria, or loss of stomach acid, is common in older patients and also causes deficiency by preventing binding of B_{12} to intrinsic factor. Colchicine and neomycin can also block B_{12} absorption. B_{12} deficiency can also cause any combination of nausea, heartburn, vague abdominal pain, or subacute neurologic disease (e.g., dementia, dorsal and lateral column defects).

Why does chronic disease cause anemia?

Anemia of chronic disease, also known as *inflammatory block,* is a mild-to-moderate anemia resulting from an

TABLE 8-1

Causes of Hypoproliferative Anemia by MCV

MCV	COMMON CAUSES	LESS COMMON CAUSES
MCV <80 Microcytosis	Iron deficiency	Thalassemia Anemia of chronic disease Hemoglobin E
MCV 80-95 Normocytosis	Anemic of chronic disease Acute bleeding	Bone marrow suppression, fibrosis, or infiltration
MCV >95 Macrocytosis	Alcohol	Vitamin B_{12} deficiency Folate deficiency Hypothyroidism Reticulocytosis

inability to utilize iron. Inflammatory mediators prevent the normal transfer of iron from bone marrow stores into hemoglobin. This type of anemia is associated with chronic inflammatory conditions, such as rheumatoid arthritis (RA) or systemic lupus erythematosus (SLE), and chronic infection, such as osteomyelitis.

What causes hemolysis?

Hemolysis can be categorized according to where the hemolysis occurs. In *intravascular* hemolysis, red cells are broken down directly in the blood vessels. Examples include red cell fragmentation across mechanical heart valves or over fibrin strands in disseminated intravascular coagulopathy (DIC). By contrast, in *extravascular* hemolysis, abnormal red cells are lysed in the reticuloendothelial system (RES) of the spleen or liver. Red cells are recognized as abnormal by the RES, due to attached antibodies, such as in autoimmune hemolysis or infection, or membrane or hemoglobin defects, such as sickle cell anemia or thalassemia.

EVALUATION

In whom should I suspect anemia?

Mild anemia is asymptomatic and is often discovered accidentally as part of routine blood work. Asymptomatic patients should not be screened for anemia. Symptoms of anemia are nonspecific and reflect inadequate oxygen delivery. Symptoms are also dependent on the abruptness of onset, severity, and age and cardiopulmonary reserve of the patient. In general, you should suspect anemia as a contributing factor in patients with fatigue, shortness of breath, dyspnea on exertion, dizziness, pallor, or tachycardia.

What medications cause anemia?

Medications can cause anemia by a variety of mechanisms. Always review a patient's medication list in un-

explained anemia. Common drugs associated with anemia are anticonvulsants, colchicine, trimethoprim, chloroquine, and certain antibiotics. Other medications cause macrocytosis by altering DNA synthesis directly; for example, chemotherapy agents, anticonvulsants, trimethoprim, and sulfasalazine.

What should I look for when I evaluate patients with anemia?

General findings in patients with significant anemia include tachycardia; cardiac flow murmur; and pale conjunctivae, palmar creases, and nail beds. A history of chest pain, light-headedness, or shortness of breath indicates possible end-organ hypoxia and should prompt rapid evaluation.

What tests are key in differentiating types of anemia?

Order a hematocrit or hemoglobin to confirm the diagnosis of anemia. Reticulocyte count, MCV, and peripheral smear will help further guide diagnosis (Figure 8-1).

If I suspect hemolysis, what tests are helpful?

Peripheral smear differentiates between intravascular and extravascular hemolysis. Spherocytes are formed during extravascular hemolysis because abnormal membrane is removed by the RES. Irregularly shaped red cell fragments, or schistocytes, are seen only in the case of intravascular hemolysis. Regardless of the site of hemolysis, red cell destruction results in reticulocytosis, elevated indirect bilirubin, elevated LDH, and decreased haptoglobin. Measurable haptoglobin drops because it binds to the hemoglobin released from hemolyzed red cells.

If I suspect iron deficiency, what else should I look for?

Ask about heavy menses, bloody or black stool, fatigue, and pica (i.e., eating dirt, a rare sign of iron deficiency).

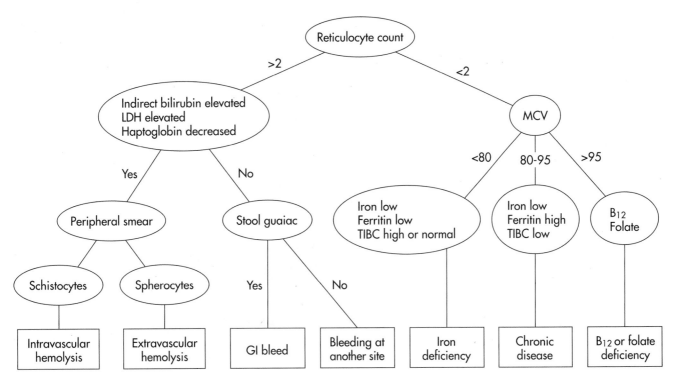

Figure 8-1 Diagnostic workup for common causes of anemia (sequence of testing may vary depending on the clinical situation).

Look for spoon nails (koilonychia); a smooth, red tongue (atrophic glossitis); or guaiac-positive stool, further signs of iron deficiency. Obtain serum iron, total iron-binding capacity (TIBC), and ferritin. Iron deficiency initially results in a normocytic anemia and low ferritin. Subsequently, serum iron falls and TIBC rises. With severe deficiency, hemoglobin falls and microcytosis develops, causing a low MCV. If the laboratory test results suggest iron deficiency, you need to find the source of blood loss. In addition to guaiac testing, endoscopy may be necessary.

The MCV is low and labs have ruled out iron deficiency. What do I do next?

If the MCV is low and iron deficiency is not apparent, consider either anemia of chronic disease or thalassemia. In anemia of chronic disease the ferritin, an acute-phase reactant, is often high and TIBC and serum iron are low. Despite low serum iron, iron replacement is of no benefit because of the inflammatory block. Thalassemia is a genetic disease of globin chains seen in patients with Mediterranean, African, or Asian heritage. Patients with thalassemia have a very low MCV in the 60 to 70 range, out of proportion to a mild anemia (Hct 33-40). Often target cells are seen on peripheral smear. Confirm β-thalassemia with hemoglobin electrophoresis. If the diagnosis remains unclear after full laboratory workup, consider a bone marrow biopsy and iron stain.

What should I do next if my patient has normocytic anemia (MCV 80–95)?

Review the history for medications that could suppress the bone marrow, such as antibiotics or chemotherapeutic agents. Additionally, check for signs or symptoms of neoplastic disease, such as anorexia, weight loss, or night sweats. Peripheral smear may suggest hemolysis or sickle cell disease, or may show tear drops in the case of marrow fibrosis or infiltration. Because normocytic anemia can result from early iron deficiency, iron studies may be helpful in differentiating iron deficiency from the anemia of chronic disease. Other specific studies for hemolysis, chronic renal failure, or thyroid disease may be warranted. Bone marrow biopsy can rule out myelodysplasia, infiltration, or bone marrow fibrosis.

What tests should I get if my patient has macrocytic anemia (MCV >95)?

Review history for alcohol or medication use, risk factors for vitamin B_{12} deficiency (e.g., gastric surgery, vitiligo, paresthesias in the feet), symptoms of hypothyroidism, or chronic liver disease. Also, look for signs or symptoms of acute bleeding or hemolysis because reticulocytes are larger than mature red cells and will raise the MCV. Examine the patient for signs of B_{12} deficiency, such as beefy red tongue and decreased peripheral vibratory or position sense, or for findings of end-stage liver disease. Review the smear for hypersegmented neutrophils and macroovalocytes, megaloblastic changes that are caused by abnormal DNA synthesis, and delayed nuclear maturation of erythrocyte precursors. Red blood cell folate and serum B_{12} levels may reveal the cause. If no obvious diagnosis is apparent, consider getting a bone marrow biopsy.

TREATMENT

In general, the underlying cause of the anemia should be identified and treated. Rarely, outpatients will need to be hospitalized or transfused for their anemia alone.

How do I treat iron deficiency anemia, and what response should I expect from treatment?

The goals of treatment are to: (1) identify and treat the cause of iron deficiency and (2) give sufficient iron to correct the anemia and replenish stores. With few exceptions, replace iron orally. Compliance can be difficult because about 25% of patients have side effects when they take iron on an empty stomach (i.e., nausea, epigastric pain, constipation, diarrhea). Although absorption is decreased 40% when iron is taken with food, this may be a necessary compromise. Start with 325 mg of ferrous sulfate once a day and advance to twice a day as tolerated. Ferrous gluconate and elixir preparations are available as well. The hematocrit should increase by 2 points every 3 to 4 weeks. A reticulocytosis is the first sign of response and is evident after 10 days.

When should I hospitalize a patient with anemia?

Hospitalize patients with anemia when they have a declining hematocrit resulting from ongoing blood loss or rapid hemolysis, or when cardiac or pulmonary symptoms occur.

Key Points

- Anemia is never normal—seek a cause in all patients who are anemic.
- History and examination are key in narrowing the differential diagnosis of anemia.
- Carefully review medications for a cause of anemia.
- Begin laboratory evaluation with a hematocrit, MCV, reticulocyte count, and smear.
- For iron deficiency anemia, start with low-dose iron replacement (325 mg PO qd).

CASE 8-1

A 26-year-old Vietnamese woman with bipolar disorder is referred from psychiatry for evaluation of her anemia. A routine CBC show Hct 35 and MCV 65. History and review of systems are negative except her psychiatric disease. She is on lithium and oral contraceptives and has very scant, regular periods.

A. What do you expect to see on peripheral smear?
B. What test(s) would you order next?
C. How would you treat this patient?

CASE 8-2

A 58-year-old alcoholic patient complains of fatigue. He takes phenytoin for seizures. He denies other symptoms, including melena or prior GI bleeding. He usually eats one meal a day at the neighborhood bar. His examination is normal except for mild hepatomegaly. His Hct is 33 with an MCV of 110 and corrected reticulocyte index of 1.7%. Several polymorphonuclear neutrophils (PMNs) with six lobes are seen on peripheral smear.

A. What are the possible causes of his anemia?
B. What test(s) would you order next?

9

Chest Pain

ETIOLOGY

What are the common causes of mild-to-moderate chest pain in clinic patients?

Chronic angina, esophageal reflux or dysmotility, and musculoskeletal pain (including costochondritis) are common. Less common causes are panic disorder and viral or bacterial infection causing pleural irritation. Rarely, biliary, gastric, or pancreatic disease cause chest pain.

What are life-threatening causes of chest pain that I shouldn't miss?

Acute aortic dissection, unstable or acute angina pectoris, MI, mediastinitis, pneumothorax, pericarditis, and PE should not be missed. Aortic dissection occurs when the aorta tears, allowing blood to dissect between layers of the vessel wall. Angina is chest pain resulting from insufficient oxygen supply to the heart muscle for the level of cardiac work (ischemia), seen particularly in patients with cardiac risk factors, such as hypertension, diabetes, cigarette use, family history of early cardiac disease, menopause, and dyslipidemia. MI occurs when angina persists long enough to cause cell death (infarction). Mediastinitis is an infection of the mediastinum, usually caused by esophageal rupture. PE occurs when a clot from the venous circulation lodges in a pulmonary artery.

EVALUATION

What pertinent history helps determine if chest pain is angina?

Ask all patients with chest pain about cardiac risk factors, character and distribution of pain, and associated symptoms. Angina is a heavy, tight, or squeezing retrosternal pain that often radiates to the neck, jaw, shoulders, or left arm. Associated symptoms are dyspnea, di-

aphoresis, nausea, vomiting, light-headedness, or palpitations. Usually, angina is brought on by exertion, stress, or large meals and is relieved by rest or sublingual nitrates. Atypical presentations are common, especially in women, the elderly, and patients with diabetes. Atypical angina may present as burning or sharp pain in atypical locations, such as the arm, neck, jaw, shoulder, or abdomen, or with isolated nausea, dyspnea, or wheezing (also called cardiac asthma). Unstable angina refers to an escalating pattern of angina, that is, angina occurring more often and/or with milder degrees of exertion. MI, which generally lasts longer than 30 minutes, causes similar but more severe pain than angina and stops once heart muscle is dead. Nonischemic causes of chest pain present with other clues (Table 9-1).

What features in history are seen in patients with acute aortic dissection?

Aortic dissection causes abrupt-onset tearing chest pain radiating to the back. Complications are life-threatening. Ask patients about neurologic deficits in addition to the usual questions about dyspnea, exercise intolerance, orthopnea (CHF, MI), nausea, or diaphoresis (MI).

What pertinent questions should I ask to explore the possibility of PE?

Ask about the triad of predisposing factors: (1) hypercoagulable states, such as cancer or family history of hypercoagulability; (2) prolonged stasis, such as with airplane trips, surgery, or immobility; and (3) vessel injury with recent surgery or trauma. Ask about unilateral leg swelling because this may reveal the embolic source. Other pertinent questions are similar to those for angina. Massive embolism can stretch a pulmonary artery, mimicking angina or causing actual right ventricular ischemia. In contrast, smaller PEs may produce lung infarcts at the pleural surface, causing sharp pleuritic pains. Isolated dyspnea without pain is the more common presentation. Syncope occurs in about 10% of PE and is a sign of a large embolus.

TABLE 9-1
Clues to Nonischemic Causes of Chest Pain

DIAGNOSIS	HISTORY	PHYSICAL EXAMINATION	DIAGNOSTIC TESTS
Costochondritis	Recent viral illness	Tender to palpation just lateral to sternum	None
Mediastinitis	Dyspnea, vomiting, recent esophageal instrumentation	Subcutaneous emphysema, "Hammon's crunch" (crepitus with heartbeat)	CXR: mediastinal air, pleural effusion (usually left-sided)
Musculoskeletal pain	Worse with motion or breath, history of trauma or cancer with metastases	Pain reproduced by palpation	Physical examination, CXR
Pericarditis	Sharp pain improved by leaning forward, recent viral illness	Pericardial friction rub, JVD, pulsus paradoxus* (with large pericardial effusion)	ECG: diffuse ST elevation, PR depression
Pneumonia	Fever, cough, dyspnea, purulent sputum, pleuritic pain	Rhonchi, egophony over involved lung, rales	CXR: pulmonary infiltrate
Pneumothorax	Pleuritic pain, dyspnea	Hyperresonance over one lung field, decreased breath sounds, tracheal shift	CXR: loss of lung markings outside sharp pleural line
Pleurisy	Pleuritic pain, dyspnea, recent viral illness, autoimmune disease	Pleural friction rub	CXR: normal, ± small effusion

JVD, Jugular venous distention; *CXR,* chest x-ray.
*Pulsus paradoxus is a drop in systolic blood pressure of more than 10 points with inspiration, caused by pericardial fluid compressing the right ventricle. You can palpate this at the radial pulse in dramatic cases of tamponade. To measure it more exactly, inflate a blood pressure cuff above systolic pressure, let air out slowly until you just begin to hear beats only during patient's expiration, and remember that value. Then let out more air until you hear all the beats through both inspiration and expiration. Subtract this pressure from the first; if it is greater than 10 mm Hg, you have pulsus paradoxus, indicating cardiac tamponade. Significant pulmonary obstructive disease also causes pulsus paradoxus.

What pertinent history should I ask to reveal an esophageal source of pain?

Historical clues to esophageal pain from acid reflux include food or acid regurgitation, pain worse with lying down, relief with antacids, delayed response (>10 minutes) to nitroglycerin, and absence of relation to exertion. However, the quality of chest pain of esophageal origin may mimic angina exactly. In fact, up to 30% of patients undergoing coronary angiography for suspected angina have normal coronary arteries, and in up to 50% of these, an esophageal cause for their pain is discovered. Esophageal spasm mimics angina, even reversing with nitroglycerin, and may be due to reflux esophagitis or other esophageal dysfunction.

How does pericarditis differ from angina in its presentation?

Pain from pericarditis is worse lying down, better leaning forward, and unimproved by rest. Risk factors for pericarditis include recent viral syndrome and renal failure.

What should I look for on examination?

Hypertension, though nonspecific, often accompanies angina and aortic dissection. Check blood pressure in both arms because they are unequal when dissection interrupts vascular supply to one side. Listen for new murmurs: Aortic insufficiency (diastolic murmur at the sternal border) suggests dissection involving the aortic valve, whereas mitral regurgitation (systolic murmur at the apex) suggests MI involving the mitral valve papillary muscle. Listen for rubs: A pulmonary friction rub timed with inspiration suggests pulmonary infarct resulting from PE or viral pleuritis, whereas a rub with each heartbeat suggests pericarditis. Palpate the chest wall to reproduce musculoskeletal pain.

What diagnostic tests do I order in an outpatient with chest pain?

Obtain current and old ECG and chest film in all patients with acute chest pain. Look on the ECG for the focal ST changes of angina or MI, or more diffuse ST elevations and PR depressions of pericarditis. Chest film can reveal CHF; pneumonia; pulmonary infarction; pneumothorax; and chest wall processes, such as rib fractures or lytic bone lesions. A widened mediastinum on chest film is a sign of possible aortic dissection, although 20% of dissections have a normal mediastinal width. Therapeutic trials performed in the clinic or at home may also aid in making a diagnosis: Relief with antacids suggests GERD or PUD, whereas relief with sublingual nitroglycerin suggests cardiac ischemia. Refer patients with stable episodes of angina-like symptoms for outpatient exercise treadmill testing (ETT) to assess for fixed coronary artery narrowing. For women (in whom ETT has low sensitivity) and for patients unable to walk, alternatives to ETT include nuclear medicine tests or stress echocardiogram.

What tests are appropriate for patients hospitalized because of chest pain?

In addition to ECG and chest film, obtain serial cardiac enzymes (see Ischemic Heart Disease section in Chapter 23 for details). Because of the high mortality of acute aortic dissection, with any suspicion obtain a transesophageal echocardiogram (TEE). If TEE is not available, chest CT is a second choice for imaging but is not as quick and cannot be done at the bedside. Also, do not forget that CHF and MI can accompany aortic dissection, and thrombolytics for MI are likely fatal if given to patients with concurrent aortic dissection. Obtain other basic laboratory tests: complete blood count with differential to look for anemia or infection; platelets, prothrombin and partial thromboplastin times for coagulopathy; and chemistry panel.

My clinic patient "ruled out" for MI but still has pain. What other tests are useful?

Patients "rule out" for MI when 24 hours of hospital monitoring and serial enzymes fail to reveal heart muscle damage. Coronary artery disease (CAD) is still possible even after ruling out and can be diagnosed by ETT or other imaging (see Ischemic Heart Disease section in Chapter 23). An outpatient GI evaluation may include a trial of proton pump inhibitors, the more invasive and expensive esophagogastroduodenoscopy (EGD) to look for esophageal or gastric lesions, or 24-hour esophageal pH monitoring to confirm GERD. Further evaluation for esophageal dysmotility may include barium swallow, balloon distention of the esophagus, or esophageal pressure monitoring.

TREATMENT

When should patients be hospitalized for chest pain?

Hospitalize and start continuous cardiac monitoring when you cannot exclude cardiac ischemia or other life-threatening illness. Recently, some centers have developed rapid diagnostic protocols for emergency-room–based evaluation of chest pain in low-risk patients with no history of CAD or other heart disease and no severe comorbidity who are able to perform ETT. These patients are evaluated over 12 hours with clinical assessment, ECG, and cardiac enzymes followed by exercise testing, which may obviate the need for admission in some patients.

What specific treatments are available for common causes of chest pain?

See Ischemic Heart Disease section in Chapter 23 for treatment of ischemia and Table 9-2 for other causes.

What is the prognosis for patients with "noncardiac" chest pain?

Normal angiography is associated with a 7-year mortality of less than 1%. Unfortunately, chest pain of unclear cause can develop into a chronic pain syndrome, causing patients significant morbidity and cost. These patients are best managed by primary care physicians with continued vigilance for the possibility of CAD (especially in the elderly), selected evaluation for esophageal or psychiatric disease, judicious use of medications for symptom control, and reassurance.

Key Points ·····································

- Consider life-threatening causes in all patients with chest pain, and use focused history, examination, and studies to rapidly find or exclude them.
- If ischemic cardiac chest pain is a reasonable possibility, admit for monitoring and serial cardiac enzyme testing.
- Pericarditis causes pain relieved by leaning forward and diffuse PR depression or ST elevation on ECG.
- Aortic dissection causes pain radiating to the back, unequal pulses, and widened mediastinum, and it may have associated neurologic deficits or MI.

TABLE 9-2

Therapeutic Options for Noncardiac Causes of Chest Pain

CAUSE OF CHEST PAIN	TREATMENT OPTIONS
Acute aortic dissection	Blood pressure control, surgical repair
Costochondritis	NSAIDs or acetaminophen, time
Gastroesophageal reflux	Proton pump inhibitors, lifestyle modification, surgical fundoplication
Esophageal spasm	Calcium channel blocker, nitroglycerin
Musculoskeletal pain	Rest, stretching, physical therapy, NSAIDs or acetaminophen
Pericarditis	NSAIDs
Pneumonia	Antibiotics, oxygen, chest physiotherapy
Pneumothorax	If tension pneumothorax, urgent decompression by angiocatheter, chest tube

CASE 9-1

A 28-year-old man presents to the emergency room complaining of 24 hours of increasing chest pain. The pain is sharp, substernal, and pleuritic in nature. He felt well until 2 days ago, when he developed low-grade fever, sore throat, and a dry cough. On examination, he is leaning forward clutching his chest. Vitals are T 37.5° C, P 90, BP 125/80, and RR 18.

A. What is your differential diagnosis?
B. The nurse hands you his ECG (Figure 9-1). What is the most likely diagnosis?
C. What would you expect on physical examination?
D. What is the likely cause for this patient's syndrome?
E. How should he be treated?

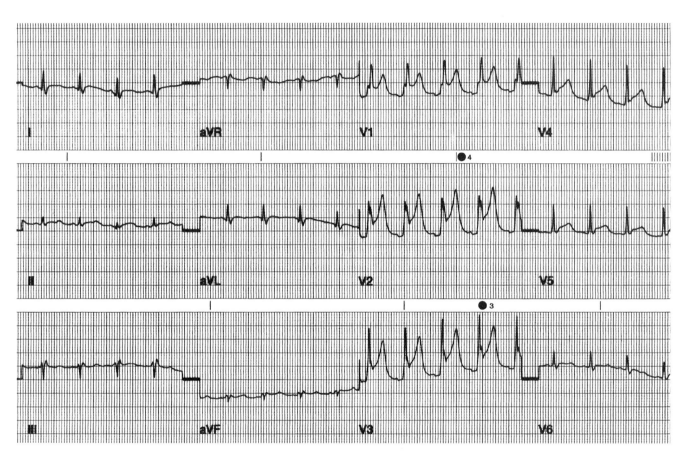

Figure 9-1 Electrocardiogram for patient in Case 9-1. *(From Davidson R:* Electrocardiography in acute care medicine, *St Louis, 1995, Mosby.)*

CASE 9-2

A 65-year-old woman presents with complaints of acute chest pain that began 30 minutes ago. The pain is squeezing, substernal pain radiating to the jaw and back of the neck, associated with dyspnea. She has type II diabetes and hypertension. Fasting lipid panel 1 year ago revealed low-density lipoprotein (LDL) of 130 and HDL of 25. She is postmenopausal. Her brother had a heart attack at age 50. Medications are NPH insulin and felodipine. On examination, she is a morbidly obese, di-

aphoretic woman. Vitals are T 36.8° C, P 105, BP 158/92, RR 20. Chest is clear. Cardiac examination reveals no murmurs, rubs, or gallops.

A. List this patient's CAD risk factors.
B. Create a differential diagnosis for her chest pain.
C. Her ECG is shown (Figure 9-2). What is the most likely diagnosis?
D. What pertinent negatives on history, examination, or chest film make aortic dissection less likely?

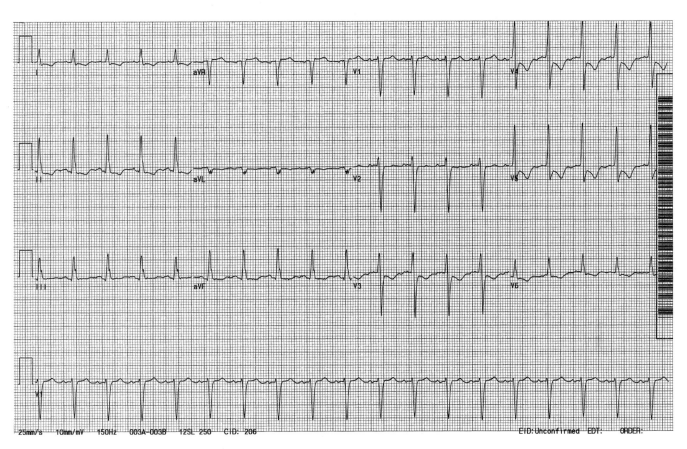

Figure 9-2 Electrocardiogram for patient in Case 9-2.

chapter

10 Cough

ETIOLOGY

What are the most common causes of cough?

Acute cough, less than 3 weeks' duration, is almost always due to infection or irritants such as cigarette smoke. *Chronic cough* (longer than 3 weeks) is most commonly caused by the conditions listed in Box 10-1. Chronic bronchitis is defined as productive cough on most days for at least 3 months of 2 consecutive years; it occurs almost exclusively in smokers. After acute viral infection, up to 40% of patients have persistent cough for several weeks resulting from transiently reactive airways. Up to 25% of cases of chronic cough have more than one cause. Angiotensin-converting enzyme (ACE) inhibitors cause cough in up to 20% of users.

What serious causes of cough should I not miss?

Cancer is always a concern in patients with chronic cough, particularly in smokers. Approximately 80% of cancer patients have other symptoms, such as weight loss or hemoptysis. CHF may present with cough. TB and pertussis, major public health risks, should always be considered. Up to 25% of adults with cough of longer than 3 weeks' duration without another cause have serologic evidence consistent with recent pertussis infection. Previous vaccination does not exclude pertussis. PE is an infrequent but serious cause of acute cough.

When cough is accompanied by hemoptysis, what should I consider?

Acute bronchitis is the most common cause of bloody sputum in the United States. Consider cancer in smokers or patients over 50 years of age. Other causes include PE and TB.

EVALUATION

What historical points and examination findings are important?

Table 10-1 lists pertinent history and examination findings to explore for each of the three common causes of chronic cough. Note medications such as ACE inhibitors. Additionally, in puzzling cases, obtain an exposure history for work or hobby hazards, such as asbestos; contact with persons with TB or pertussis; and cat or bird contact. Inhaler or antacid use suggests asthma and gastroesophageal reflux disease, respectively. Review constitutional symptoms and risk factors for cancer and human immunodeficiency virus.

What tests will help me determine benign causes of a chronic cough?

There is no standard workup. If you suspect asthma, office spirometry is reasonably specific when forced expiratory volume in 1 second (FEV1) is less than 80% predicted or the forced expiratory volume/forced vital capacity ratio (FEV1/FVC) is less than 75%. Normal spirometry does not rule out asthma. The most sensitive diagnostic test for cough-variant asthma is the methacholine challenge test, an inhalant that induces bronchospasm in these patients. If you suspect gastroesophageal reflux disease, a barium swallow may show hiatal hernia or reflux (make sure that you indicate that you suspect reflux on the radiology requisition). The gold standard is esophageal pH probe testing. In reality, most of these conditions are suggested by history and confirmed by an empiric treatment trial.

BOX 10-1 Common Causes of Chronic Cough

Postnasal drip	Cough-variant asthma
Gastroesophageal reflux disease	Chronic bronchitis

TABLE 10-1
History and Examination Findings in Common Causes of Chronic Cough

CAUSE	HISTORY	EXAMINATION
Asthma	Recent viral infection Cold/exercise provoke cough Aspirin or NSAID sensitivity Family or personal history of asthma/allergies Wheezing	Eczema Wheezing (rare) Prolonged forced expiration
Postnasal drip	Nasal drainage Early morning productive cough Throat clearing	Conjunctival irritation Pharyngeal cobblestoning Pale and boggy nasal mucosa Mucus in posterior pharynx
GERD	Heartburn Acid or food regurgitation Cough after meals Symptoms worse when supine Obesity Hoarseness Calcium channel blocker use	Obesity Hoarseness

How can I use therapeutic trials to diagnose these three common conditions?

With an empiric trial of therapy, the cough should improve significantly. These trials are not rapid; allow 4 to 6 weeks before you assess the impact. If you suspect postnasal drip (PND) or allergic rhinitis, try decongestants; antihistamines, such as diphenhydramine or chlorpheniramine, that promote nasal mucosal drying; and/or nasal steroids, particularly if allergic rhinitis is suspected. If GERD is suspected, begin by eliminating substances that relax the gastroesophageal sphincter, such as cigarettes, alcohol, spicy foods, chocolate, and peppermint. Raise the head of the bed 6 inches with blocks or bricks (pillows do not work because they bend the patient at the waist, increasing pressure on the stomach). Add empiric proton pump inhibitor therapy. If the cost is prohibitive, histamine$_2$ blockers (H$_2$ blockers) can be tried (e.g., ranitidine) but may fail to relieve the cough. Treat patients with symptoms suggestive of cough-variant asthma with β-agonist inhalers. If the patient already uses β-agonists, add a steroid inhaler. Steroid inhalers can irritate airways, so do not start them during acute infection.

When should I obtain a chest film or other more specialized invasive tests?

Get a chest film in patients with acute cough with high fever, tachycardia, history concerning for pulmonary embolism, abnormal lung examination, or hypoxia on pulse oximetry. For chronic cough patients, if history, examination, and empiric trial do not elucidate a cause, or if constitutional symptoms or cancer risk factors are present, get a chest film. Because of low sensitivity, sputum cytology cannot be used to rule out cancer. A chest film should be considered early in the workup if the patient has a history of cigarette abuse, concerning occupational exposure, or risks for TB or HIV.

TREATMENT

How do I manage acute infectious cough?

Sinusitis, bronchitis, and viral respiratory infections often do not require antibiotic treatment. Community-acquired pneumonia should be treated with appropriate antibiotics (see Chapter 29).

What are some ways to relieve symptoms for cough patients?

Prescribe β-agonist inhalers for cough caused by postviral reactive airways. Eliminate irritants, especially cigarette smoke. Counsel about smoking cessation. Advise adequate hydration and humidity. Many patients expect a prescription for cough syrup, but only prescribe codeine if cough interferes with sleeping or eating. Start with 15 to 30 mg of codeine every 2 to 4 hours as needed. Otherwise, recommend over-the-counter preparations with only one or two active ingredients, such as guaifenesin (expectorant) or dextromethorphan (suppressant). "Cold" and "flu" preparations are best avoided because the number of active ingredients may double or interact with other medicines.

When should I refer?

Refer to a pulmonologist when the cause of cough is unclear and/or empiric therapy has not helped; when bronchoscopy is indicated to rule out TB, cancer, or other rare disease; or when specialized intervention is required (e.g., interstitial lung disease, cancer). For suspected reflux that does not respond to proton pump inhibitor, refer to a gastroenterologist. In addition to your own counseling regarding cigarette use, smoking cessation clinics can be useful. If occupational exposure is possible, refer for occupational medicine evaluation.

Key Points

- Acute cough is almost always infectious or caused by airway irritants.
- Chronic cough is often due to PND, GERD, or bronchospasm (postinfectious or asthma). Empiric therapy is often helpful.

CASE 10-1

A 30-year-old woman had an upper respiratory illness several weeks ago and has been coughing since then, especially in the morning when she wakes up or when she goes jogging. She has no personal history of asthma but does recall coughing when she competed in college crew. She has seasonal allergies and an allergy to cats. She recently moved into a new, carpeted apartment. Her job is office-based. She takes no medications.

  A. What is your differential diagnosis?
  B. What history or physical findings might assist your diagnostic evaluation?
  C. What tests do you order?
  D. What treatment do you pick?

CASE 10-2

A 65-year-old woman seeks your opinion regarding a cough she has had for 6 months. She started an ACE inhibitor 3 months ago for hypertension. She has a morning cough with throat clearing and slight sputum production, and minimal symptoms during the day. However, for the past 1 to 2 months she has been coughing much more frequently and having difficulty sleeping. She does not smoke and has no wheezing or heartburn.

  A. What is your differential diagnosis?
  B. What history or physical findings might assist your diagnosis?
  C. What further interventions will be helpful with diagnosis?
  D. How would your answers change if an S_3 and lung crackles are found on examination?

11

Diarrhea

ETIOLOGY

Does my patient really have diarrhea?

Diarrhea is an increase in stool water or a stool weight greater than 200 g/day. If stool takes the shape of the container it is in, the patient probably has diarrhea. Chronic diarrhea lasts longer than 3 weeks.

Why does diarrhea occur?

Three main pathologic processes cause diarrhea (Table 11-1). In *secretory* diarrhea, intact intestinal cells produce excess fluid, usually from a toxin effect. In *osmotic* diarrhea, poor absorption of osmotic agents increases stool volume. In *inflammatory* diarrhea, intestinal lining cells are destroyed, so red and white blood cells are evident in the stool. Any of these may coexist. For example, inflammatory diarrhea can result in lactose intolerance (osmotic diarrhea).

What are the common causes of acute diarrhea?

Viral infections cause most acute diarrhea (usually Norwalk agent or rotavirus). Bacteria and parasites are less common culprits. Transmission occurs via the fecal-oral route by ingestion of contaminated food or water or sexual activity. Less common causes include leakage around a fecal impaction, narcotic withdrawal, diverticulitis, and medications (Box 11-1).

What causes bloody diarrhea?

Bloody diarrhea indicates inflammation, most commonly from invasive enteric pathogens, such as *Campylobacter*, *Shigella*, *Salmonella*, and *Escherichia coli* O157:H7. Inflammatory bowel disease (Crohn's disease and ulcerative colitis) may also present this way, usually in young adults. Other causes of bloody diarrhea include ischemic colitis, radiation injury, and GI bleed.

Is antibiotic-associated diarrhea always due to *Clostridium difficile* overgrowth?

Antibiotic-associated diarrhea is generally mild, dose-related, without a causative agent, and resolves when antibiotics are stopped. *Clostridium difficile* causes 25% of antibiotic-associated diarrhea.

What are the common causes of chronic or recurring diarrhea?

Lactose intolerance, indolent infection, and irritable bowel syndrome (IBS) are the most common causes. Lactose intolerance, an acquired lactase deficiency, occurs in greater than 75% of African-Americans and Asian-Americans and up to 20% of Caucasians. Undigested lactose after milk-product ingestion causes flatulence, bloating, and diarrhea. Infections with *Giardia lamblia* or *C. difficile* may be recurrent or chronic. *Giardia* is most notable for foul-smelling flatulence and steatorrhea. None of these conditions causes nocturnal diarrhea or bloody stool, so evaluate further if these symptoms are present.

What is the difference between irritable bowel syndrome (IBS) and inflammatory bowel disease (IBD)?

IBS is a common alteration in intestinal motility with enhanced visceral sensitivity. Both IBS and inflammatory bowel disease can cause intermittent abdominal pain, cramping, and alternating diarrhea and constipation over many years. IBS has specific diagnostic criteria (Box 11-2). Inflammatory bowel disease (Crohn's and ulcerative colitis) is due to bowel wall inflammation of unclear cause, with peak incidence in 15- to 35-year-olds. In addition to diarrhea, patients with inflammatory bowel disease may have bloody stool, tenesmus (if the rectum is involved), or weight loss. Crohn's disease causes transmural inflammation and involves any part of the bowel from oral mucosa to rectum in discontinuous patches. Ulcerative colitis causes more superficial inflammation of the bowel

TABLE 11-1

Patterns Suggesting the Underlying Pathologic Process in Patients With Diarrhea

CAUSE	STOOL PATTERN	COMMON SYMPTOMS
SECRETORY		
Rotavirus	Watery	Low-grade fever, myalgias
Cholera	Watery, large volume	Severe dehydration
Hormone-producing tumors	Watery	Persists with fasting
MALABSORPTIVE/ OSMOTIC		
Lactose intolerance	Loose	Bloating, cramping, flatulence
Pancreatic insufficiency	Loose	Greasy (floats like oil in water)
INFLAMMATORY		
Ulcerative colitis	Bloody	Tenesmus, weight loss
Enteric pathogens	Bloody	Higher fever, myalgias, cramping

BOX 11-1   Common Medications That Can Cause Diarrhea

Alcohol
Antibiotics
Antihypertensives: β-blockers, furosemide, hydralazine
Antiinflammatory medications: ibuprofen, colchicine
Caffeine
Digoxin
Laxatives
Magnesium-containing antacids
Serotonin reuptake inhibitor antidepressants
Sorbitol: cough drops, sugarless gum

BOX 11-2   Criteria for the Diagnosis of Irritable Bowel Syndrome

A. Must have one of these for at least 3 months:
  • Persistent or intermittent abdominal pain or discomfort relieved with defecation, or
  • Persistent or intermittent change in stool frequency or consistency
B. Must also have two of these in addition to a criterion from list A:
  • Altered stool frequency of greater than 3 bowel movements per day or less than 3 per week
  • Altered stool form, either hard or loose
  • Altered stool passage with straining, urgency, or feeling of incomplete evacuation
  • Passage of mucus
  • Bloating or feeling of abdominal distention

TABLE 11-2

Pertinent Questions Regarding Diarrhea

QUESTION	CAUSE SUGGESTED BY POSITIVE ANSWER
Bloody stool, mucus	Inflammatory cause
Fever	Infection (viral, bacterial), IBD
Greasy stools	Fat malabsorption (sprue, pancreatic insufficiency)
Nocturnal symptoms	Concerning for pathologic cause, IBS unlikely
Persistence with 24-hour fast	Secretory cause (VIP-oma)
Recent antibiotics, institutionalization	*C. difficile*
Camping, day care exposures	*G. lamblia*

VIP-oma, Vasoactive intestinal polypeptide secreting tumor.

or Crohn's ileitis, fat-soluble vitamins A, D, E, and K can become deficient, causing vision problems (vitamin A), bone thinning (vitamin D), or coagulopathy (vitamin K). Vitamin B_{12} deficiency can also develop with malabsorption in the terminal ileum.

EVALUATION

What questions should I ask my patient with diarrhea?

Many patients cannot specifically characterize their diarrhea. Prompt them to describe frequency, volume, and appearance of the diarrhea to assess severity of their illness and identify likely causes. Attempt to categorize the diarrhea as acute or chronic based on duration of symp-

wall, begins at the rectum, and affects a continuous section of colon.

Why is malabsorption important?

Clinically significant malabsorptive syndromes can cause deficiencies of nutrients and/or vitamins. This can occur with intestinal cell injury or loss of digestive enzymes. If fat is malabsorbed, as with bile salt depletion

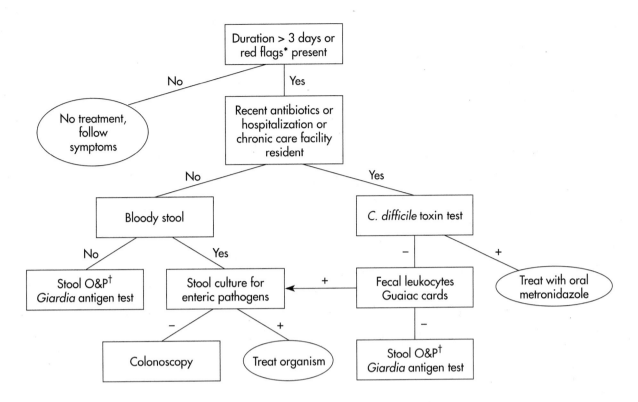

* Red flags: high fever, bloody diarrhea, severe volume depletion, severe abdominal pain, or immunocompromise. †In travelers.

Figure 11-1 Workup of acute diarrhea.

toms. Further, try to categorize diarrhea as inflammatory by presence of blood and mucus, secretory by watery stool, or malabsorptive by looseness without blood or water. Other pertinent details to ask about are included in Table 11-2.

What history suggests an infectious cause?

Acute onset, fevers, chills, or myalgias suggest infection. Patients at high risk include children in day care centers and their household contacts, travelers, institutionalized or hospitalized patients, patients who are immunocompromised or recently on antibiotics, and people who have anal sex.

What diagnostic tests should I order in a patient with acute diarrhea?

Most episodes of diarrhea are self-limited and require no tests. Although many tests are available, their indiscriminate use is unproductive and costly. For example, routine stool cultures for enteric pathogens in patients with diarrhea are positive only 2% of the time. Consider further testing when the patient has any of the following: symptoms longer than 3 days, temperature higher than 38.5° C, bloody diarrhea, severe volume depletion, severe abdominal pain, or immunocompromise (Figure 11-1).

When should I test for *C. difficile* or *Giardia*?

Obtain *C. difficile* toxin with recent antibiotic use, in recently hospitalized patients, or in chronic care facility residents. *C. difficile* toxin testing identifies clinical disease, whereas cultures will be positive with asymptomatic colonization, as seen in up to 20% of inpatients. The test for *Giardia* antigen has good sensitivity (>92%) and specificity (95%) to pick up this infection and should be obtained in campers and day care workers with persistent diarrhea.

What diagnostic tests should I order for chronic diarrhea?

Confirm the presence of diarrhea with a 24-hour stool collection because 40% of patients referred for diarrhea have fecal weights less than 200 g per day. Discontinue loperamide before testing. Consider IBS in patients who do not have true diarrhea. Obtain complete blood count (CBC) to look for infection or blood loss; ESR, electrolytes, albumin, stool guaiac, and fecal leukocytes to look for inflammation; and *C. difficile* toxin and *Giardia* antigen in patients at risk. If signs of malabsorption are present, such as weight loss, anemia, low albumin, ecchymoses, or neuropathy, obtain qualitative fecal fat and prothrombin time (for vitamin K deficiency). A successful trial of a lactose-free diet diagnoses lactose intolerance. A 24-hour fast helps distinguish between malabsorption of ingested material (diarrhea abates) and secretory diarrhea (diarrhea continues). If parasitic infections are suspected, in travelers or those engaging in anal sex, obtain three stool samples for ova and parasite studies.

How do I test for irritable bowel syndrome?

IBS is a functional disorder, meaning there are symptoms without objective abnormalities. Like many other clinical syndromes, there is no diagnostic test and clinical criteria assist in making the diagnosis.

When should I refer to a gastroenterologist?

Refer patients in whom the cause of documented diarrhea is unclear, for endoscopic procedures (e.g., malabsorption, inflammatory diarrhea without infectious cause), and for treatment of advanced cases of inflammatory bowel disease.

TREATMENT

Who needs antibiotics?

Antibiotics are not required for most cases of acute infectious diarrhea. Treat *Giardia* and *C. difficile* with oral metronidazole. Refractory or recurrent *C. difficile* may require oral vancomycin (very expensive). Severe traveler's diarrhea, often caused by an enteric pathogen, can be treated with a quinolone to reduce severity and duration. Finally, give antibiotics if there is high fever, leukocytosis, and frequent stools (almost always resulting from an enteric pathogen). *Campylobacter jejuni* and *Giardia* relapse in about 20% of cases, so consider re-treating for recurrent symptoms.

Which medications decrease the symptoms of diarrhea?

Treat volume depletion: for mild orthostasis, caffeine-free glucose–containing beverages are adequate; for more severe depletion, use oral rehydration solutions (i.e., sports drinks). Bismuth subsalicylate can reduce by 50% the number of unformed stools through antibacterial, antiinflammatory, and antisecretory action. Opiate derivatives, such as loperamide, slow intestinal motility and reduce the number of stools by 80%. Beware, however,

that antimotility agents can prolong the course of invasive bacteria and are not used in IBD. Rule out *C. difficile* if this is a possibility before starting loperamide because of the risk for toxic megacolon and rupture.

How do I treat IBS?

An effective physician-patient relationship is important for reassurance and for education about the chronic nature of symptoms, dietary modification (high-fiber, low-fat), and exercise. Treat the predominant symptom: hyoscyamine for abdominal cramping, loperamide for diarrhea, and high fiber to even out alternating constipation and diarrhea.

When should I hospitalize a patient with diarrhea?

Hospitalize patients with severe dehydration (>20% of volume lost) or significant emesis preventing oral rehydration for IV fluids and electrolytes. Patients with severe GI bleeding as from a flare of IBD may need hospitalization for stabilization and initiation of IV nutrition or steroids.

Key Points
- Acute diarrhea is usually self-limited, requiring rehydration without further workup.
- Confirm the presence of chronic diarrhea by measuring stool volume first.
- Use history and physical examination to distinguish inflammatory, osmotic, or secretory diarrhea.

CASE 11-1

A 78-year-old woman presents with diarrhea. She was healthy until 4 weeks earlier, when she was hospitalized for angina. She started aspirin and atenolol and was treated for a urinary tract infection. Since discharge, she reports 3 to 4 soft, watery stools daily with mild left lower quadrant cramping. She denies fever, melena, or hematochezia. On examination, she is afebrile and guaiac negative and has mild abdominal pain to deep palpation of the left lower quadrant.
 A. *What are possible causes of her diarrhea?*
 B. *What laboratory tests would you order, if any?*
 C. *Would you start any treatment at this point?*

chapter

12

Dizziness and Syncope

ETIOLOGY

How do I categorize causes of dizziness?

It is most useful to place the dizziness into one of three broad categories: vertigo, presyncope, or other. Ask the patient to describe the sensation without using the word "dizzy." *Vertigo* is an illusory sense that either the room or the patient is moving; this implicates the central or peripheral vestibular system. *Presyncope* is often described as light-headedness, "seeing stars," "blacking out," or impending fainting. This sensation implies cerebral dysfunction resulting from decreased perfusion, such as from low blood pressure or arrhythmia. One large study found that nearly half of the patients complaining of dizziness had more than one cause.

What are the causes of vertigo?

Vertigo is the most common type of dizziness, accounting for 40% to 60% of all patients presenting with the complaint. Causes are divided by anatomic source: *peripheral*, located in 8th nerve or inner ear, which are very common and often benign, or *central*, located in the cerebellum or brainstem, which are more worrisome (Table 12-1). Select findings can help distinguish the location. These include latency (the time to onset of symptoms after aggravating maneuver—such as head movement), whether the symptoms are fatigable (get better with repeated maneuvers), the pattern of onset, and whether nystagmus is prominent (Table 12-2).

What are the causes of presyncope and syncope?

Presyncope and syncope are caused by decreased cerebral perfusion. The main classes are *decreased intravascular volume* (bleeding, diarrhea, diuretic overuse), *neurally mediated* (loss of vascular tone and/or bradycardia), and *cardiac* (organic heart disease or arrhythmia). Neurally mediated causes include situational, micturition, and vasovagal syncope. Patients frequently experience

nausea and warmth before their light-headedness or syncope. These reflex-mediated problems are more common in younger patients (i.e., younger than 60 years of age). Elderly patients have a different set of neurally mediated causes, including an exaggerated carotid sinus reflex and autonomic neuropathy. The elderly are also more sensitive to medications (e.g., nitroglycerin, antihypertensive agents, and antidepressants), which can lead to chronic postural light-headedness or syncope.

What suggests a cardiac cause of syncope?

When symptoms occur without warning or with exertion, cardiac syncope is more likely. Cardiac syncope is more common in patients older than 60 years of age. It may be due to ischemia, arrhythmia, or structural problems, for example, critical aortic stenosis or hypertrophic cardiomyopathy. A PE can suddenly drop left ventricular filling and cardiac output, leading to syncope. Consider PE in any syncope that sounds cardiac but occurs in patients with low cardiac risk or high deep venous thrombosis risk (e.g., pregnant women or oral contraceptive pill users).

What are some other important causes of dizziness?

Three other causes to keep in mind are early pregnancy, hyperventilation, and multiple sensory deficits. Hyperventilation is a common cause of a dysphoric light-headed feeling, often accompanied by circumoral or extremity tingling and numbness. A common combination is hyperventilation exacerbating benign positional vertigo. Reproducing the symptoms after forced hyperventilation makes the diagnosis and reassures the patient. Multiple sensory deficits are common in elderly patients with dizziness. Minor dysfunction in two or three of the spatial orientation systems (vestibular, visual, and proprioceptive) can cause significant lack of confidence and an unsteady sensation. In addition, "polypharmacy" likely exacerbates problems with dizziness.

TABLE 12-1

Clinical Features and Frequency of Selected Causes of Vertigo

CAUSE	CLINICAL FEATURES	FREQUENCY
CENTRAL		
Cerebellar hemorrhage	*Life-threatening!* Abnormal finger-to-nose or heel-to-shin exam	Very rare
Brainstem ischemia	Usually accompanied by other brainstem findings (diplopia, weakness or numbness of extremities, dysarthria)	Rare
PERIPHERAL		
BPV	Moderate to severe, brief spells (often <1 min) Most pronounced with position changes (getting out of bed) Occurs after age 50, younger if history of head trauma	25%-30% of all vertigo
Vestibulitis/neuritis	Sudden onset, severe, lasting days to weeks Often follows viral illness and can occur in clusters	10%-15% of all vertigo
Meniere's syndrome	Triad of: (1) Recurrent vertigo spells lasting minutes to hours, not days (2) Tinnitus (3) Low frequency hearing loss	10% of all vertigo
CENTRAL + PERIPHERAL		
Acoustic neuroma	Presents as peripheral cause initially, then insidiously progresses to central pattern May involve 5th and 7th cranial nerves	Very rare

BPV, Benign positional vertigo.

TABLE 12-2

Features That Help Distinguish Peripheral From Central Causes of Vertigo

FINDINGS	CENTRAL	PERIPHERAL
Latency (time to onset of symptoms after perturbation, i.e., moving the head)	None	3-20 seconds
Fatigable (decreases with successive trials)	—	+++
Onset	Insidious	Sudden
Nystagmus	Marked (enhanced with fixation)	Minimal (decreased with fixation)

EVALUATION

What questions should I ask the patient with dizziness or syncope?

- Possibility of pregnancy
- Current medications (nitroglycerin, antihypertensive agents, and antidepressants)
- Timing, chronicity, onset, and prior episodes
- Effect of physical factors (position, movement, stress, or micturition)
- Presence of hearing loss (suggests Meniere's disease or acoustic neuroma)
- History of ear infections, head trauma, or barotrauma (suggests benign positional vertigo [BPV])
- Ototoxic drugs (aminoglycosides, loop diuretics, salicylates, quinine, or quinidine)
- Brainstem symptoms (double vision, dysarthria, weakness, or numbness in face or extremities suggest worrisome central causes)
- Palpitations, chest pain, or shortness of breath (suggests cardiac cause)

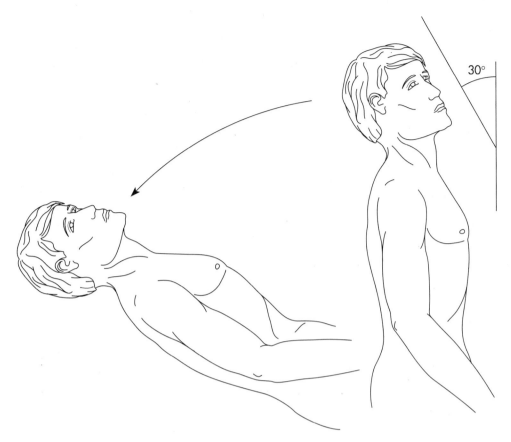

Figure 12-1 The Dix-Hallpike (or Nylen-Bárany) maneuver: Have the patient sit up with the head tilting back 30 degrees and to the side 30 degrees. Lie the patient rapidly backwards while maintaining the same head position relative to the body (i.e., so the head ends up tipped 30 degrees below the plane of the table). Have the patient keep eyes open and look for nystagmus and reproduction of symptoms. The nystagmus may be subtle and horizontal or rotary. The best place to look for it is a blood vessel at the edge of the limbus. Repeat the test, tilting the head to the other side.

What should I look for on the physical examination?

Vital signs: Postural changes, irregular pulse, normal gross visual acuity, tachypnea

HEENT: Ear canals, carotid bruit and upstrokes, carotid sinus massage if older than 60 years old (unless they have a bruit, history of ventricular tachycardia, or recent MI or cerebrovascular accident [CVA])

Lungs: Rales (indicating possible CHF)

Heart: Rate, intensity of first and second heart sounds, murmur

Rectal: Occult blood (if volume depleted)

Neurologic: Cranial nerves (especially hearing, subtle diplopia, or loss of facial sensation), cerebellar function (finger-to-nose, rapid alternating movement, heel-to-shin), general screen of strength, sensation (especially vibration and proprioception in feet looking for peripheral neuropathy), and reflexes

Other: Three minutes of forced hyperventilation (if no other clear cause is identified); Dix-Hallpike maneuver when suspecting benign positional vertigo (Figure 12-1)

What tests should be obtained routinely?

Obtain ECG for any case of syncope or if cardiopulmonary review and examination suggest a cardiac cause of dizziness. Obtain hematocrit if volume depleted or guaiac positive.

TREATMENT

What can I try before using medications?

Most peripheral causes of vertigo are fatigable; that is, the patients get better with repeated provocation. For example, ask your patient to repeat whatever physical maneuver reproduces their vertigo until they no longer get symptoms (5 to 10 repetitions) about 4 times per day. If the patient can tolerate this, it is an excellent therapy. Hyperventilation is made better by breath-holding or bag-breathing exercises. Multiple sensory deficits may improve with eyeglasses, hearing aids, or a cane. Loose-necked shirts and avoiding neckties may help people with overactive carotid sinus reflexes.

What are useful medications?

Antidizziness drugs treat symptoms and generally fall into four categories: neuroleptics (e.g., prochlorperazine, droperidol, promethazine), antihistamines (especially meclizine and cyclizine), anticholinergics (e.g., scopolamine, dramamine), and sympathomimetics (e.g., pseudoephedrine). Pseudoephedrine is useful in combination with antihistamines or anticholinergics because it helps counter their sedation. Occasionally, a patient might need benzodiazepines (e.g., diazepam) for severe vertigo, tricyclic antidepressants for hyperventilation, or thiazide diuretics for Meniere's disease.

When should I admit or refer?

Obviously, the five life-threatening causes (arrhythmia, cardiac outflow obstruction, cerebellar hemorrhage, pulmonary embolus, and significant blood loss) require immediate attention and referral/admission (Table 12-3). All central causes of vertigo should be further evaluated by imaging techniques (CT, MRI), audiology evaluation, and/or ENT referral and may require admission, depending on severity. Patients who have a first syncope with clinical suspicion for organic heart disease should be admitted. Referral for echocardiogram, Holter monitor, treadmill, and/or cardiology evaluation may be required, depending on clinical findings. Some patients with hyperventilation, especially those with associated panic symptoms, may benefit from psychiatric referral.

Key Points

- Dizziness is common, is usually self-limited, and should be separated by history into vertigo, presyncope/syncope, and other causes.
- Quickly screen for life-threatening causes: arrhythmia, cardiac outflow obstruction, cerebellar hemorrhage, pulmonary embolus, or significant blood loss.
- Treat most patients with nonpharmacologic measures and medications, such as meclizine.
- Ask patients to call if symptoms get worse, if new symptoms develop, or if the symptoms have not resolved in 2 weeks.

CASE 12-1

A 35-year-old woman was well until this morning when she had the sudden onset of very severe dizziness described as "the room spinning out of control." She has vomited twice since the onset. On examination, she has spontaneous horizontal nystagmus and is holding her head perfectly still. She states that head movement makes it much worse. Her pulse is regular and normal. Her cardiac examination is normal, and she has no abnormal cerebellar findings. On questioning, she remembers stuffiness and nasal congestion beginning 2 to 3 days ago.

What is the most likely cause of her symptoms?

TABLE 12-3
Life-Threatening Causes of Dizziness or Syncope

CONDITION	FINDINGS
Cardiac arrhythmia	History of palpitations
	Irregular pulse
Cardiac outflow obstruction	Systolic murmur
Aortic stenosis	Delayed carotid upstrokes
Hypertrophic cardiomyopathy	Abnormal splitting of the S_2
Cerebellar hemorrhage	Abnormal neurologic exam
Pulmonary embolus	Risk for deep venous thrombosis
	Loud S_2
Significant blood loss	History of bleeding
	Orthostatic hypotension
	Guaiac-positive stool
	Low hematocrit

CASE 12-2

A 76-year-old man with peptic ulcer disease, diabetes with retinopathy (with baseline 20/200 vision corrected), nephropathy (creatinine 1.7 mg/dl), and peripheral neuropathy reports gastroenteritis for 4 days with moderate diarrhea. This is now resolving, but he is afraid to walk because he states he feels "unsteady and light-headed." His stool is guaiac positive. His pulse is regular and rapid. He has a soft systolic murmur at the base and left sternal border. He has no abnormal cerebellar findings.

A. *What are four things that could be contributing to his dizziness?*

B. *What additional history and physical examination would be most helpful?*

C. *If you could order only one test, what should it be?*

13

Dyspepsia

ETIOLOGY

What is dyspepsia?

Dyspepsia is defined as persistent and recurrent upper abdominal or epigastric pain that may be associated with nausea, bloating, or postprandial fullness. It affects up to one fourth of the U.S. population and represents one of the most frequent reasons for outpatient visits in adult medicine.

What causes dyspepsia?

Up to 40% of patients presenting with dyspepsia have either gastroesophageal reflux disease (GERD) or peptic ulcer disease (PUD). Duodenal ulcer disease is almost always due to the bacterium *Helicobacter pylori*. Gastric ulcers can be caused by nonsteroidal antiinflammatory use alone. The risk of NSAID-induced ulcer increases with age, and concomitant *H. pylori* makes a gastric ulcer even more likely. Another 50% of cases of dyspepsia arise from lactose intolerance, irritable bowel syndrome, and nonulcer dyspepsia. Irritable bowel syndrome and nonulcer dyspepsia are functional diagnoses; that is, no pathophysiologic basis can be found. Although gastric cancer, biliary disease, and pancreatic disease are important to exclude, they only cause 2% of dyspepsia. Other rare causes include atypical presentations of cardiac ischemia and musculoskeletal and endocrine causes, such as diabetic gastroparesis and hypercalcemia.

What is the role of *H. pylori* in dyspepsia?

Up to 90% of patients with PUD have *H. pylori* infection. However, colonization is present in approximately 10% of the general population, most of whom do not have ulcer disease. Therefore only some patients are susceptible to ulcer formation with *H. pylori* infection. Factors such as host response, strain variability, and luminal milieu play important roles in ulcer pathogenesis. *H. pylori* eradication reduces recurrence of PUD but does not reduce symptoms of GERD or nonulcer dyspepsia.

EVALUATION

How do I recognize GERD and PUD as causes of dyspepsia?

Obtain a thorough history of pain characteristics, including location, precipitating factors, and alleviating factors. Patients with GERD classically present with epigastric burning pain or heartburn exacerbated by large or fatty meals and by lying down. Risk factors for reflux include obesity, smoking, eating meals just before bedtime, and use of calcium channel blockers. Many patients also complain of transient regurgitation of gastric contents. On the other hand, PUD tends to present as a persistent, dull, gnawing pain in the epigastrium, which is relieved by taking antacids or eating a meal. Factors aggravating PUD include NSAIDs, alcohol, and nicotine. Include a careful examination on initial evaluation. Obtain stool guaiac and CBC to exclude ongoing significant blood loss.

How can I be certain I am not missing an important diagnosis (e.g., cancer)?

Every patient being evaluated for dyspepsia should be asked about the presence of "red flags," or worrisome signs (Box 13-1). These red flags help identify individuals who may have a more serious underlying condition, such as cancer.

What initial testing is appropriate for dyspepsia?

If the patient has no red flags by history or on examination, there is no need for initial testing. For suspected GERD and PUD, the approach is essentially the same: begin with an empiric trial to confirm the diagnosis (see below). With good response, further testing is not necessary. The only divergence between the evaluation of the two conditions is that with PUD, a blood test for *H. pylori* antibodies is an important step when empiric therapy fails, whereas with GERD there is no need to test for *H. pylori* because it is not a causative factor (Figure 13-1).

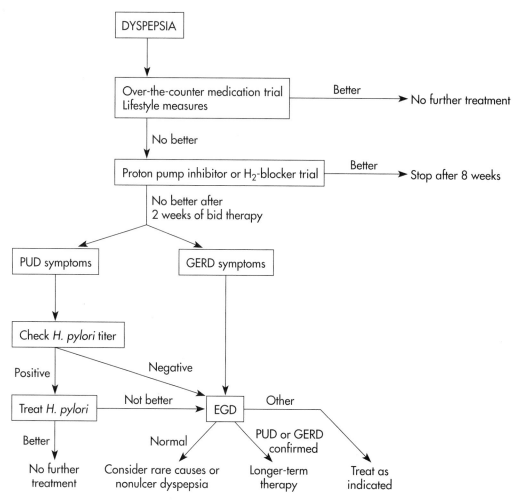

Figure 13-1 Dyspepsia workup and therapeutic algorithm.

What empiric medications are used to help diagnose suspected PUD?

Although antacids such as calcium carbonate (Tums) can provide symptomatic relief, a full 6- to 8-week course of prescription-strength H_2-blockers or proton pump inhibitor is warranted; healing of an ulcer is expected after 6 to 8 weeks. Stop NSAIDs, cigarettes, and alcohol if possible. Most patients with PUD respond,

thus confirming the diagnosis. Close follow-up is key to ensuring that symptoms resolve.

When patient history suggests GERD, what empiric trial confirms the diagnosis?

Diagnosis can begin with lifestyle modification, which should be continued even if medication is added to the regimen to minimize the dosage. Advise patients to elevate the head of the bed on blocks (Figure 13-2); not to eat 2 to 4 hours before bed; and to avoid caffeine, peppermint, fatty meals, acidic or spicy foods, tobacco, and alcohol. Use antacids for symptom relief. When patients find little improvement with these measures, quickly proceed to a trial of a proton pump inhibitor to confirm GERD. Both lansoprazole and omeprazole are frequently used.

What tests are warranted if the patient does not respond to treatment?

Further testing is indicated for patients whose symptoms persist after 2 weeks of maximal-strength proton pump inhibitor therapy, or in whom symptoms recur

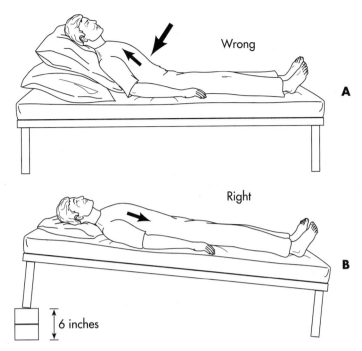

Wrong

A

Right

B

6 inches

Figure 13-2 Appropriate bed elevation for GERD prevention. **A,** Sleeping on pillows actually increases intraabdominal pressure, leading to increased reflux. **B,** Elevating the head of the bed on blocks allows gravity to help reduce reflux.

after an 8-week course (see Figure 13-1). In GERD, referral for esophagogastroduodenoscopy (EGD) is warranted. In suspected PUD, testing for *H. pylori* is the next step. If *H. pylori* antibody is negative, refer for EGD; if positive, treat for *H. pylori.*

What is the best test for *H. pylori?*

Testing for immunoglobulin G (IgG) antibodies to *H. pylori* is currently the most widespread noninvasive method for determining exposure. This may be falsely positive in the elderly or in patients from third-world countries, who are more likely to have been exposed in the past. Urease breath testing gives a more accurate indication of disease activity but is less available and may be falsely negative with proton pump inhibitor use. Definitive diagnosis is by biopsy obtained during EDG.

What is the role of EGD and upper GI series?

EGD, also called upper endoscopy, is used most frequently for evaluation of dyspepsia that fails empiric treatment. It allows for direct visualization and thus can definitively rule out PUD, esophagitis, or esophageal stricture from chronic inflammation. In addition, biopsies can be obtained to evaluate for *H. pylori* infection or cancer. However, endoscopy is invasive and uncomfortable with significant risk of aspiration of gastric contents. Upper GI barium series is less invasive but of limited use, identifying deep ulcers in the gastric or esophageal mucosa or esophageal strictures. Reflux of barium into the

esophagus does not correlate with GERD symptom severity, so it is not a helpful finding diagnostically. Acid perfusion (Bernstein test) and 24-hour pH monitoring are used to diagnose GERD; however, these tests are also invasive and cumbersome. Patients with chronic GERD require intermittent EGD to screen for Barrett's esophagus, a precancerous condition caused by chronic reflux.

What are the complications of PUD?

Complications of PUD include upper gastrointestinal tract bleeding (UGIB), which can be life-threatening. More rarely, gastric outlet obstruction and gastric perforation can occur. Individuals who have multiple ulcers or recurrent episodes of UGIB from PUD should be considered for work-up of Zollinger-Ellison syndrome (gastrin-producing tumor).

What complications can be seen with GERD?

Esophageal ulceration and stricture occur from chronic esophageal acid exposure and inflammation. Reactive airway disease is also associated with acid reflux into the lower esophagus, even in the absence of actual aspiration. Prolonged irritation of the esophagus with gastric reflux can also lead to Barrett's metaplasia, in which the normal squamous epithelial lining of the esophagus is replaced by columnar epithelium. Barrett's esophagus is a precancerous condition, with a 10% chance of progression to esophageal carcinoma. These patients require close surveillance with frequent endoscopy.

TREATMENT

What are the long-term treatment options for PUD and GERD?

For persistent symptoms in patients with a definitive diagnosis of either PUD or GERD, continue ongoing lifestyle modifications and avoidance of aggravating activities. PUD typically resolves with an 8-week course of antisecretory drugs and *H. pylori* treatment when indicated. GERD, on the other hand, often requires chronic medication. For patients with GERD, attempt to taper therapy to the lowest-cost regimen that eradicates symptoms. For persistent symptoms on maximal proton pump inhibitor therapy, consider adding a promotility drug to increase gastric emptying (Table 13-1) or referring for fundoplication surgery.

How is *H. pylori* treated?

Treat patients who test positive for *H. pylori* with a combination antibiotic and acid-reducing regimen (Table 13-2). Approximately 30% of patients experience resolution of symptoms, thus eliminating the need for endoscopy. However, up to 70% of patients fail treatment, suggesting conditions unresponsive to *H. pylori* eradication, such as nonulcer dyspepsia.

When is referral for surgery indicated?

Emergent partial gastrectomy may be necessary when catastrophic gastrointestinal bleeding unresponsive to EGD maneuvers occurs, usually as a result of PUD. GERD is rarely the source of significant bleeding from erosions. Refer patients with chronic GERD unresponsive to medical treatment for Nissen fundoplication, now increasingly performed by laparoscopic techniques. Complications from antireflux surgery include dysphagia, inability to belch, and splenic trauma. Patients who have multiple comorbid conditions, impaired motility, and unclear diagnoses are not good candidates for surgery.

TABLE 13-1
Drugs Used to Treat GERD

DRUG	DOSE	COST
Lansoprazole	15 or 30 mg bid	$$$$
Omeprazole	20 mg bid	$$$$
Sucralfate	1000 mg qid	$$$
H$_2$-blocker	150 mg bid	$$$
Metoclopramide (add to acid-reducing agent)	10 mg tid	$$

TABLE 13-2
Two Possible Treatment Regimens for *H. pylori*

DRUGS	DOSES	CURE RATE
Omeprazole	20 mg bid × 10 days	89%
Amoxicillin	1000 mg bid × 10 days	
Clarithromycin	500 mg bid × 10 days	
Bismuth	2 tabs qid × 14 days	90%
Metronidazole	500 mg tid × 14 days	
Tetracycline	500 mg qid × 14 days	
Ranitidine	150 mg bid × 8 weeks	

CASE 13-1

A 34-year-old man presents with 1 week of upper abdominal pain. He has been using aspirin for knee pain, which developed while he was training for an upcoming marathon. He denies any dysphagia or nausea. Examination and hematocrit are normal.
  A. What do you recommend for diagnosis/treatment?
  B. What else can you suggest if initial intervention does not work?
  C. Will he ever be able to take aspirin again?

Key Points

- Approach dyspepsia first by ruling out warning signs and then with an empiric trial of lifestyle modification and antacid therapy.
- Treat *H. pylori* associated with PUD with a short course of a multidrug regimen.
- GERD is a chronic disease, usually requiring long-term therapy.
- Surgery for GERD is reserved for those who fail maximal medical intervention.

CASE 13-2

A 42-year-old woman complains of heartburn, for which she takes nearly 2 bottles of Mylanta every day. She recently got divorced and is under a lot of stress because she is trying to find a better job. She drinks coffee all day long in the diner where she waitresses, and she smokes 2 packs of cigarettes a day. She usually does not have time to eat dinner until work is over at 10 PM, and then she is up all night with heartburn, even though she sleeps on 3 pillows to keep her head up.
  What intervention(s) do you recommend?

chapter 14

Dyspnea

ETIOLOGY

What causes dyspnea?

A combination of mechanical receptors in the upper airway, lungs, and chest wall, as well as chemoreceptors in the carotid arteries, aorta, and medulla, appear to mediate the uncomfortable sensation of breathing experienced as dyspnea. Hypoxia, hypercapnia (elevated P_{CO_2}), and increased work of breathing can all contribute to dyspnea.

What are common causes of chronic dyspnea?

Although there are numerous causes of dyspnea, four conditions cause 70% of chronic dyspnea: asthma, chronic obstructive pulmonary disease (COPD), congestive heart failure (CHF), and interstitial lung disease (Box 14-1). Deconditioning is another frequent cause of chronic exertional dyspnea. Less common causes of chronic dyspnea include anemia, neoplasms, hyperthyroidism, and recurrent pulmonary emboli.

What are common causes for dyspnea of recent onset?

Patients with recent-onset dyspnea often have exacerbations of one of three chronic conditions (asthma, COPD, or CHF) or are found to have pneumonia (Box 14-2). Patients with bronchitis or other upper respiratory infections sometimes complain of dyspnea. This is generally mild unless they have an underlying pulmonary problem, such as asthma or COPD. Dyspnea is commonly associated with chest pain in patients with angina. Important but less common reasons for acute dyspnea include pulmonary embolus, tachyarrhythmia, and pneumothorax. Dyspnea without chest pain (silent ischemia) resulting from coronary artery disease sometimes occurs and is more common in patients with diabetes. Recurrent dyspnea associated with anxiety is often due to panic attacks; however, tachyarrhythmias can sometimes produce symptoms similar to panic attacks.

EVALUATION

How helpful is the history in the evaluation of dyspnea?

In one study of 146 patients admitted with dyspnea, 74% were correctly diagnosed after a 5- to 15-minute history. Important features of the history in a patient with dyspnea include duration, severity, exacerbating and relieving factors, associated symptoms, medication use (especially whether medications such as diuretics or inhalers have been used as prescribed), past medical history (particularly of cardiac and pulmonary diseases), environmental exposures, and any history of trauma. It can be helpful to ask a patient how far he or she can walk or how many flights of stairs he or she can climb, and have the patient compare this to his or her exercise tolerance at some time in the past.

Which symptoms are commonly associated with important causes of dyspnea?

Symptoms provide clues to diagnosis (Table 14-1).

Which elements of the physical examination are most important in evaluating a patient with dyspnea?

General appearance provides excellent information about the severity of the condition, including how hard a patient is working to breathe, the presence or absence of cyanosis, and the ability to speak a full sentence before taking a breath. Vital signs give information about the likelihood of an infection and hemodynamic stability. Consider repeating a respiratory rate on a dyspneic patient because this is frequently recorded incorrectly. Inspect the chest, looking for intercostal, subcostal, and supraclavicular retractions, and for abnormalities of the chest wall. Percuss, listening for dullness resulting from an effusion or area of consolidation or for the hyperresonance of a pneumothorax. Auscultate for wheezes, rales, rhonchi, or rubs; for symmetry of breath sounds; and for abnormal prolongation of the expiratory phase.

Remember that patients with an exacerbation of congestive heart failure may have wheezes, or "cardiac asthma," rather than a predominance of rales. Also beware that absence of wheezes in an acutely dyspneic patient with asthma or COPD may be an ominous sign of a serious limitation of airflow. In examining the heart, note the presence of any murmurs or an S₃ gallop of severe congestive heart failure. Inspect the neck veins to determine the jugular venous pressure (JVP). Assess for edema and unilateral calf swelling or tenderness. If a PE is being considered, measure calf diameters at an equal distance from the distal edge of the patella.

BOX 14-1   Common Causes of Chronic Dyspnea

Asthma
Chronic obstructive pulmonary disease
Congestive heart failure
Interstitial lung disease

BOX 14-2   Common Causes of Acute Dyspnea

Pneumonia
Exacerbations of:
    CHF
    Asthma
    COPD

Which tests are most helpful in evaluating the patient with dyspnea?

Selection of appropriate tests in a patient with dyspnea depends on the diagnostic hypotheses generated during the initial history and physical examination. A chest x-ray is useful in most patients who are moderately or severely symptomatic and can be helpful in mildly symptomatic patients in whom the reason for their dyspnea is unclear. Oximetry at rest and/or with exercise can be helpful. Spirometry or peak flow measurements provide information about the presence and severity of airflow obstruction. Perform an electrocardiogram on any patient who might have a cardiac cause for their dyspnea. A hematocrit and thyroid-stimulating hormone (TSH) test should be considered in any patient whose diagnosis remains unclear after the initial history and physical examination. In patients with

---

TABLE 14-1
Symptoms and Examination Findings in Important Causes of Dyspnea

CONDITION	SYMPTOMS	EXAM FINDINGS
CHF	Orthopnea (dyspnea when supine) Paroxysmal nocturnal dyspnea (awakening short of breath) Increase in leg edema	Elevated jugular venous pressure Crackles at lung bases Leg edema Third heart sound (S₃)
COPD or asthma exacerbation	Productive cough Wheezing	Increased expiratory-to-inspiratory ratio Supraclavicular retraction Wheezing
Pneumonia	Productive cough Fever Pleuritic chest pain	Tachycardia Egophony Decreased breath sounds
Pulmonary embolus	Abrupt onset dyspnea Calf pain or swelling Pleuritic chest pain	Pleural rub Unilateral calf swelling Tachycardia
Cardiac ischemia	Chest pressure or discomfort Nausea or diaphoresis	Tachycardia and hypertension Diaphoresis
Pneumothorax	Abrupt-onset dyspnea Severe pleuritic chest pain	Deviated trachea Hyperresonance on affected side Decreased breath sounds on affected side
Hyperventilation	Anxiety Palpitations Paresthesias, distal extremities or perioral	Normal exam

chronic dyspnea, pulmonary function testing with measurement of pulmonary diffusion capacity (DLCO) can be used to determine if a patient has interstitial lung disease. Cardiopulmonary exercise testing can be useful in some patients to clarify the cardiac and pulmonary components of their dyspnea and to determine the relative contribution of deconditioning. Echocardiography can be helpful in evaluating patients with dyspnea thought to be associated with valvular heart disease and/or CHF.

How do I evaluate a patient with suspected pulmonary emboli?

Pulmonary emboli can mimic many cardiac and pulmonary problems. Dyspnea is the most common symptom in patients with large pulmonary emboli, but patients with small emboli may present with pleuritic chest pain or hemoptysis. (See Pulmonary Embolism in Chapter 33).

What are typical symptoms in a patient whose dyspnea is due to panic attacks?

Patients with panic attacks experience episodes in which they have some combination of dyspnea, chest pain, palpitations, dizziness, and anxiety. During an acute episode, patients often benefit from reassurance and advice to slow their breathing. Patients who fail to respond to this can be asked to breathe into a paper bag. This helps increase their PCO_2 level, which has been lowered by hyperventilation. Sometimes patients with tachyarrhythmias will have symptoms similar to those of patients with panic attacks. If it is unclear whether a patient is having panic attacks or tachyarrhythmias, an event monitor, which records a tracing of a patient's heart during a period of symptoms, can be a useful way of distinguishing between the two.

When is dyspnea most likely to be life-threatening?

When evaluating a patient with dyspnea, it is important to keep in mind those causes that may put a patient at risk for a life-threatening outcome. In cases of recent-onset unexplained dyspnea, be alert for the possibility of a PE or silent ischemia. Assessing a patient's oxygenation with oximetry or arterial blood gas analysis, if needed, will identify patients at risk for cardiac or neurologic compromise caused by hypoxia. Assess the ventilatory status (how effectively they can exhale CO_2) of the acutely dyspneic patient by examination (work of breathing, level of alertness) and with an arterial blood gas measurement to identify elevated PCO_2 as a sign of impending respiratory arrest. Remember that normal oxygenation in an acutely dyspneic asthmatic patient does not exclude retention of CO_2, which puts the patient at increased risk for a respiratory arrest resulting from fatigue from excessive work of breathing.

TREATMENT

How do I treat dyspnea?

If possible, identify and treat the underlying cause. Some causes of dyspnea, such as asthma and CHF, may respond well to treatment directed at the underlying problem. Other causes, such as COPD or interstitial lung disease, may have a limited response to treatment. Opiates and benzodiazepines have been shown to reduce dyspnea but should generally be avoided because of the risk of dependence and respiratory depression.

Which patients with dyspnea should receive supplemental oxygen?

Supplemental oxygen has been shown to improve survival for patients with chronic dyspnea and a PO_2 less than or equal to 55. Currently, Medicare will pay for supplemental oxygen if patients have a PO_2 less than or equal to 55 or if they have a PO_2 less than or equal to 60 concomitant with a condition worsened by low oxygen levels, such as cor pulmonale (elevated right heart pressures associated with hypoxia), or if they have an O_2 saturation by oximetry less than or equal to 88%. Patients with acute dyspnea who are moderately to severely symptomatic or who have oxygen saturations below 90% to 91% should receive supplemental oxygen pending further evaluation and treatment. The caveat to this recommendation is patients with severe COPD, in whom CO_2 retention can be worsened with oxygen administration.

Which patients with dyspnea should be hospitalized?

Patients with chronic dyspnea can generally be evaluated as outpatients. Patients with acute dyspnea caused by an exacerbation of asthma or COPD can sometimes be treated with inhaled bronchodilators in a clinic or emergency room and will improve sufficiently to be discharged home. These patients are often discharged with a short course of steroids to decrease airway inflammation. Patients with acute dyspnea of unclear cause, those who require supplemental oxygen, or those who have potentially unstable cardiac or respiratory status should be hospitalized.

Key Points

- Most patients with dyspnea can be correctly diagnosed by taking a careful history.
- Asthma, COPD, CHF, and interstitial lung disease are the most common causes of chronic dyspnea.
- Pneumonia and exacerbations of asthma, COPD, and CHF are common causes for recent-onset dyspnea.
- Consider PE in any patient with recent-onset dyspnea who does not have a clear explanation for his or her symptoms.

CASE 14-1

A 21-year-old woman complains of 4 months of exertional dyspnea that she especially notices when she plays basketball. Her breathing is worsened by cold weather. She complains of a nonproductive cough for 2 months. She is a nonsmoker and is a college student. Past history is notable for eczema. Family history is negative for any pulmonary conditions. She has had no fevers or weight loss and denies postnasal drip. Examination is notable for a clear chest.

A. What is the most likely diagnosis in this patient?

B. What tests, if any, should be ordered?

C. What treatment should be instituted?

CASE 14-2

An 82-year-old woman with a history of hypertension and mild CHF comes to clinic reporting 2 weeks of exertional dyspnea. She was initially evaluated in an emergency room and was thought to have rales at her lung bases on examination. Her furosemide was increased from 40 to 80 mg/day, but her dyspnea has not improved. She states that she first noticed her dyspnea on awakening 2 weeks ago. She has a nonproductive cough. She can walk up half a flight of stairs at present but could climb two flights of stairs a month ago. She has no chest pain, hemoptysis, melena, or calf swelling and is taking her furosemide as prescribed. She is a nonsmoker. She is breathing comfortably at rest and has normal vital signs, a clear chest, no murmurs or gallops, no jugular venous distention, and no edema or calf swelling.

A. Which test would you order first? Which other tests would you consider?

B. If her chest film showed a normal heart size and a peripheral small opacity consistent with infection, fluid, or a pulmonary infarct, which test or tests would you order next?

15

Fatigue

ETIOLOGY

How common is fatigue?

Twenty-five percent of primary care patients report fatigue, and 5% of all office visits to primary care physicians are for a chief complaint of tiredness.

What causes fatigue?

Over half of fatigue is due to a psychologic cause, usually depression. Up to 30% is due to a diagnosable medical illness. No cause is found in about 20% of cases. Common physical causes include viral infection, metabolic disorders, and medications (Box 15-1). Duration is important: fatigue present for longer than 4 months is 75% psychiatric, whereas fatigue present for less than 4 weeks has physical cause determined in 70% of cases.

What are dangerous causes of fatigue that I shouldn't miss?

Fatigue can be the presenting symptom for a vast array of diseases, including depression; infection (TB, HIV, hepatitis); cancer; renal failure; and endocrine (diabetes, thyroid disease), neuromuscular (multiple sclerosis), and inflammatory diseases (sarcoidosis, rheumatoid arthritis).

What is chronic fatigue syndrome?

This is a symptom complex whose main feature is chronic or recurrent debilitating fatigue. Only 5% of chronically fatigued patients meet criteria. To make the diagnosis, exclude known causes of fatigue. Further, at least four of eight possible symptoms must be present: impaired memory or concentration, sore throat, tender cervical or axillary lymph nodes, muscle pain, joint pain, new headaches, nonrestorative sleep, or postexertional malaise. Although the cause is unknown, many etiologies have been proposed, including chronic viral infection, hypothalamic dysfunction, and disordered autonomic regulation. A significant psychiatric component is often present, confounded by the fact that chronic fatigue can be depressing in itself. Treatment includes adjustment of maladaptive coping strategies, antidepressants, and a low-level exercise program.

EVALUATION

What are the key parts of the history?

Ask the patient what he or she thinks is the cause of the fatigue. This provides useful clues and the opportunity to allay fears. Question the duration and progress of symptoms. Take a good sleep history, including initiation and maintenance of sleep, history of snoring (sleep apnea), and energy on awakening. In contrast to fatigue from physical causes, fatigue resulting from psychologic causes is unimproved by sleep, is worse in the morning, and improves throughout the day (Table 15-1). Review medications, especially recent additions. Ask a thorough social history, including about work, substance use, sexual history, history of physical or sexual abuse, and recent major stressors (e.g., career changes, deaths, or relocation). With a careful review of systems, identify new neurologic, pulmonary, cardiac, or gastrointestinal symptoms. Pay particular attention to constitutional symptoms because fevers, night sweats, or unexplained weight loss suggest infection or tumor. When patients answer yes to most questions, review again for abuse because a significant proportion of patients with multiple complaints have a history of domestic violence. Once you have reviewed physical symptoms, be sure to address possible depression in a direct and open manner. For example, you could say: "Many times fatigue is a sign of depression. I'd like to ask you about some of the other physical manifestations of depression." Ask about sleep, eating, anhedonia (loss of the ability to enjoy anything), sadness, feelings of guilt or loss, thoughts about death or suicide, or difficulty concentrating as other clues to depression.

TABLE 15-1
Comparing Features of Fatigue From Psychologic and Physical Causes

	PSYCHOLOGIC	PHYSICAL
Onset	Coincides with stress, psychologic disruption, conflict	Coincides with onset of a physical disease, e.g., respiratory infection, dental extraction
Duration	Chronic	Recent onset, parallels course of underlying disease
Progression	Fluctuates; worse with distasteful activity or stress; may not progress	Progresses as disease worsens Relieved by sleep
Effect of sleep	Sleep is nonrestorative	Better in AM
Diurnal pattern	Worse in AM Better as day progresses	Worsens as day progresses

BOX 15-1 Common Causes of Fatigue

MEDICATIONS
β-blockers
Sedatives, psychotropics

METABOLIC DISORDERS
Thyroid disease

PSYCHIATRIC
Anxiety
Depression
Somatization

VIRAL INFECTION
Epstein-Barr virus
Hepatitis viruses
HIV

What is an appropriate physical examination?

Perform a complete examination, with special attention to the most bothersome associated symptoms. Although the diagnostic yield compared with history is low, examination may confirm suspicions raised by the history, and the examination itself reassures patients that their concerns are being taken seriously.

What studies should I order?

Blood tests are appropriate for evaluation of new fatigue or worsening symptoms. Order a CBC with differential, basic chemistry panel of electrolytes with glucose and renal function, ESR, liver transaminases, and TSH. Other tests may be indicated (chest x-ray, ECG, urinalysis, other endocrine tests) as suggested by history and examination. Epstein-Barr virus (EBV) titers are not useful and should not be ordered. With risk factors such as

unprotected sex or intravenous drug use, test for HIV, hepatitis viruses, and syphilis (Venereal Disease Research Laboratory [VDRL] or rapid plasma reagin [RPR] tests). For homeless, incarcerated, or HIV-infected patients, look for tuberculosis by placing a purified protein derivative (PPD) with controls and consider ordering a chest film. Consider a pregnancy test in young women.

What if the results do not point to any specific abnormality?

Emphasize the positive, that there is no evidence of a life-threatening disease. Reassure the patient that you still are concerned about the symptoms and want to see him or her back. Help the patient problem-solve to improve coping with the symptoms. If there is personal turmoil, empathize that these upheavals can be exhausting. If you think your patient is depressed, find out what he or she thinks about this assessment. If the patient has trouble accepting this diagnosis, acknowledge that, because depression has such a stigma associated with it, the symptoms may show up in the body before people recognize its effect on their mood. Finally, recognize that you have begun to address a problem whose solution may be beyond the time frame of a single visit. You can ask patients to keep a diary of symptoms, activities, and degree of fatigue for review at the next visit.

TREATMENT

Treat any underlying physical cause found during evaluation. If you suspect depression, you may wish to recommend antidepressant therapy or psychiatry referral, emphasizing that even if depression is not the foundation of the problem, having fatigue for such a long time could by itself result in depression.

Key Points

- The duration, associated symptoms, progression, effect of sleep, and diurnal variation of fatigue help indicate whether the fatigue has a physical or psychologic cause.
- Fatigue of recent onset or with new associated symptoms is concerning for medical disease.
- A trusting therapeutic relationship is the cornerstone of therapy for fatigue of unclear origin.

CASE 15-2

A 65-year-old man with diet-controlled type II diabetes says he has been "feeling run down all the time" for almost 9 months. This has progressed to the point that he just does not feel like getting out of bed any more; he is sleeping poorly and does not feel refreshed. Along with these complaints, he notes listlessness, decreased interest in his usual activities, some mild aches and pains in his joints, poor appetite, and a 5-pound weight loss.

A. *What are the red flags in this history?*
B. *What other history do you need?*
C. *What should your initial workup be?*

CASE 15-1

A 30-year-old woman has worsening fatigue over the past 2 months. About 1 month ago, she developed an intermittent dry cough and felt "warmer than usual" several times but has not taken her temperature. Over the past week, she had two episodes of night sweats.

A. *What features in this history are concerning for potential serious disease?*
B. *What other questions would you like her to answer?*
C. *What is your initial workup?*

Gastrointestinal Bleeding

ETIOLOGY

What are the most common causes of gastrointestinal (GI) bleeding?

Divide GI bleeding into upper and lower, based on whether the bleeding originates above or below the ligament of Treitz in the distal duodenum. The most common causes of *upper GI bleeding* are peptic ulcer disease, gastritis, and esophageal varices related to cirrhosis and portal hypertension. Common causes of *lower GI bleeding* include diverticulosis and angiodysplasia, a condition of disordered vessel growth in the bowel wall (Box 16-1).

EVALUATION

What pertinent history should I elicit when a patient has GI bleeding?

Use history to tell whether the source of bleeding is from the upper or lower GI tract. Generally, upper GI bleeds present with hematemesis, or coffee ground emesis. The stool is usually melenic (i.e., black) resulting from prolonged transit time in the bowel, which oxidizes the blood. By contrast, lower GI bleeding produces hematochezia (maroon stools) or bright red blood per rectum. The caveat to this distinction is that a brisk upper GI bleed can cause hematochezia as a result of the cathartic effects of fast bleeding. Patients with rapid, severe bleeding may report dizziness, weakness, confusion, or syncope related to volume depletion. A slow or chronic bleed from any source can lead to fatigue and dyspnea on exertion as anemia progresses. Most GI bleeding is painless, although bleeding from peptic ulcers may be preceded by days to weeks of burning epigastric pain. Risk factors for peptic ulcer disease include NSAIDs, steroids, and alcohol use. If tenesmus is present, rectal inflammation is likely, as from ulcerative colitis. Weight loss suggests neoplasm. Fever suggests infectious or inflammatory disorders. Alcohol use and/or chronic liver disease are risks for esophageal varices. Older age is a risk factor for angiodysplasia or diverticulitis. Patients with diverticular bleeds may have a history of prior episodes of painful diverticulitis.

How does physical examination help me evaluate my patient with bloody stools?

Examination should help you judge the severity of bleeding. Orthostatic vital signs are key. Tachycardia and hypotension are worrisome for a large amount of bleeding. Orthostasis, that is, an increase in pulse or drop in blood pressure of greater than 20 points from lying to standing, indicates volume loss of 20% or greater. Pallor, cool skin, and poor capillary refill are also signs of severe blood loss and volume depletion. Conjunctival pallor and pale palmar creases indicate a hematocrit in the low 20s or less. If signs of chronic liver disease are present, suspect esophageal varices. These examination findings include spider telangiectasias, ascites, jaundice, asterixis, hepatomegaly and/or splenomegaly, palmar erythema, Terry's nails, and gynecomastia. Parotid or lacrimal gland enlargement, testicular atrophy, or Dupuytren's contractures of flexor tendons in the hand suggest alcohol abuse, which increases risk for gastritis, peptic ulcer disease, or cirrhosis-related esophageal varices.

When is anoscopy or nasogastric lavage helpful?

Perform anoscopy and digital rectal examination in patients with bright red blood per rectum to distinguish hemorrhoidal bleeding from other more proximal sources. Perform nasogastric (NG) lavage to confirm upper GI bleeding. Bloody NG aspirate diagnoses an upper GI bleed. The amount of saline lavage required to clear all blood from the NG aspirate correlates with the rapidity of bleeding. NG lavage containing bile rules out an upper GI bleed. Clear NG aspirate rules out a gastric bleed but not a duodenal bleed because, without bile, it is not clear whether the duodenum has been sampled.

What studies are standard in a patient with a GI bleed?

Repeat hematocrits every 4 hours until you are sure the patient is not acutely bleeding. Remember, however, that a fall in hematocrit may lag behind blood loss by several hours. Order blood type and cross-match, and 2 to 4 units of blood to be kept "in house" in the event of catastrophic bleeding. Check chemistry panel for renal function and electrolytes; BUN may rise with upper GI bleeding because of absorption of blood in gut. Glucose may be low with severe liver disease and may provide a clue to presence of varices or gastritis. Check liver function values to screen for liver dysfunction and prothrombin, partial thromboplastin times, and platelets for a coagulopathy that could worsen blood loss. Follow calcium in patients receiving transfusions because the citrate preservative may cause calcium to fall.

Are x-rays or other diagnostic imaging studies useful?

Plain films are relatively unhelpful except to rule out perforation with an upright view. Endoscopy for suspected upper bleeding often identifies the cause of bleeding, can be used to take biopsies for diagnosis of *Helicobacter pylori* or tumor, and may be used therapeutically to sclerose or ligate varices. Selective arteriography or nuclear medicine labeled red blood cell (RBC) scan may identify the source of lower GI bleeding if the rate of bleeding is brisk.

BOX 16-1 Common Causes of GI Bleeding

UPPER GI BLEEDING
Gastritis
Mallory-Weiss tear from retching
Nose bleed
Peptic ulcer disease
Varices: esophageal, gastric

LOWER GI BLEEDING
Angiodysplasia
Brisk upper GI bleeding
Colitis: infectious, inflammatory, or ischemic
Colon cancer or polyp
Diverticulosis

TABLE 16-1
Presentation, Diagnosis, and Treatment Options of Common Causes of GI Bleeding

CAUSE	PRESENTATION	DIAGNOSIS	TREATMENT OPTIONS
Angiodysplasia	Elderly patients Slow, occult bleeding Anemia and fatigue	Colonoscopy; angiography if bleeding brisk	Surgical removal of involved bowel
Colon cancer	Elderly patients Slow, occult bleeding Anemia and fatigue Weight loss Change in caliber of stool, new constipation	Colonoscopy; if lesion extensive, CT scan for staging disease	Surgical removal if cancer isolated to the bowel
Diverticulosis	Acute, rapid bleed Painless Prior diverticulitis	Colonoscopy, selective arteriography, or labeled RBC scan if bleeding brisk	80% of bleeding resolves with bowel rest alone; surgical excision if persists
Ischemic bowel	Elderly patients Risk factors for atherosclerosis or emboli Midabdominal pain Postprandial pain	Plain radiographs or CT scan to identify edematous bowel and to rule out perforation	Surgical excision if patient stable enough for surgery
PUD/gastritis	Preceding episodes of epigastric pain NSAIDs, alcohol, caffeine, steroids, or cigarette use	EGD with biopsy or serology for *H. pylori*	H_2-blocker, proton pump inhibitor; antibiotics for *H. pylori;* discontinue NSAIDs, caffeine, alcohol
Mallory-Weiss tear	Retching preceding hematemesis Usually painless	EGD	Antiemetics, supportive care
Varices	Hematemesis in patient with cirrhosis and portal hypertension Usually painless	EGD	EGD banding, octreotide, Sengstaken-Blakemore tube, β-blockers for prophylaxis, TIPS

TIPS, Transjugular intrahepatic portosystemic shunt.

TREATMENT

Treat the underlying cause of bleeding (Table 16-1).

My patient is orthostatic and vomiting up blood. What should I do?

Begin with urgent resuscitation. Obtain rapid intravenous access, usually two IV catheters, 16 gauge or larger, or a central line. Administer normal saline to maximize the portion that stays in the intravascular compartment. Packed RBCs or whole blood are better than saline for expanding the intravascular volume but take longer to obtain. Replace factors or platelets as indicated by severe coagulopathy. Order 2 to 6 units of blood in house (pick the number of units based on severity of bleeding) so that you can quickly transfuse rapidly bleeding patients. Consult GI and surgery early for almost all patients with GI bleeding. GI consultants can assist with diagnostic and possibly therapeutic endoscopy. Surgical colleagues prefer knowing as early as possible about patients who may require surgery if bleeding is refractory to medical therapy.

Key Points

- Evaluation should determine if the bleed is from the upper or the lower GI tract to guide differential diagnosis and workup.
- Call GI and surgical consultants early.
- Obtain adequate IV access, type and cross, serial hematocrits, and reassess frequently.

CASE 16-1

A 68-year-old man has history of colon cancer resected 3 years ago, diverticulosis noted on previous colonoscopy, osteoarthritis, and hypothyroidism. He presents with 1 day of hematochezia and dizziness, without abdominal pain or vomiting. His medications include levothyroxine, piroxicam, psyllium, trazodone, and vitamin E. On examination, BP is 90/60, pulse is 120, skin is cool and moist, mouth is without lesions, heart exam reveals a 2/6 systolic murmur at the right upper sternal border without radiation, abdomen is soft and nontender, and rectal exam reveals grossly bloody stool. Laboratory tests show hemoglobin of 10, hematocrit of 30, MCV 86, white blood cell count 11, BUN 45, creatinine 1.0, sodium 136, potassium 3.3, and chloride 98.

A. Where do you think is the most likely site of bleeding?

B. What are the most common causes of lower GI bleeding?

C. What can be done to prevent NSAID-induced ulcers?

CASE 16-2

A 47-year-old man with alcoholic liver disease presents with hematemesis, light-headedness, and confusion. On examination, BP is 80/60; pulse is 140; skin reveals spider angiomata on the upper chest; abdomen is distended with shifting dullness; and extremities show palmar erythema, Dupuytren's contractures, and Terry's nails. Upper endoscopy reveals bleeding esophageal varices.

A. What are the physical findings of liver disease, and which findings suggest alcoholism?

B. What should you do to immediately stabilize this patient?

C. What is the most useful medication to administer?

D. What additional nonpharmacologic intervention might be useful?

17

Headache

ETIOLOGY

What causes headaches?

Approximately 99% of all headaches are recurrent benign headaches and are either tension-type, migraine, or cluster headaches. Rare causes not to miss are subarachnoid hemorrhage (SAH), meningitis, and cancer.

What distinguishes tension-type headaches from migraine headaches?

Patients with tension-type headaches classically describe a "bandlike pressure" around the skull that is mild to moderate in severity but does not prevent daily activities (Box 17-1). Migraines are usually unilateral, throbbing, associated with nausea and/or vomiting, and frequently disabling, with sufferers often retiring to bed in a dark, quiet room. An aura may precede the headache, most commonly visual scintillations. Effective clinical criteria make the diagnosis (Box 17-2).

What describes a chronic daily headache patient?

A subset of headache patients has chronic daily headaches, sharing the following features: family history of headaches (90%), sleep disturbances (close to 100%), analgesic overuse (NSAIDs, ergotamine, and particularly narcotics, such as codeine), and depression.

What are cluster headaches?

These occur predominately in middle-aged men and are severe, unilateral, retroorbital, and often described as stabbing in quality. Often, cluster headaches are accompanied by unilateral nasal congestion or lacrimation. These headaches recur over consecutive days to weeks and then remit, hence the term cluster headaches.

EVALUATION

My patient has recurring headaches. What questions should I ask?

The basic goal of evaluation is to determine the type and severity of the headache. History should be directed at pattern and location, previous headaches and treatment, preceding and accompanying symptoms (e.g., nausea, vomiting, visual changes, photophobia), triggering factors, severity and progression, medication use, and family history.

What are clues to ominous headaches versus benign ones?

Although the cause of most headaches is benign, it is important to recognize signs that suggest an ominous cause for headache (Box 17-3).

What should I look for on examination?

Perform a good general examination, with a complete neurologic evaluation, including cranial nerve testing and mental status assessment. Conduct additional examination as suggested by the patient's history. For example, if you suspect meningitis, check vital signs, mental status, and nuchal rigidity. If you are concerned about sinus infection, look for maxillary tenderness, purulent discharge, and poor transillumination of the sinuses. If you are concerned about temporal arteritis, palpate the temporal arteries.

My patient requests a CT scan or an MRI. Should I get one?

Probably not. Headache is, for the most part, a clinical diagnosis. Several studies have demonstrated that imaging will not add anything to the diagnosis *if* the person with a headache does not have any of the warning signs mentioned above and has a normal neurologic examination. The great majority of patients fall into this category. Longitudinal care will help with diagnosis; if the patient develops suspicious symptoms, has a mental status change, or does not get better as you expect, go back and revisit your original diagnostic assumptions and reconsider further evaluation.

What if I suspect a subarachnoid hemorrhage (SAH)? Which do I order—CT scan or MRI?

SAH usually presents suddenly, often as "the worst headache ever." The purpose of imaging is to detect the blood. The sensitivity of the CT scan depends on the presence of fresh bleeding. In the first 24 hours, CT detects 95% of SAHs. If the CT scan is negative, and you still suspect SAH, perform a lumbar puncture (LP) to detect the 5% of bleeds missed by CT scan. Look for xanthochromia, a yellow pigmentation to the spinal fluid, indicating the breakdown of blood in the CSF. If the suspected bleed occurred over a week before, an MRI is more sensitive.

How will I know if my patient has a brain tumor?

This is often the patient's fear as well. Although the headache of brain tumor has been described as a morning headache associated with nausea and vomiting, in reality most brain tumor–associated headaches do not fit this picture. Unfortunately, there is no typical brain tumor headache. Again, any warning signs listed above indicate the need for further evaluation. If none of those signs are present, longitudinal care will reveal progression of symptoms or neurologic changes, indicating the need for more extensive evaluation, including imaging.

TREATMENT

How should I treat migraines and tension-type headaches?

Before adding a medication, make sure your patient is not using any medications that might induce headaches, including birth control pills, caffeine, alcohol, antidepressants, and H_2-blockers. Headaches can also be due to daily withdrawal symptoms from medications initially used to treat headaches, including NSAIDs or aspirin. Have the patient look for other triggers (e.g., wine, cheese, too much sleep) and remove them.

What medications are useful?

Medications to treat recurrent benign headaches fall into two categories: abortive and prophylactic. Abortive treatment is given at the time of the headache to try to stop it. Prophylactic treatment is used for headaches occurring more than 4 times a month. For abortive therapy, many people respond to aspirin; NSAIDs, such as naproxen (500-1000 mg is effective 70% to 75% of the time); or acetaminophen. Cafergot, a combination of ergotamine and caffeine, is effective 60% of the time. Because gastroparesis accompanies headache, particularly migraine, concomitant use of promotility agents, such as metoclopramide or cisapride, can improve the absorption and the effect of the analgesic medication. Triptans are successful in 70% to 80% of cases and are available by oral formulations, nasal spray, or subcutaneous injection (Table 17-1). Both ergotamines and triptans can cause vasoconstriction and may induce angina or myocardial infarction, so do not use these in patients with atherosclerotic disease.

BOX 17-1   Clinical Diagnosis of Tension-Type Headache

Mild-to-moderate tightness, bandlike pressure
Lasts 30 minutes to 7 days
Not worsened by daily activity
Lacks photophobia plus phonophobia (one may be present)
Ten previous episodes

BOX 17-2   Clinical Diagnosis of Migraine Headache

Requires any two of the following:
  Unilateral site
  Throbbing quality
  Nausea
  Photophobia or phonophobia

BOX 17-3   Danger Signs Suggesting an Ominous Cause of Headache

First headache, or marked change in chronic headache
Onset after age 50
Sudden onset or worst headache ever
Onset during exertion
Accompanied by fever
Abnormal neurologic examination, including mental status
Neck stiffness

If abortive therapy for migraine is not effective, what next?

Patients with severe migraines often come to the emergency room or clinic having failed to get relief from the above therapies. For these patients, consider the following: sumatriptan is 80% effective when given subcutaneously, but headaches recur in one third of patients. IV prochlorperazine is particularly suited to nauseated migraine patients, improving nausea and aborting 80% of headaches. Dihydroergotamine (IV or subcutaneous) is as effective as sumatriptan but may cause nausea. Narcotics, such as IV meperidine (Demerol), should be reserved as a last resort.

What should I do if the headaches are frequent?

If your patient has bothersome headaches more than 4 times a month, ensure that basic measures have been taken: regulate sleep patterns, avoid food triggers, and eliminate caffeine. Review medications to detect causes for withdrawal headaches. If these measures are to no avail, consider prophylactic treatment. Low-dose tricyclic antidepressants are especially effective for tension-type headaches but also work for migraines. Calcium channel blockers and β-blockers, especially nonselective propanolol and nadolol, are effective for preventing migraine headaches. If possible, choose a medication that treats a concurrent medical condition. For example, in a patient with hypertension, β-blockers might be your first choice.

How do I treat chronic daily headaches and cluster headaches?

The only treatment for chronic daily headaches is to get the patient off all analgesics and start from scratch. Unmedicated patients with chronic daily headaches may respond to tricyclic antidepressants. For cluster headaches, lithium, ergotamine, and 100% oxygen are effective.

How often should my patient follow up, and what should I review at appointments?

Headaches are a chronic condition. While you are initiating or changing therapy, every 4 to 6 weeks is a good interval. Once the patient is stable, the frequency is dictated by the frequency of complaints. At each appointment, review the type and frequency of headaches, triggers, compliance, and side effects. Strategize with the patient regarding avoidance or elimination of triggers. Review the treatment plan, and change medications if the current regimen is ineffective. If a compliant patient is not getting better as you would expect or develops a new, different headache, reassess your diagnosis and consider further evaluation or referral to a neurologist.

Key Points
- Most headaches are benign.
- The diagnosis of a headache is clinically based on accurate history and examination.
- Look for warning signs suggesting an ominous cause.
- Review medications for those causing headache by side effect or withdrawal.

CASE 17-1

A 25-year-old woman reports headache, nausea, and phonophobia for 24 hours. She has had 3 previous episodes in the past 2 years. She has partial relief with extra-strength Tylenol. Her neurologic examination, including mental status, is normal.
- A. What is your differential diagnosis?
- B. What imaging technique do you recommend?
- C. What treatment do you recommend?
- D. If her symptoms recur every week, what treatment would you recommend?

CASE 17-2

A 26-year-old orthopedic surgery resident presents with a sudden, severe headache while weight lifting. Neurologic examination is normal, including normal CT. He is fine until his next call night, when he collapses with a severe headache.
- A. What is the most likely diagnosis?
- B. What testing do you recommend?

TABLE 17-1
Triptans Used to Treat Headache*

DRUG	ROUTE	ONSET	DOSE (MG)
Sumatriptan	Subcutaneous	10-15 min	6
	Nasal spray	15-20 min	5-20
	Oral tablet	1-2 hrs	50
Naratriptan	Oral tablet	1-3 hrs	2.5
Rizatriptan	Oral tablet	30-60 min	10
	MLT (melt) tablet	30-60 min	10
Zolmitriptan	Oral tablet	45 min	2.5

*Contraindications are coronary artery disease, uncontrolled hypertension, and basilar migraines.

18

Healthy Patients

DISEASE PREVENTION AND SCREENING

What is preventive medicine?

Preventive medicine attempts to decrease disease and increase health. Prevention assumes that clinical disease is a cumulative process and that interventions can prevent, stop, or slow that process. The process includes three stages: health before disease; preclinical disease, in which biologic changes have occurred but disease is not apparent; and clinically overt disease. Examples of preventive interventions include screening tests; immunizations; counseling and behavioral changes; and chemoprophylaxis, such as postmenopausal hormone replacement therapy.

What are primary and secondary prevention?

These terms refer to the stage of the disease process during which the intervention occurs. In *primary prevention,* interventions are begun in asymptomatic patients before disease is present to alter susceptibility or reduce exposure. Good examples are classes for smoking prevention or cessation, nutrition counseling, and immunization. *Secondary prevention* attempts to detect disease in preclinical or beginning stages, such as in screening programs for cervical or breast cancer (Pap smears and mammography, respectively). *Tertiary prevention* attempts to restore function and alleviate disability from disease (e.g., cardiac rehabilitation after heart attack). The distinction is important because the risk-to-benefit ratio and cost-effectiveness of an intervention differ, depending on the stage of disease it targets. For example, lowering cholesterol in people who already have had an MI may be worth the cost and potential side effects of 3-hydroxy-3-methylglutaryl coenzyme A (HMG CoA) reductase inhibitors. In comparison, primary prevention with HMG CoA reductase inhibitors in healthy

people may be too costly or may cause too many side effects for the smaller benefit gained.

Why do we screen for some diseases and not for others?

Certain criteria must be met before screening is considered worthwhile. This varies according to the treatment of the disease, the test, and the patient population (Box 18-1).

Why are some screening tests controversial?

Prostate-specific antigen (PSA) is an example of a screening test for prostate cancer that was clinically available before the implication of its use was clearly understood. There are several problems with it as a screening test. First of all, PSA has poor sensitivity and specificity: it can be elevated in the absence of prostate cancer or can be normal in cancer's presence. Second, cancer identified by an elevated PSA may not be clinically significant (i.e., will the patient die from the cancer or die with the cancer but from another cause?). Third, the effectiveness of treatment for prostate cancer is debated. A Swedish study suggests that watchful waiting has the same mortality rate as surgery without the perioperative risk or complications of urinary incontinence or impotence.

Preventive health practices differ for age and gender. How can I know what to do?

In general, address the health issues specific to that age and gender. Some preventive measures apply to all adults: immunization (Table 18-1); blood pressure screening; and counseling for healthy diet and exercise, smoking cessation, and use of seat belts (Boxes 18-2 and 18-3). Other interventions are based on age or gender, such as Pap smears, mammography, or fecal occult blood testing (Table 18-2). Certain measures are directed only to high-risk populations, for example, aspirin for heart disease. For more specific guidance, consult available references. One of the most widely used is the U.S. Preventive Services Task Force (USPSTF) Guide to Clinical Preventive Services. This guide provides evidence-based recommendations for groups of people based on age, gender, and risk factors. The need to base recommendations on well-designed outcome studies is especially important in preventive medicine, in which you may be recommending an intervention to a currently healthy patient that, in itself, carries risk of complication.

BOX 18-1 Criteria for Judging Whether Screening Is Worthwhile

DISEASE CHARACTERISTICS
Has negative effect on quality or quantity of life
Has asymptomatic period
Effective prevention or treatment possible
Early detection improves outcomes

TEST CHARACTERISTICS
Has adequate sensitivity and specificity
Benefits of test outweigh risks

POPULATION CHARACTERISTICS
Sufficient incidence to justify cost
Population screened will live long enough to benefit
Intervention acceptable to and used by population

BOX 18-2 Suggested Periodic Health Examination for Adults

Height, weight, blood pressure, and symptom-focused examination
Age 18-39: Every 3-5 years
Age ≥40: Annual

BOX 18-3 Suggested Preventive Counseling for Adults

INJURY PREVENTION
Automobile lap/shoulder belts
Bicycle helmets
Smoke detectors

DIET AND EXERCISE
Limit fat and cholesterol
Adequate calcium intake
Regular aerobic activity

SAFE SEXUAL PRACTICE
STD prevention

SUBSTANCE USE
Tobacco cessation
Problem alcohol use
Illicit drug use

TABLE 18-1
Suggested Routine Immunization for Adults

DISEASE	RECOMMENDATION
Tetanus-diphtheria (Td)	Two booster strategies are equivalent: Td boosters every 10 years throughout life *or* Single booster at age 50 for individuals who received 3-dose pediatric series and teenage booster
Measles-mumps-rubella	Single dose for adults born after 1956 without proof of immunity or documentation of previous immunization Second dose for college students, health care workers, and foreign travelers
Hepatitis B	Recommended for all young adults and older adults at high risk Assess serologic response in persons older than 30 years
Hepatitis A	Recommended for adults at risk: foreign travelers, injection drug users, multiple sexual partners, day care workers, patients with chronic liver disease
Influenza	Give annually to all adults age 65 or older, younger if at risk Consider for all healthy adults
Invasive pneumococcal disease	Recommended for all adults at age 65, younger if at risk Reimmunization recommended for high-risk adults at age 65 who received vaccine >5 years earlier, asplenic or immunocompromised adults 5 years after first dose

TABLE 18-2
Suggested Screening for Adults

DISEASE	INTERVENTION	RECOMMENDED SCHEDULE	STRENGTH OF EVIDENCE
Breast cancer	Mammography	Annual for women ages 50-69 Consider for ages 40-49 Reasonable to continue beyond age 69	Good
Cervical cancer	Papanicolaou smear	Every 1-3 years from age 18 or onset of sexual activity Stop after hysterectomy for benign disease or at age 65 if repeatedly normal	Good
Colorectal cancer	Fecal occult blood testing (FOBT) Flexible sigmoidoscopy	Screen beginning at age 50 Perform annual FOBT *or* sigmoidoscopy every 3-5 years *or both*	Fair
High blood cholesterol	Total cholesterol	Men aged 35-65 and women aged 45-65	Fair
Pelvic inflammatory disease	Chlamydia screening	Women younger than 25 with multiple sexual partners at highest risk	Fair
Prostate cancer	PSA	Discuss possible benefits and known risks of screening with patient before testing Men aged 50-69 most likely to benefit	Poor

Key Points ···

- Prevention saves lives, decreases disease, and increases health.
- Because prevention is aimed at healthy people, the evidence must be compelling that the benefits outweigh the risks.
- Evidence-based recommendations geared to specific age and gender are available, most notably in the USPSTF Guide to Clinical Preventive Services.

CASE 18-1

A 22-year-old apparently healthy man is in clinic for a routine visit.
A. What general counseling should you offer?
B. What specific immunizations are indicated?
C. Is prostate screening needed?

CHANGING HARMFUL HEALTH HABITS

Is it possible to get someone to quit smoking or lose weight?

Studies of how people change provide a model that divides the process into clinically useful stages: (1) precontemplation, (2) contemplation, (3) determination, (4) action, and (5) maintenance. Relapse often occurs, reinitiating the cycle (Figure 18-1). By identifying which

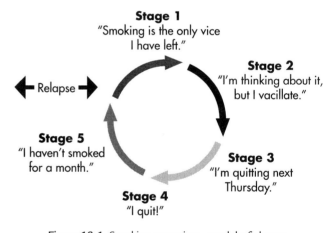

Figure 18-1 Smoking cessation—model of change.

stage the patient has achieved, you can target your efforts to help the patient reach the next stage. Thus the focus is on moving the patient closer to change rather than an "all or nothing" outcome.

What is an example of using this model in patient care?

The example below follows a patient through smoking cessation.

Stage 1: Precontemplation
In this stage, the patient is not consciously thinking of quitting. Studies show that simple physician advice and encouragement to consider quitting have an effect, although the results are not immediately obvious. Maintain an empathetic and nonjudgmental approach while

making a clear statement: "I think it is important for you to quit smoking. In fact, this is the most important thing you can do for your health."

Stage 2: Contemplation

The patient is now considering quitting smoking. Ask questions at each visit to help the patient identify reasons and barriers to quitting. Personalize your motivation: "You had one heart attack already—another and you might not be around to enjoy your new promotion." Make sure the motivation fits the particular age, gender, and individual. For example, adolescents tend to "bum" cigarettes, so arguments about cost are ineffective, but it may work to say, "If you quit smoking, you will be able to breathe better, and that will help your soccer game."

Stage 3: Determination

The patient has decided to quit smoking. Problem-solve with the patient about what has worked in the past and what led to failure to quit. Address the patient's concerns about possible negative consequences of quitting, including weight gain, bad moods, and issues of peer nonsupport. Offer a support system: intensive smoking cessation program; nicotine replacement therapy, such as gums, patch, or nasal spray; and other pharmacologic aids, such as bupropion.

Stage 4: Action

The patient quits! Schedule a series of biweekly or monthly visits, beginning 1 week after the quit date. Express continuing care and support.

Stage 5: Maintenance and relapse

Congratulate patient on the successes and reinforce the benefits of not smoking. Anticipate relapses. Reframe these as positive learning experiences and plan how to restart the cessation process.

Is this model of change applicable to all behavioral changes?

Yes. Ambulatory medicine offers you a longitudinal relationship with a patient, allowing you to address these issues repeatedly, a little bit at a time. As you get to know your patients, you can help them recognize opportunities for and benefits of prevention that matter to them, whether it is being able to breathe easier when playing with their grandchildren since they quit smoking or their improved job performance since they quit drinking. Seeing the benefits of change is reinforcing for patients.

Key Points ···

- There is a cycle of change that occurs in predictable stages: precontemplation, contemplation, determination, action, and maintenance.
- Providers can assist patients in moving from one stage to the next.
- Providers should inquire about harmful health habits, advise patients to change them, and offer continuing support in a nonjudgmental, empathetic manner.

CASE 18-2

A 35-year-old man wants to lose weight. He has tried several times in the past but failed and states that he has "given up."

A. In which stage is he?

B. What questions should you ask?

C. He decides to try to lose weight. What follow-up should you plan?

19

Joint and Muscular Pain

JOINT PAIN

ETIOLOGY

What causes joint pain?

The causes of joint pain can be divided roughly into two categories: mechanical and inflammatory (Figure 19-1). Mechanical processes are much more common and arise from wear and tear on the joint or overuse syndromes affecting surrounding structures. Frequently a single joint is affected. Inflammatory causes of joint pain are autoimmune disease, crystal-induced disease, and infection. These can involve few or multiple joints, often in a characteristic pattern. The autoimmune arthropathies, systemic lupus erythematosus (SLE), and rheumatoid arthritis (RA) affect small and large joints, as well as multiple organs. In gout, few joints are involved. Septic arthritis affects a single joint, unless disseminated gonococcal infection is present. Occasionally, patients and physicians confuse muscular pain with joint pain.

What causes of joint pain should I not miss?

Do not miss septic arthritis, malignancy, or osteonecrosis. Clues to these include rest pain; delayed response to therapy; risk factors, such as prior malignancy; or systemic signs, such as fever, chills, or weight loss. Osteonecrosis (death of bone resulting from vascular insufficiency) is seen in the hip or proximal tibia, particularly with long-term steroid use, sickle cell anemia, or vasculitis.

Why is septic arthritis important?

Septic arthritis is a medical emergency requiring rapid diagnosis and treatment, including possible surgical débridement to avoid joint destruction. Onset is acute, with marked synovitis, effusion, and extreme pain with movement. Approximately 80% of cases involve one joint, usually the knee. Infectious agents in adults are *Staphylococcus aureus,* other gram-positive organisms, and *Neisseria gonorrhoeae* (a gram-negative coccus). *S. aureus* is especially common in septic arthritis superimposed on RA. This is particularly tricky because a clinician may believe the inflammation is due to RA alone. Suspect gonorrhea in young, sexually active adults, and remember that disseminated infection can rarely affect multiple joints.

What is osteoarthritis?

Synonyms include *degenerative arthritis* and *mechanical arthritis.* This condition occurs as a consequence of wear and tear on the joints, which generates low-grade inflammation. Prevalence is high in patients over age 55 or when joints are heavily used, such as hip degenerative arthritis in a construction worker. Obesity or prior trauma also predisposes to early osteoarthritis.

Does patient age change the likely cause of joint pain?

Patients over age 55 are much more likely to have degenerative arthritis, gout, or bursitis. Autoimmune arthropathies are more common in younger patients (especially women), as are trauma and overuse syndromes, such as ligament injury or tendinitis.

For major joints, what are the common causes of joint pain?

Degenerative arthritis occurs predominately in high-use joints, such as the hands, and in weight-bearing joints, so knees and hips are frequently affected, while the shoulder and elbow are often spared. All joints are subject to tendinitis and bursitis (Table 19-1 and Figure 19-2).

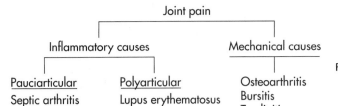

Joint pain

Inflammatory causes   Mechanical causes

Pauciarticular   Polyarticular

Septic arthritis   Lupus erythematosus   Osteoarthritis
Crystal-induced   Rheumatoid arthritis   Bursitis
    arthritis   Tendinitis
                                                   Trauma

Figure 19-1 Classification of joint pain.

TABLE 19-1
Common Conditions Afflicting Major Joints

LOCATION	CONDITION	FINDINGS
Hip	Degenerative arthritis	Pain in groin, medial thigh
		Pain with internal and external hip rotation
	Trochanteric bursitis	Pain in lateral thigh
		Point tenderness on greater trochanter
Knee	Degenerative arthritis	Pain deep to patella
		Joint line tenderness
		Effusion without heat
	Prepatellar bursitis	Pain over patella when kneeling
		Heat, swelling anterior to patella
	Patellar femoral syndrome	Pain with deep knee bend, walking upstairs, prolonged sitting with knees bent
	Baker's cyst	Fullness behind knee, lower extremity swelling if ruptures
Shoulder	Rotator cuff tendinitis	Weakness if rotator cuff tear present
		Pain when rolling onto shoulder at night
		Decreased internal range of motion
	Frozen shoulder	Pain as above, markedly limited range of motion
	Trauma	Point tenderness, history of trauma, deformity with dislocation or fracture
Elbow	Lateral epicondylitis (tennis elbow)	Lateral elbow pain with wrist supination or extension
	Olecranon bursitis	Swelling and tenderness over olecranon process

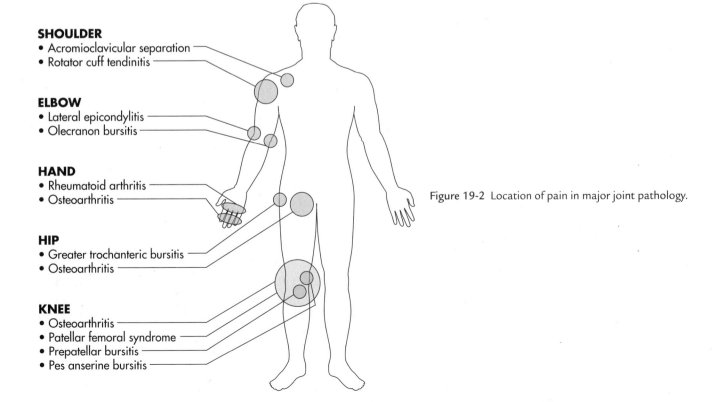

SHOULDER
• Acromioclavicular separation
• Rotator cuff tendinitis

ELBOW
• Lateral epicondylitis
• Olecranon bursitis

HAND
• Rheumatoid arthritis
• Osteoarthritis

HIP
• Greater trochanteric bursitis
• Osteoarthritis

KNEE
• Osteoarthritis
• Patellar femoral syndrome
• Prepatellar bursitis
• Pes anserine bursitis

Figure 19-2 Location of pain in major joint pathology.

What is rotator cuff tendinitis?

The rotator cuff is made of four muscles that rotate and stabilize the humeral head. The subacromial bursa lies between the cuff muscles and acromial process. Varying terms are used to describe disorders that affect this cluster of muscles and surrounding structures, including *rotator cuff tendinitis, subacromial bursitis, frozen shoulder,* and *impingement syndrome.* The primary complaint of these conditions is pain and limited range of motion.

EVALUATION

How can I distinguish mechanical from inflammatory causes of joint pain?

The presentation of these conditions can overlap. Aside from acute trauma, mechanical causes of joint pain tend to be gradual in onset with minimal obvious inflammation. By contrast, inflammatory causes of joint pain often come on rapidly, but synovitis is usually present with joint erythema, pain, swelling, and loss of function. These findings indicate either a vigorous inflammatory arthritis, such as gout or SLE, or possibly septic arthritis. Another key historical distinction is "gelling." In inflammatory arthritis, symptoms worsen with rest as the joint "gels" resulting in prolonged stiffness longer than 1 hour after a period of rest; in mechanical arthritis, the pain improves with rest, and stiffness is worked out of the joint over minutes.

How is degenerative arthritis different from bursitis or tendinitis on examination?

The primary distinction is the anatomic location of the pain. A good example is the knee. In degenerative arthritis, the pain is localized behind the patella within the joint space. In prepatellar bursitis, the pain is localized anterior to the patella. Similarly, in the hip, degenerative arthritis symptoms are deep in the groin and anterior thigh and are reproduced with hip range of motion. Greater trochanteric bursitis produces point tenderness over the bursa with deep palpation over the lateral aspect of the hip.

When evaluating joint pain, what are key points on the physical examination?

Nothing replaces a solid knowledge of the musculoskeletal system, with particular attention to the location of bursae. Examine joints for focal tenderness, range of motion, synovitis (spongy synovial hypertrophy), effusions, crepitus, clicking or locking (suggests cartilage injury), or deformity. Examine soft tissue for ligamentous laxity, muscle weakness, or tender points (as with fibromyalgia).

How can I evaluate shoulder pain for presence of bursitis versus rotator cuff tear?

Rotator cuff tendinitis and subacromial bursitis present with shoulder pain in the deltoid distribution, exacerbated at night when rolling over onto the affected shoulder. On examination, pain is reproduced with arm abduction in an arc between 80 and 120 degrees and with internal or external rotation (reaching hands behind the back). Range of motion is not significantly limited. In frozen shoulder, calcification of the tendon limits motion both passively and actively, and pain is more severe. Rotator cuff tear is distinguished by weakness, particularly with abduction, although passive range of motion is often pain-free. Pain and an inability to relax may confound the examination. A lidocaine injection into the subacromial bursa may be necessary to allow evaluation for true weakness.

Is x-ray helpful in the diagnosis of joint pain?

Degenerative arthritis causes joint space narrowing and sclerosis (i.e., diffuse bone thickening seen as a bright whiteness at the joint surface). RA and gout can cause characteristic erosions that may be absent in the initial phases of disease (see Chapter 34). If the evaluation is consistent with a chronic mechanical cause, films do not add much information. If, on the other hand, recent trauma or concern for cancer are present, an x-ray can help rule out fracture or lytic disease. For suspected rotator cuff tear, obtain ultrasound or MRI to confirm diagnosis.

What blood tests should I order?

Given a history and examination consistent with mechanical cause of joint pain, no further blood tests are needed. For suspected gout, obtain a serum uric acid, although this may be normal. For any acutely inflamed single joint, or if disseminated gonococcal infection is suspected, obtain a CBC (elevated WBC in infection, anemia in autoimmune disease), BUN/creatinine (looking for abnormal renal function in autoimmune disease or gout), uric acid (gout), and C-reactive protein or sedimentation rate (general assessment for inflammation). Use of antinuclear antibody (ANA) reflexive panel and rheumatoid factor are outlined in Chapter 34.

When is arthrocentesis required?

A synovial fluid tap is imperative if septic arthritis is suspected by presence of fever, monoarticular synovitis in a young person, or worsening monarticular inflammation in the setting of stable polyarticular disease. Undiagnosed synovitis requires arthrocentesis. Send fluid for culture, cell count, crystal evaluation, and glucose to distinguish among gout (birefringent crystals), inflammatory arthritis (WBC 2000-75,000), and septic arthritis (WBC >75,000 with low glucose, although lower counts of 30,000-60,000 can occur).

TREATMENT

How are bursitis and tendinitis treated?

Maintaining range of motion and function is the overall goal. Instructions in strengthening exercises are helpful, either by handout or through personal instruction from a physical therapist. Short-term NSAIDs diminish pain and inflammation. For severe cases, consider steroid injection into the inflamed bursa or tendon. Do not inject more often than every 3 months for a total of three shots because this can weaken tendons and muscles.

What is the appropriate treatment for osteoarthritis?

Avoid aggravating activities. Physical therapy and low-impact strengthening exercises are effective. Acetaminophen is the first-line treatment for both pain and inflammation with fewer side effects than NSAIDs. The most common error is inadequate dosing; aim for up to 4000 mg per day, assuming normal liver function. NSAIDs are second-line therapy and have more side effects, particularly gastrointestinal bleeding. Chondroitin sulfate and glucosamine, cartilage derivatives, may be beneficial. These are not controlled by the U.S. Food and Drug Administration (FDA) (dosing depends on manufacturer's recommendations) and effects take 6 to 8 weeks, so warn patients to expect delayed response. For severe rest pain or limitation of daily activities, refer for joint replacement.

When does joint pain require referral?

Refer for orthopedic evaluation any patient with joint dysfunction, such as locking or giving way, joint instability, or inability to bear weight. These symptoms suggest significant meniscal tear, ligamentous injury, or unsuspected fracture or osteonecrosis. Suspected septic arthritis requires immediate orthopedic evaluation and treatment. For patients with degenerative arthritis and pain significantly limiting daily activities, an orthopedic evaluation for joint replacement is indicated. Rheumatologists are particularly skilled at the management of systemic arthropathies, particularly RA and SLE. Further, in any patient with persistent, unexplained symptoms, a subspecialty referral is indicated.

How should the inflammatory causes of joint pain be treated?

Septic arthritis is a surgical emergency. Treatment includes broad-spectrum antibiotics and joint space drainage. Once an organism is identified, the coverage can be narrowed. Repeated aspiration may be adequate, but often surgical drainage is required. For treatment of SLE, RA, and gout, see Chapter 34.

When should I hospitalize a patient with joint pain?

Any patient with a septic joint needs immediate hospitalization.

MUSCULAR PAIN

ETIOLOGY

What causes diffuse persistent muscular pain?

Common causes are fibromyalgia; polymyalgia rheumatica (PMR); and hormonal conditions, such as cortisol excess and thyroid aberrations. Less commonly, myositis with primary muscle inflammation is caused by autoimmune disease or as a medication side effect, for example, with HMG CoA reductase inhibitors.

EVALUATION

How are fibromyalgia, PMR, and polymyositis different?

Fibromyalgia is a syndrome of diffuse muscle and joint pain without any identifiable underlying pathology or inflammation. Criteria for diagnosis include widespread pain and presence of 11 of 18 tender points on examination (Figure 19-3). Stiffness and sleep disturbance are common. *Polymyalgia rheumatica* also presents with diffuse muscle pain, particularly in the proximal limb muscles of elderly patients. In contrast to fibromyalgia, PMR causes elevated ESR and is associated with temporal arteritis, a vasculitis that can cause blindness or stroke. In both fibromyalgia and PMR, the muscle fibers themselves are not damaged, so muscle strength and enzymes are normal. Myositis, as the name implies, results in inflammation and destruction of muscle fibers with resulting weakness and elevated creatine phosphokinase (CPK) and aldolase. When polymyositis occurs with a heliotrope rash (violaceous discoloration of the eyelids) and Gottron's papules (plaquelike eruptions over the joints), the condition is called dermatomyositis.

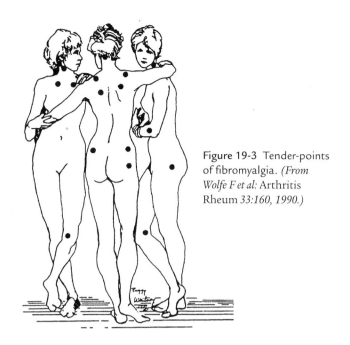

Figure 19-3 Tender-points of fibromyalgia. *(From Wolfe F et al:* Arthritis Rheum *33:160, 1990.)*

TREATMENT

Treatment depends on the underlying disorder (Table 19-2).

Key Points ··

- Generally, mechanical causes of joint pain occur gradually and with minimal inflammation.
- Inflammatory joint conditions cause prolonged stiffness after rest and marked synovitis.
- Septic arthritis is a medical emergency.
- Consider muscular causes for joint pain.

TABLE 19-2
Common Causes, Findings, and Treatment of Diffuse Muscular Pain

CAUSE	FINDINGS	TREATMENT
Fibromyalgia	Nonrestorative sleep, tender points, normal blood tests, normal strength	Exercise, NSAIDs, tricyclic antidepressants, improved sleep
Polymyalgia rheumatica	Diffuse aches, worse in AM, elevated ESR, associated temporal arteritis with jaw claudication, normal strength	Low-dose prednisone, high dose if temporal arteritis present
Polymyositis	Muscle weakness and tenderness on examination, elevated CPK and aldolase	Prednisone, methotrexate if needed
Hormones: hypothyroidism, hyperthyroidism, Cushing's disease	High or low TSH, high 24-hour urine cortisol, may have muscle weakness, CPK elevated in hypothyroidism only	Hormone replacement or identification and removal of site of overproduction

CASE 19-1

A 45-year-old woman reports diffuse, constant joint aches and fatigue. She has a history of depression, poor sleep, and thyroid disease. Review of systems (ROS) is otherwise negative. Examination reveals normal joints without pain on range of motion, normal muscle strength, and multiple tender points.

A. What is your differential diagnosis?

B. Would you order an ANA test?

C. What is appropriate therapy?

CASE 19-2

An 85-year-old woman presents with right shoulder pain. It is worse at night, and some morning stiffness occurs, which improves in a half-hour. She can no longer brush her hair. She reports a 10-pound weight loss. She is otherwise in good health. Examination findings include decreased passive and active range of motion on right shoulder abduction and point tenderness under the acromial process on right.

A. What is the differential diagnosis?

B. What evaluation is indicated?

C. Does this patient have a rotator cuff tear?

20

Low Back Pain

ETIOLOGY

What causes acute low back pain?

Over 95% of all low back pain arises from relatively benign changes to musculoskeletal structures in the low back. Degenerative arthritis, lumbosacral strain, bulging vertebral disks, sciatic nerve irritation, and spinal stenosis all cause low back pain. Pinpointing the anatomic source of the pain is often difficult and in fact does not correlate with prognosis. Fortunately, the great majority of low back pain will resolve with a conservative approach of brief rest, antiinflammatories, and gradual return to previous activity. Your job is to reassure the patient and yourself that another condition does not exist, and to monitor the patient's progress.

What is sciatica?

Sciatica refers to pain radiating in the sciatic nerve distribution down the back of the leg. Although classically associated with a herniated disk, many other conditions can cause this pain syndrome (e.g., spinal stenosis, sacroiliitis).

What are the "red flags" for dangerous causes of low back pain?

Warning signs for potentially serious causes of back pain are listed in Box 20-1.

EVALUATION

Is the patient's description of the pain helpful?

Most back pain is nonspecific and does not lead reliably to a diagnosis. The following generalizations may be useful. *Radicular pain,* that is, pain in a nerve distribution, extends from the back or buttock past the knee and suggests impingement of a nerve as it exits the spinal canal. In contrast, pain that goes from the back to the thigh or hip, but not past the knee, is *radiating pain* and is less worrisome for neuropathic cause. Rest pain and/or progressive pain may indicate cancer or abscess. Pain with cough, bowel movement, or sneeze is consistent with disk herniation because increased pressure through Valsalva's maneuver worsens this condition.

How is the history for spinal stenosis different from other causes of low back pain?

Spinal stenosis is narrowing of the spinal canal usually associated with arthritis. It causes pain in the thighs and buttocks with walking or standing that is relieved by sitting.

What is an appropriate neurologic examination for low back pain?

For low back pain, a good neurologic examination is your best tool. This does not mean an exhaustive examination. Over 90% of neurologic sequelae of back disease occur in the L5-S1 region, so your examination can focus primarily on the foot. (The exception is the patient with bowel or bladder symptoms, symptoms of possible acute cord compression. In those cases, you need to check perianal sensation and rectal tone.) The top of the foot allows you to test the three sensory distributions L4-S1. A helpful mnemonic is S1 = Small toe, L4 = Large toe. Reflexes are technically difficult to reproduce. This does not mean that you should not do them, but realize that they may not be accurate. Motor weakness should be obvious; a good screening test is great toe dorsiflexion, L5, and plantar flexion, S1 (Figure 20-1).

What is the best test for nerve impingement as the cause of acute low back pain?

The best test is the straight leg raise. With the patient lying on his or her back, elevate the straight leg. A positive test reproduces radicular pain with the leg 70 de-

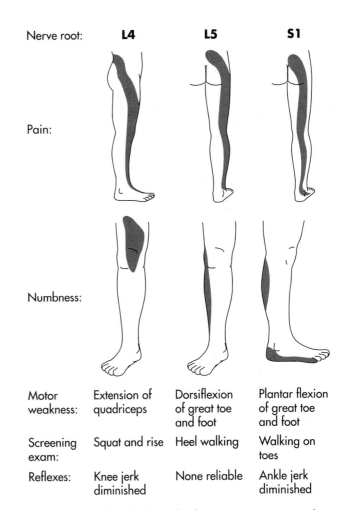

Figure 20-1 Findings localizing lumbar nerve root compromise.

Nerve root:	**L4**	**L5**	**S1**
Motor weakness:	Extension of quadriceps	Dorsiflexion of great toe and foot	Plantar flexion of great toe and foot
Screening exam:	Squat and rise	Heel walking	Walking on toes
Reflexes:	Knee jerk diminished	None reliable	Ankle jerk diminished

---

grees or less from horizontal, indicating tension in the L5/S1 nerve root. Pain produced in the low back or hip does not qualify as a positive test.

If the neurologic examination is abnormal, what should I do?

This is a red flag. Major motor weakness, such as absent dorsiflexion of the great toe, traditionally requires imaging. However, here is a refinement on this rule: a patient with mild disk herniation may have slight numbness or even weakness by history and examination. This mild degree of symptoms can be managed conservatively for 2 to 4 weeks. If the patient's numbness persists, obtain a CT or MRI and electromyography (EMG) as evaluation for potential surgery.

How do red flags help me decide what further studies to order?

If no red flags are present, no further workup is needed. When any red flag is present, start with an ESR and lumbosacral spine film. If history suggests infection, obtain a CBC and/or urinalysis. Although you may be tempted to obtain a CT scan early in your evaluation, remember that CT and MRI are very sensitive modalities but are extremely nonspecific. These studies reveal disk bulging in up to 60% of the normal population. In asymptomatic elderly patients, frank disk herniation is seen in 30%. Reserve these studies for symptoms or signs of cord compression (see below), when you suspect spinal stenosis, when there is an abnormal x-ray or sedimentation rate, or for preoperative evaluation.

What are potential low back pain emergencies?

The spinal cord sits within a confined space, defined by the surrounding vertebral bone structure. If the cord is compressed, paralysis can occur. The main causes of acute spinal cord compression are epidural abscess (an infection in the epidural space surrounding or next to the cord), encroaching tumor, and, rarely, massive disk herniation. Acute neurologic change or progressive neurologic symptoms, particularly in high-risk patients with IV drug use or known cancer, should alert you to this possibility. If you suspect one of these conditions, the patient requires emergent imaging and neurosurgical evaluation. The quicker the treatment, the more complete the recovery.

What is the cauda equina syndrome?

The cauda equina is the "horse's tail" of sacral nerves that travel in the distal spinal canal. This syndrome is a description of acute cord compression, such as with disk herniation, of these distal sacral nerves, causing bowel and bladder dysfunction of either marked constipation or incontinence, and sacral nerve numbness in the perianal distribution.

TREATMENT

How do I treat acute low back pain?

When red flags are absent, use conservative therapy (Box 20-2).

Do I manage acute and chronic low back pain differently?

A repeat episode of acute low back pain is managed just like a first episode. Chronic back pain present for several months is a different problem. First, review your history and physical for red flags, and consider further studies if the patient has not responded as you would have expected. Second, screen your patient carefully for depression. This condition is common among patients with chronic pain. Antidepressants serve a dual function in these cases, improving both chronic pain and depression. Pending legal action predicts poorer prognosis.

How do I fill out disability forms?

Describe objectively what you see on examination. You do not have to determine disability; that is the job of the Department of Labor and Industry. Often there is a section asking how many pounds the patient can lift. A general guideline follows symptom severity (Table 20-1).

Is there a role for chiropractic or acupuncture?

In a nonblinded study, 400 men with acute back pain improved over controls with chiropractor intervention in the first 2 weeks after acute back pain. There is no evidence supporting more frequent weekly chiropractic intervention or acupuncture. Nonetheless, some patients swear by chiropractors and acupuncture.

What if my patient has a true disk herniation?

If the patient has acute radicular pain, a positive straight leg raise, and none of the historical red flags, he or she most likely has a herniated disk. However, 80% to 90% of patients with disk herniation will be back to normal after 1 month without any specific intervention. Therefore unless the patient has significant neurologic symptoms or signs, you can watch and wait. If symptoms persist, it is reasonable to obtain a CT or MRI and refer to a neurosurgeon.

BOX 20-2	Elements of "Conservative Therapy" for Acute Low Back Pain

NSAIDs: No evidence for one over another
From 2 to 3 days of bed rest: Longer worsens outcomes
Return to previous activities: As soon as tolerable, except heavy lifting
Physical therapy/back exercises: When the acute episode resolves

---

TABLE 20-1
Weight-Lifting Limitations by Symptom Severity

SYMPTOM SEVERITY	WOMEN	MEN
Moderate to severe	20 lb	20 lb
Mild	35 lb	60 lb
None	40 lb	80 lb

BOX 20-3	Criteria for Surgical Intervention in Back Pain Patients

Epidural abscess
Cauda equina syndrome
Cord compression
Persistent nerve root compromise
Severe spinal stenosis

What surgeries are done for back pain? Do they work?

With the exception of catastrophic herniations, most disk herniations resolve on their own. Although initial response to surgery may be good, at 4 years, there is little difference in conservative versus surgical management. Various surgical techniques have been developed, including open diskectomy (in which the surgeon exposes the disk space and removes herniated disk material) and endoscopic diskectomy (analogous to laparoscopic gallbladder removal: less invasive, leaves smaller scar). The least invasive procedure is chymopapain injections, in which a proteolytic enzyme is injected into the disk and causes reduction in the disk size. Unfortunately, this has been associated with anaphylaxis and transverse myelitis, so it is out of favor in the United States. Surgery should only be considered if the patient has appropriate criteria (Box 20-3).

Key Points

- Most back pain, although bothersome to patients, is benign and self-limited.
- Red flags for pathology will dictate when to get further studies.
- With few exceptions, conservative therapy is the appropriate first step.

CASE 20-1

A 45-year-old laborer has severe low back pain after lifting a concrete pipe. He has never had back pain before. He smokes and is obese. On examination, he has no weakness or numbness but has a positive straight leg raise.

A. Do you want any further tests, and if so, what tests?
B. What do you recommend for treatment?
C. When can he return to work?
D. How soon should he feel better?

CASE 20-2

A 56-year-old diabetic office worker comes in with low back pain after working in her garden this weekend. She was pulling some weeds and developed acute pain in her back. Her pain is steady but has improved with ibuprofen. She states that her diabetes is under good control. She has had some difficulty with recurrent urinary tract infections. On examination, she has decreased sensation in both feet across her toes and her straight leg test causes pain in her low back.

A. What are the red flags in her history?
B. Do you want any further tests, and if so, what tests?
C. What is the significance of her straight leg raise and her distal numbness?

chapter

21

Lower Extremity Pain, Swelling, and Ulcers

LOWER EXTREMITY PAIN

ETIOLOGY

What are common causes of lower extremity pain?

Common causes are peripheral vascular disease (PVD, also known as arterial insufficiency), peripheral neuropathy (PN), radiculopathy, venous obstruction, and nocturnal cramps.

Are there any emergencies that cause lower extremity pain?

Compartment syndrome and arterial occlusion from thromboembolism are rare emergencies. Compartment syndrome occurs when tissue swelling or hematoma in a muscle compartment raises pressures above arterial pressure, occludes blood flow, and causes tissue necrosis. Arterial occlusion causes acute onset of the five Ps: pain, paresthesias, paralysis, pulselessness, and pallor.

EVALUATION

How do symptoms distinguish between the common causes of leg pain?

Patients with PVD report claudication with exertion that resolves with rest. The pain is aching or cramping and occurs predictably in leg muscles with exercise. Pain from spinal stenosis, also called *pseudoclaudication,* can be very similar. Unlike true claudication, spinal stenosis may be accompanied by back pain, does not resolve with standing, and requires sitting for several minutes. PN pain occurs in a stocking-glove distribution and is described variably as burning, tingling, a "pins and needles" sensation, or numbness. It is often worse at night.

Radiculopathy is often worse with sitting and relieved by standing. Pain from venous obstruction may be worse when legs are dependent and improved with leg elevation. Nocturnal muscle cramps occur suddenly and only at night, are not exertional, and are relieved with massage or stretching.

What physical findings help with diagnosis?

With PVD you may hear bruits; find weak or absent pulses; or see loss of leg hair, dependent rubor, pallor with elevation, or delayed capillary refill. With PN, look for decreases in proprioception, light touch and sharp sensation, and deep tendon reflexes. PVD and PN are usually bilateral, although they may be worse on one side. Radiculopathy is usually unilateral and may give focal loss of a reflex or strength or shooting pain down the leg with straight leg raise (see Chapter 20).

What does the ankle-brachial index mean?

The ankle-brachial index (ABI) assesses severity of PVD, as estimated by ankle systolic pressure divided by brachial artery systolic pressure. To measure ankle systolic pressure, inflate a cuff around the calf and palpate the systolic pressure at the dorsalis pedis or posterior tibialis artery. Normal values are 0.9 to 1.2. ABI greater than 0.9 generally rules out arterial insufficiency. ABI of 0.6 to 0.8 is usual with one-block claudication. A ratio less than 0.4 indicates limb-threatening ischemia, and patients often have leg pain at rest and/or ischemic non-healing ulcers. Obtain arterial duplex when the ratio is less than 0.9. ABIs may be difficult to measure in diabetic patients because of noncompressible calcified arteries.

What tests are appropriate for patients with a PN?

Most patients with PN have diabetes and require no further workup. If diabetes is absent, you need to consider

---

BOX 21-1   Causes of Peripheral Neuropathy

COMMON CAUSES
Metabolic
Diabetes
Alcohol use

Medications
Didanosine (ddI)
Zalcitabine (ddC)
Stavudine (d4T)
Isoniazid (INH) (if vitamin B$_6$ not replaced)

LESS COMMON CAUSES
Metabolic
Malnutrition
Hypothyroidism
Renal insufficiency
Vitamin B$_{12}$ deficiency

Medications
Metronidazole
Pyridoxine
Simvastatin
Hydralazine
Colchicine
Vincristine
Cisplatinum

Infections
HIV
Lyme disease
Syphilis
Leprosy

Immunologic
Multiple myeloma
Paraneoplastic syndromes
Vasculitis

Metals/industrial chemicals
Lead
Arsenic
Solvents (toluene, hexane)

TABLE 21-1
Treatment Strategies for Common
Causes of Lower Extremity Pain

CAUSE	TREATMENT
Peripheral neuropathy	Tight glycemic control in diabetes
	Tricyclic antidepressants, SSRIs
	Anticonvulsants (gabapentin, carbamazepine)
	Topical capsaicin
	Foot care for ulcer prevention (shoes, lanolin to prevent cracks)
Peripheral vascular disease	Risk factor reduction (smoking, hypertension, lipids, diabetes)
	Exercise
	Angioplasty or surgery for claudication at rest
Nocturnal cramps	Quinine, calf stretching during day

---

other causes (Box 21-1). A complete history, including alcohol use, diet, toxin exposures, medications, and family history, helps direct evaluation. In patients without diabetes, start with CBC, B$_{12}$, TSH, creatinine, serum protein electrophoresis, and ANA. EMG and nerve conduction studies confirm PN and assess its severity. Nerve biopsies are rarely indicated.

TREATMENT

Table 21-1 lists treatment options for lower extremity pain.

LOWER EXTREMITY SWELLING

ETIOLOGY

What causes swelling in the lower extremities?

Swelling is often due to edema, the accumulation of fluid in the interstitial tissue. Edema is pitting when skin remains indented after pressure has been applied. Nonpitting edema does not indent and implies inflammation or infiltration. Edema may signal significant systemic illness.

What diseases cause unilateral lower extremity edema?

This depends on how rapidly the edema develops. Acute edema occurring over hours to days is often associated with pain and inflammatory signs, such as increased warmth and erythema. Common causes of acute unilateral edema are deep venous thrombosis (DVT), cellulitis, Baker's cyst rupture, superficial thrombophlebitis, and trauma. Chronic unilateral edema accumulates over weeks to months without accompanying inflammatory signs and is usually caused by venous insufficiency or lymphatic obstruction. Lymphatic obstruction, also called *lymphedema*, may be idiopathic or secondary to tumor, infection, or scarring from previous surgery or radiation.

BOX 21-2   Systemic Causes of Bilateral Lower Extremity Edema

CONDITIONS ASSOCIATED WITH FLUID RETENTION
Congestive heart failure
Renal insufficiency
Hypothyroidism

CONDITIONS ASSOCIATED WITH HYPOALBUMINEMIA
Hepatic cirrhosis
Nephrotic syndrome
Malnutrition
Protein-losing enteropathies

MEDICATIONS
Nifedipine, felodipine, amlodipine
Corticosteroids
Estrogen, progesterone, testosterone
Nonsteroidal antiinflammatory agents

What is a Baker's cyst?

A Baker's cyst is accumulation of excess synovial fluid in a pouch of synovium that extrudes from the knee joint into the popliteal fossa. It is related to underlying joint inflammation (osteoarthritis, rheumatoid arthritis, meniscal tear, trauma, or crystalline arthropathy).

What diseases cause bilateral lower extremity edema?

Causes of bilateral edema are venous insufficiency or systemic diseases that cause fluid retention or low albumin. Medications are a common cause of edema unresponsive to diuretics (Box 21-2).

EVALUATION

What features of the history and examination distinguish a DVT?

All causes of acute unilateral edema can present exactly the same way (erythema, swelling, and pain developing over hours). Because DVT can cause life-threatening pulmonary embolism, it is imperative to exclude this first. Ask about DVT risk factors (i.e., oral contraceptive pills, recent period of prolonged inactivity, pregnancy, postpartum, recent major surgery, family history of hypercoagulability, paresis, history of DVT). On examination of the leg, look for a palpable cord (indurated vein) or positive Homans' sign (pain elicited in popliteal region with ankle dorsiflexion of the flexed knee), al-

though neither finding is very sensitive or specific. Examination may only reveal mild unilateral calf swelling confirmed by measuring bilateral calf diameters. Duplex ultrasound is highly sensitive (>98%) and specific (>97%) for clots above the knee.

How do I distinguish among Baker's cyst, DVT, cellulitis, and superficial thrombophlebitis?

A Baker's cyst presents as a bulge on the medial aspect of the popliteal fossa and often is diagnosed by examination alone. Cyst rupture may create ankle or foot ecchymoses, differentiating it from a DVT. With cellulitis, pain, lymphangitis (red streaking along a lymph vessel), ipsilateral groin lymphadenopathy, chills, or fever may be present. About 50% of the time, a portal of entry for bacteria can be identified, usually maceration from tinea pedis infection. Superficial thrombophlebitis causes a localized tender vein, without lymphangitis, adenopathy, or palpable cord. If you are not convinced that it is not a DVT, obtain duplex ultrasound to be sure.

When should I look for a systemic cause of edema?

Bilateral lower extremity or generalized edema suggests systemic cause. Obtain thorough history and examination. Ask about signs of CHF: fatigue, dyspnea on exertion, orthopnea, and paroxysmal nocturnal dyspnea. Examination findings suggesting left heart failure include tachypnea, tachycardia, rales, and S_3. Signs of right heart failure include distended neck veins and hepatojugular reflux (see Chapter 23, Congestive Heart Failure section). Renal insufficiency and nephrotic syndrome may not be apparent on history or examination. Hypothyroidism and low albumin states, such as nephrotic syndrome, can cause periorbital edema. Hypothyroidism is usually accompanied by other symptoms, such as fatigue, weight gain, cold intolerance, or hair, voice or skin changes (see Chapter 25, Thyroid Disease section).

What laboratory tests or imaging studies are helpful?

Kidney disease may not be evident by history or examination, so obtain a serum creatinine, BUN, and urinalysis, looking for renal insufficiency or nephrotic syndrome in patients with new bilateral edema. Obtain renal ultrasound if creatinine is high to distinguish acute from chronic insufficiency. Many patients with nephrotic syndrome have normal creatinine, so if proteinuria is present on urinalysis, obtain serum albumin and a 24-hour urine protein. Low serum albumin without proteinuria suggests malnutrition or liver disease, so reexamine for ascites and consider liver function tests and abdominal imaging. If you suspect left ventricular heart failure, obtain chest x-ray and consider ECG and echocardiogram. Obtain TSH when you suspect hypothyroidism, and obtain 24-hour urine cortisol when you suspect Cushing's syndrome.

TREATMENT

How do I manage fluid retention in the legs?

General treatments include lower extremity elevation, salt restriction, elastic support stockings, and low-dose diuretics (hydrochlorothiazide 12.5 mg/day). Avoid medications that cause edema, such as calcium channel blockers. Treat underlying systemic diseases when present.

How do I treat a DVT?

Clotting at or above the popliteal fossa increases risk for pulmonary embolus. Identify and address any underlying risk factors, and if none are found, draw blood looking for a hypercoagulable state before starting anticoagulants (see Chapter 28, Bleeding Disorders section). Hospitalize for intravenous heparin. Start oral warfarin to overlap with heparin (duration of overlap is debated). The goal of warfarin is to raise the protime INR to a therapeutic range of 2 to 3. Some physicians now use low-molecular-weight heparins (LMWH) in place of standard heparin. LMWH is given subcutaneously and can be used at home without monitoring, so it shortens hospital stay. Continue anticoagulation for 3 to 6 months. Anticoagulation is not indicated for a clot isolated to the calf because these are unlikely to embolize; they require serial duplexes to monitor for proximal migration.

How do I treat a Baker's cyst?

Observe smaller cysts. Aspirate cysts when they are large or interfering with knee function. Submit synovial fluid for crystal analysis and cell count. NSAIDs and intraarticular steroids can decrease inflammation. Recurrent problems may warrant MRI to look for a meniscal tear.

Is there an effective treatment for lymphedema?

Address treatable obstructive processes (pelvic mass, infection). Treatment options are limited when lymphedema is idiopathic or caused by postsurgical scarring or radiation. Compression garments and home lymphapress machines may be helpful. Diuretics are not useful. Because lymphedema places patients at risk for cellulitis and recurrent cellulitis worsens lymphatic obstruction, prevent cellulitis by treating tinea and moisturize skin to prevent cracking.

How do I treat cellulitis and superficial thrombophlebitis?

Treat cellulitis with oral dicloxacillin or cephalexin. Patients with diabetes may need broader coverage. Arrange close follow-up. Hospitalize for IV antibiotics if response is inadequate. Treat superficial thrombophlebitis with warm compresses, elevation, and NSAIDs. Symptoms should resolve or improve significantly within a week. If not, obtain a duplex.

LOWER EXTREMITY ULCERS

ETIOLOGY

What predisposes patients to ulceration?

Main causes of lower extremity ulcers are venous insufficiency (90%), sensory peripheral neuropathy, and arterial insufficiency secondary to peripheral vascular disease. Pyoderma gangrenosum is an unusual cause associated with inflammatory bowel disease.

EVALUATION

What distinguishing examination features help with diagnosis?

Venous insufficiency ulcers generally are painless; are abrupt in onset, located on the medial malleolus; and are accompanied by edema, stasis dermatitis, and superficial varicosities. Neuropathic ulcers are painless, sharply marginated, and found at plantar pressure points (metatarsal heads, distal phalanges, heels). Ulcers from arterial insufficiency or ischemia occur distal to the ankle joint, often at the tips of the toes; have a punched-out appearance; and are exquisitely painful. Associated findings include dependent rubor, nonpalpable pulses, delayed capillary refill, and loss of hair growth. Pyoderma gangrenosum ulcers are sharply demarcated; exudative; and have heaped-up, boggy, violaceous edges that are often undermined.

How do I know if the ulcer or underlying bone is infected?

This can be difficult to determine. All ulcers are colonized with bacteria, and therefore cultures are unhelpful. A yellow/green discharge is common, even in non-infected wounds. Débride and probe all ulcers to determine their depth. If the bone can be probed, osteomyelitis is likely. If there are systemic symptoms (fever, chills, sweats) or local signs of cellulitis (warmth, erythema and swelling), presume the ulcer is infected and give antibiotics. X-ray may be helpful to screen for a foreign body, gangrene (gas), or late osteomyelitis (periosteal elevation). If you are highly suspicious of osteomyelitis, check sedimentation rate and obtain MRI, bone scan, or bone biopsy.

TREATMENT

Are all ulcers treated the same?

Some general wound care issues pertain to ulcers of many causes: saline wet-to-dry dressings and whirlpool treatment for débridement, synthetic occlusive dressings (DuoDERM), or Unna's paste boots. Ulcers caused by PN require a non–weight-bearing period or total contact cast in order to heal. Other specific treatment depends on the cause (Table 21-2).

TABLE 21-2
Treatments for Common Lower Extremity Ulcers

CAUSE	TREATMENT
Ischemic ulcers	Vascular surgery referral with arteriography
Peripheral neuropathy/ neuropathic ulcers	No weight bearing Good shoes Avoidance of foot trauma Meticulous foot care
Venous insufficiency/ stasis ulcers	Edema reduction (improves healing) Skin lubrication (prevent cracks, cellulitis) Topical steroids
Pyoderma gangrenosum	Oral steroids

Key Points

- Rule out DVT with any case of new, acute unilateral peripheral edema.
- Bilateral lower extremity edema warrants an investigation for systemic diseases.
- Patients with diabetes, PN, and ulcers require a non–weight-bearing period in order to heal.
- Lymphedema will not respond to diuretic therapy.

CASE 21-1

A 50-year-old woman with type II diabetes reports a painless ulcer on her foot, present for 10 months. It has been unresponsive to antibiotics, DuoDERM dressings, whirlpool treatments, and saline wet-to-dry dressings. She denies swelling or pain with walking. On examination, she has a 1-cm ulcer on the plantar surface at the first metatarsal head, palpable posterior tibialis pulses, and decreased foot sensation. BP is 140/80, and ankle systolic pressure is 130. Foot x-ray is negative.
   A. What is her ABI, and is this helpful?
   B. Why does her ulcer not heal?
   C. How do you treat her?

CASE 21-2

A healthy 65-year-old woman presents with 2 days of right lower extremity swelling and pain, making it difficult for her to walk. Initially, she noticed swelling around her knee, but it progressed to involve her calf and distal thigh in the last day. There is no history of trauma, and she has not had knee problems in the past. On examination, she has a knee effusion and diffuse swelling and tenderness involving her ankle, calf, knee, and distal thigh.
   A. What is your differential diagnosis?
   B. Are there any tests you want to order?

22

Lymphadenopathy

ETIOLOGY

When is lymphadenopathy pathologic?

Lymph nodes are usually too small to appreciate, but not all palpable nodes are pathologic. In the neck and groin, small "shotty" nodes smaller than 1.0 cm are common and are of no consequence in someone who feels well. Nodes of any size in any patient with constitutional symptoms of fever, weight loss, fatigue, or night sweats or nodes larger than 1.5 cm need repeat physical examination to be sure they are resolving. If not, further evaluation is required (Box 22-1). Nodes larger than 3 cm suggest malignancy in an adult and should be pursued sooner. Reactive nodes, which occur in response to infection, are tender, enlarge quickly, and regress in 4 to 6 weeks. Some reactive nodes do not regress completely but remain small and palpable. Age can help distinguish whether an enlarged node is pathologic: in patients younger than 30 years old, most enlarged nodes are benign. However, in 60% of patients 50 years old and older, lymphadenopathy is due to a malignancy.

What is meant by generalized or localized lymphadenopathy?

Generalized adenopathy is present when two or more noncontiguous sites have enlarged nodes, for example, right neck and left axilla. The most common causes are infectious (Box 22-2). Localized nodes occur contiguously, suggesting an inflammatory process or malignancy in the corresponding area of drainage. A single source of infection may explain several clusters of nodes, for example, a chronic nonhealing ulcer of the left hand, causing forearm, epitrochlear, and axillary adenopathy (Figure 22-1).

What causes lymphadenopathy in the neck?

The neck is the most common site of lymphadenopathy. In most younger adults, bilateral cervical adenopathy is due to infectious mononucleosis, pharyngitis, or dental infections. Other causes of adenopathy with a mononucleosis-like illness (fever, fatigue) include primary HIV infection, cytomegalovirus (CMV) infection, toxoplasmosis, primary herpes simplex virus (HSV) infection, and secondary syphilis. Although unilateral cervical adenopathy in the younger patient is most likely to be mononucleosis or pharyngitis, more than half of Hodgkin's disease patients present with adenopathy in the neck. In older patients, cancer is more likely. Submandibular and anterior cervical nodes suggest head and neck cancer. Anterior cervical nodes can also arise from metastatic lung, breast, or thyroid cancer. Preauricular adenopathy is seen with conjunctivitis and cat-scratch disease (a self-limited disease seen mostly in children), whereas postauricular adenopathy is common with scalp infections or inflammation, such as seborrheic dermatitis.

What is Virchow's node?

Supraclavicular nodes are often pathologic, and the side of presentation suggests the cancer of origin. Virchow's node refers to any left supraclavicular node and is usually due to a gastrointestinal, renal, testicular, or ovarian malignancy. A right supraclavicular node may herald a pulmonary, mediastinal, or esophageal tumor.

What are the common causes of axillary lymphadenopathy?

The most common cause is ipsilateral injury or infection in the arm or hand. In a woman with unilateral axillary adenopathy, breast cancer must be considered.

Lymphomas such as Hodgkin's disease also present in the axilla. When a linear inflamed set of nodes leads from an open wound, group A streptococcal skin infection is the usual cause.

What causes epitrochlear lymphadenopathy?

Unilateral epitrochlear nodes suggest infection in the hand. Bilateral epitrochlear adenopathy is uncommon but is a clinical clue suggesting lupus, secondary syphilis, or sarcoidosis.

What causes hilar lymphadenopathy on chest x-ray?

Causes of bilateral hilar adenopathy include sarcoidosis; lymphoma; bronchogenic carcinoma; and infection, such as primary tuberculosis, coccidioidomycosis, and histoplasmosis. If a mediastinal mass, pleural effusion, or pulmonary mass is associated with bilateral or unilateral adenopathy, a diagnosis of cancer should be pursued. If erythema nodosum or uveitis is seen in an otherwise asymptomatic patient, sarcoidosis is the most likely cause.

BOX 22-1   Lymphadenopathy Requiring Further Evaluation

Node greater than 1.5 cm
Age greater than 40 to 50 years
Smoking or drinking history
Concerning symptoms

BOX 22-2   Causes of Generalized Lymphadenopathy

COMMONLY SEEN
Infection
    Mononucleosis
    HIV or AIDS
    Tuberculosis
Lymphoma or leukemia

LESS COMMONLY SEEN
Drugs
    Phenytoin
    Hydralazine
    Allopurinol
Sarcoidosis
Secondary syphilis
Lupus or rheumatoid arthritis
Serum sickness
Hyperthyroidism

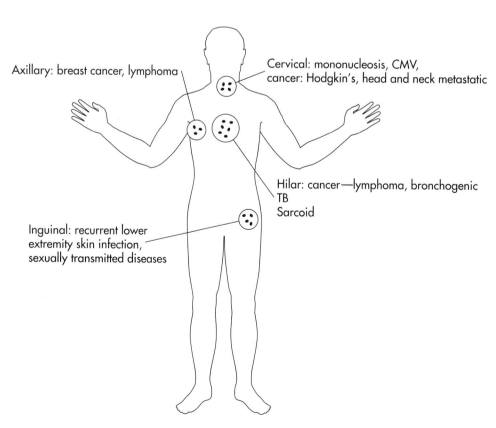

Figure 22-1 Common causes of focal lymphadenopathy.

What causes inguinal lymphadenopathy?

Chronic shotty adenopathy is common. This may be due to subclinical or low-grade infections in the lower extremities or perineum. A femoral hernia may masquerade as a single large inguinal node. More marked inguinal adenopathy often accompanies acute lower extremity infection or sexually transmitted diseases (herpes, syphilis, gonorrhea, chancroid, and lymphogranuloma venereum). A persistent or large node can result from rectal, vaginal, or cervical cancer or melanoma.

What about lymphadenopathy and HIV infection?

In HIV infection, persistent generalized lymphadenopathy occurs often before the CD4 counts drop below 200. Nodes are rarely larger than 1.5 cm. Larger nodes or asymmetric distribution should be evaluated further. Non-Hodgkin's lymphoma, Hodgkin's disease, Kaposi's sarcoma, and tuberculosis are more common in HIV-positive patients. They can occur when the CD4 is only modestly suppressed, that is, 200 to 500. If the CD4 is less than 100, rule out *Mycobacterium avium* complex, fungal, and suppurative infections.

EVALUATION

Is this lump a lymph node?

Your examination must include careful palpation of the occiput, around the ears, the entire neck, the supraclavicular fossa, the axilla, the epitrochlear space, the abdomen, and the groin. Pay attention to the quality of the node: size, mobile or matted, tender or painless, rock-hard or rubbery. Cancer tends to be painless and may or may not be matted. Infection is tender, mobile, and occasionally rubbery. The cervical node examination may be most problematic because of overlying muscle, tendon, thyroid, carotids, and salivary glands. The parotid and submandibular salivary glands can be nodelike. If their respective ducts are obstructed, inflammation or infection can occur. Parotid gland enlargement can occur with a number of conditions, such as pregnancy, eating disorders, Sjögren's disease, diabetes mellitus, alcoholism, mumps, and HIV. Any distinct mass should be referred for biopsy. Similarly, submandibular gland may be the site of infection, but masses here are even more likely to be cancer. Other findings may mimic lymphadenopathy, such as rheumatoid nodule; lipoma; sebaceous or ganglion cyst; and, even less commonly, thyroglossal duct and branchial cleft cysts.

What are pertinent clues from history of patients with generalized lymphadenopathy?

Because the causes of generalized adenopathy are limited, a focused history can quickly narrow your differential. Epidemiologic clues may provide the diagnosis before any laboratory tests return. Ask about symptoms of acute viral syndrome versus longer-term weight loss, night sweats, or fatigue. Explore risk factors for HIV exposure. Patients with secondary syphilis have constitutional symptoms and a history of a painless genital ulcer, which has healed. Review drug or serum exposure and symptoms of hyperthyroidism, rheumatoid arthritis, and lupus.

What physical examination findings are useful in the evaluation of generalized lymphadenopathy?

Skin may reveal a rash on the palms and soles (secondary syphilis) or erythema nodosum (red, tender subcutaneous nodules usually on the lower extremities that can accompany TB or sarcoidosis). Malar rash across the cheeks suggests lupus. Pharyngeal erythema or exudates can occur with mononucleosis. Oral hairy leukoplakia is found only with HIV infection (see Chapter 29, HIV Infection section). Splenomegaly occurs with mononucleosis, lymphoma, and leukemia. Synovitis suggests lupus, rheumatoid arthritis, or serum sickness. Tremor warrants investigation for hyperthyroidism.

What laboratory tests are helpful?

When the clinical picture is confusing, order a CBC, white cell differential, ESR, purified protein derivative (PPD), and chest radiography. The presence of hilar adenopathy points to granulomatous disease in a young patient and malignancy in an older patient. Atypical lymphocytes suggest mononucleosis, other viral infections, or toxoplasmosis. Extensive testing is rarely needed (Table 22-1).

When should I pursue a biopsy?

If no cause is found and the node is enlarging, refer to a surgeon. Do not delay if cancer is suspected. When history and physical suggest a viral infection, a biopsy may be confusing because the histology may mimic lymphoma. In this case, watchful waiting for 4 to 6 weeks is advisable before referral for biopsy.

Key Points

- A complete history and careful physical examination will narrow your differential diagnosis.
- Laboratory testing need not be extensive.
- When the diagnosis is uncertain and the risk for malignancy is low, careful observation for 1 month is appropriate.

TABLE 22-1

Testing in Lymphadenopathy According to Clinical Presentation

CLINICAL PRESENTATION	TESTING
Cervical adenopathy and pharyngitis	Throat culture for strep +/− gonorrhea; Monospot
Cervical adenopathy and mononucleosis-like syndrome	Monospot (negative in 10% of EBV mononucleosis); if negative, consider EBV IgM, HIV RNA, CMV, and toxoplasmosis serology
Cervical adenopathy in a patient >50 years old or with history of tobacco or alcohol	Refer for biopsy
Adenopathy and HIV risks	HIV test
Inguinal adenopathy, marked	HIV test, RPR; culture for herpes simplex and gonorrhea; chlamydia LCR
Hilar adenopathy	PPD testing, ACE level (for sarcoid)

LCR, Ligase chain reaction.

CASE 22-1

A 26-year-old man comes to clinic worried about a swelling in his neck for several days. He feels well but missed 2 days of work last week with the "flu." He has no significant past medical history. His examination is unremarkable with the exception of a 3-cm minimally tender mass anterior to the right superior sternocleidomastoid muscle.

A. What is your differential diagnosis? List five possibilities.
B. What tests should be done on the first visit?
C. One week later, all blood tests ordered are negative. What is your plan?

CASE 22-2

A 58-year-old man returns for an annual visit. He smokes 1.5 packs per day. He denies drinking problems, although his wife has asked you to ask him to cut down. He feels well. On examination, you find a new 1.5-cm node in his left anterior neck.

A. What is your differential diagnosis? How would you manage or evaluate this?
B. Are fine-needle aspiration and excisional biopsy equally preferred in this case?

3

Patients Presenting With a Known Condition

Cardiology

COMMON CARDIAC ARRHYTHMIAS

ETIOLOGY

How should I categorize arrhythmias?

Abnormal heart rhythms should be categorized by the ventricular rate and the origin of the rhythm disturbance. Rhythms with a rate greater than 100/min are called *tachycardias,* and those less than 60/min are called *bradycardias.* The origin of the abnormality may be in the atria, nodes, or ventricles (Figure 23-1). Close inspection of the ECG will usually allow specific localization (see below).

What causes a fast heart rate?

Tachycardia can originate anywhere within the heart. Fast rhythms that are initiated in the atria or AV node are collectively referred to as *supraventricular tachycardias* (SVTs). Common causes include sinus tachycardia and atrial fibrillation. Less common are atrial flutter, AV nodal reentrant tachycardia (AVNRT), and multifocal atrial tachycardia. Ventricular tachycardia (VT) originates below the AV node within abnormally functioning ventricular tissue. It occurs most commonly with cardiac ischemia but is also seen with electrolyte abnormalities, cardiomyopathy, and drug intoxication (Table 23-1). VT can rapidly deteriorate into ventricular fibrillation (completely disorganized ventricular electrical activity), a precursor to cardiac arrest.

What is the significance of sinus tachycardia?

Sinus tachycardia is sinus rhythm going faster than 100/min. It is often due to hypovolemia, anemia, hy-

perthyroidism, hypoxia, fever, or pain. Unexplained sinus tachycardia requires a search for a cause.

What is atrial fibrillation, and what causes it?

Atrial fibrillation results from completely disorganized electrical activity in the atria, causing the atrial muscle to quiver, or fibrillate. It may exist in isolation, but usually it occurs secondary to long-standing hypertension; CHF; hypoxia; valvular heart disease; hyperthyroidism; alcohol use; or hypercatecholamine states, such as acute MI or surgery. An irregularly irregular rhythm without identifiable P waves on the ECG makes the diagnosis. Atrial flutter, a related rhythm, occurs when an organized circuit of electrical activity causes a fast atrial rate. The ECG will show a regular oscillating ("saw-toothed") baseline on the ECG. Atrial flutter often degenerates into atrial fibrillation. Multifocal atrial tachycardia (MAT) is an irregularly irregular rhythm that is often confused with atrial fibrillation. In contrast, the ECG shows P waves before each QRS. To be diagnostic, there must be at least three different P-wave morphologies reflecting the multiple atrial foci (Figure 23-2).

What is AVNRT?

AVNRT is a cyclic, or reentrant, loop of electrical activity within the AV node that is conducted into the ventricles. It produces a regular tachycardia, usually at a rate of 160 to 180/min (see Figure 23-2, C). Although not a sign of underlying heart disease, AVNRT may produce ischemia, hypotension, or heart failure.

What are the causes of a slow heart rate (bradycardia)?

Bradycardia refers to any rate less than 60. Sinus bradycardia is the most common cause and is frequently seen

TABLE 23-1
Causes of Tachyarrhythmias

TACHYARRYTHMIA	ORIGINATING LOCATION	COMMON CAUSES	LESS COMMON CAUSES
Supraventricular tachycardia	Above or in AV node	Sinus tachycardia Atrial fibrillation	Atrial flutter MAT AV node reentry
Ventricular tachycardia	Below AV node	Cardiac ischemia	Electrolyte abnormalities Cardiomyopathy Drug intoxications: tricyclic antidepressants, cisapride

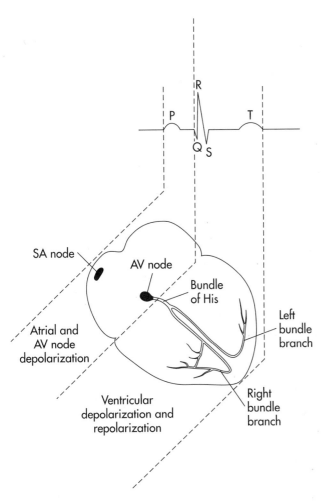

Figure 23-1 How the ECG reflects the normal sequence of heart muscle depolarization. Normal depolarization begins in the SA node and travels through the atria, causing a P wave. There is a slight delay as depolarization funnels through the AV node, reflected in the PR interval. The QRS reflects rapid depolarization by way of the bundle of His and bundle branches. The T wave reflects ventricular repolarization to resting potential.

with advanced age, athletic training, MI, hypokalemia, hypothyroidism, and drugs such as β-blockers, calcium channel blockers, and digoxin. Sinus bradycardia is simply sinus rhythm going at less than 60/min. Less common causes of bradycardia are AV node block or

sinoatrial (SA) node failure. In complete AV block and SA node failure, an ectopic ventricular focus (idioventricular rhythm) or area in the AV node (junctional rhythm) may take over pacing the ventricular beats (Figure 23-3, C).

What is AV node block?

AV block occurs as a result of impaired conduction of atrial impulses through the AV node. Cardiac ischemia and medications such as β-blockers, calcium channel blockers, and digoxin are the most common causes. AV block is subcategorized into first, second, or third degree based on the severity of the conduction abnormality (see Figure 23-3).

My patient is reporting "extra heart beats." What could be causing this?

Patients frequently report the sensation of extra heartbeats. These are usually due to premature atrial contractions (PACs) or premature ventricular contractions (PVCs). Although common, only a minority of patients notice them. PACs occur when atrial tissue outside of the SA node initiates an early beat. The ECG shows an early P wave that appears different from the preceding beats. Episodic PACs do not indicate cardiac pathology. PVCs result from the same phenomena, but the focus is in the ventricle. The ECG shows episodic wide QRS complexes without associated P waves (Figure 23-4, A). When frequent (>5/min), PVCs may be indicative of ischemic or structural heart disease.

EVALUATION

What symptoms suggest a cardiac arrhythmia?

In general, arrhythmias cause the heart to function poorly or work harder. As a result, patients with arrhythmia often present with syncope, dizziness, chest pain, palpitations, shortness of breath, or exercise intolerance. Some patients do not report symptoms at all,

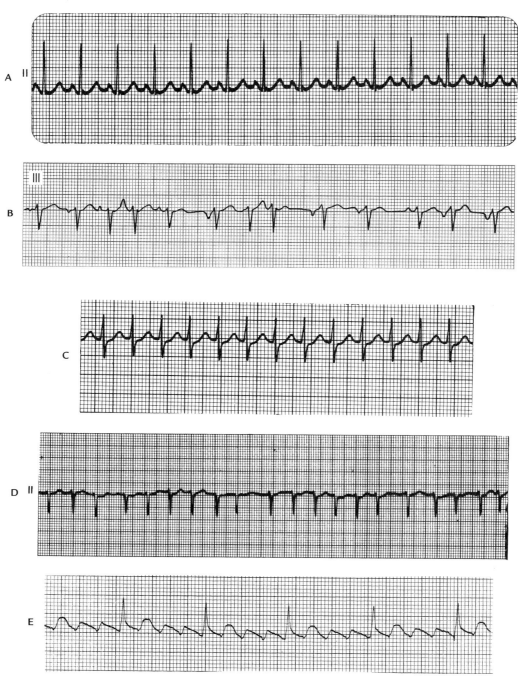

Figure 23-2 Atrial arrhythmias. **A,** *Sinus tachycardia:* Rate >100 and regular, QRS is narrow, each P wave is associated with a QRS, each QRS has a P wave, PR interval is normal in length. **B,** *Multifocal atrial tachycardia:* Irregular rhythm with a P wave before each QRS and at least three different P wave morphologies reflecting three or more atrial foci initiating beats. **C,** *Supraventricular tachycardia:* Rate >100 and regular, QRS is narrow, P waves may be absent so that PR interval cannot be determined. Cause is likely an AV nodal reentry loop (see text). **D,** *Atrial fibrillation:* Rate irregularly irregular, QRS is narrow, P waves are absent so that PR interval cannot be determined. Atrial fibrillation can be fast, regular, or slow, depending on how refractory the AV node is to passing on the erratic atrial electrical activity to the ventricles. **E,** *Atrial flutter:* Regular rate with a saw-toothed baseline of P waves going at a rate of about 300/min (one per large box), conducting every fourth P through to the ventricles (4:1 conduction). Atrial flutter can be associated with a fast or slow ventricular rate, depending on refractoriness of the AV node. *(From Goldberg AL:* Clinical electrocardiography: a simplified approach, *ed 6, St Louis, 1999, Mosby.)*

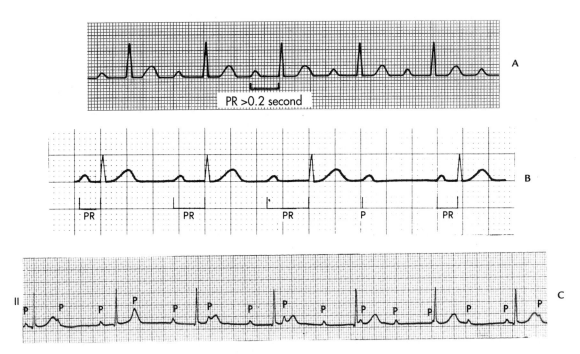

Figure 23-3 AV node blocks. **A,** *First-degree block:* PR interval uniformly prolonged longer than one big box (>0.2 seconds). **B,** *Second-degree block* type 1 (Wenckebach): A cycle of PR widening culminates in a dropped QRS, then cycle begins again. **C,** *Third-degree block:* No atrial impulses pass through the AV node, causing complete AV dissociation. AV node or ventricle may beat independently, usually at a rate far slower than 60/sec, giving AV dissociation as seen above. *(From Goldberg AL:* Clinical electrocardiography: a simplified approach, *ed 6, St Louis, 1999, Mosby.)*

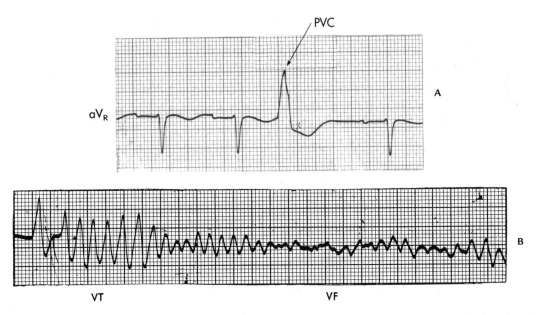

Figure 23-4 Ventricular arrhythmias. **A,** *Premature ventricular contraction:* An isolated wide QRS superimposed on the baseline sinus rhythm. **B,** *Ventricular tachycardia:* A rapid regular rhythm >100/sec with wide QRS. The rhythm degenerates into *ventricular fibrillation* (VF) in this recording. *(Goldberg AL:* Clinical electrocardiography: a simplified approach, *ed 6, St Louis, 1999, Mosby.)*

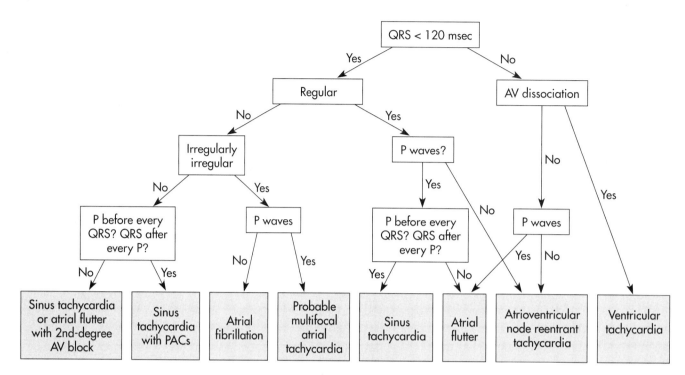

Figure 23-5 Algorithm for identifying tachycardias.

and an arrhythmia is only identified when an abnormal pulse is noted on examination.

How do I evaluate an abnormal pulse?

First, ensure clinical stability with a quick assessment of vital signs. Look for signs or symptoms of cardiac ischemia or shock. Get help immediately if the patient is unstable. If the patient is stable, inquire about prior heart problems and cardiopulmonary symptoms. A quick examination focusing on signs of cardiopulmonary disease, anemia, and thyroid abnormalities is appropriate. Characterize the pulse by rate and pattern, and obtain an ECG.

Now that I have an ECG, how do I identify the rhythm?

First, determine the *rate:* >100/min = tachycardia; <60/min = bradycardia. Second, measure the *QRS* width. A narrow QRS (<3 small boxes or 120 msec) indicates that the rhythm originates in the atria or AV node and is traveling through the ventricles via the His-Purkinje system. Conversely, a wide QRS indicates a ventricular origin. Occasionally, supraventricular rhythms will not conduct normally through the His-Purkinje system. This is called aberrancy or intraventricular conduction delay and can make distinguishing ventricular tachycardia from supraventricular tachycardia difficult. Third, compare *RR intervals* with a pair of calipers to decide if the rhythm is regular. Regular

rhythms have equal distance between each QRS complex. An irregular rhythm with no pattern to the irregularity is termed irregularly irregular and is almost always atrial fibrillation. Fourth, look for *P waves.* If absent, and the rhythm is irregular, atrial fibrillation is likely. If P waves occur in no relation to the QRS complexes, consider VT (fast, wide QRS) or AV block (slow). Examine the *PR interval* for prolongation, variability, or intermittently dropped QRS complexes suggestive of AV block. Algorithms to aid in identifying common rhythm disturbances are suggested (Figures 23-5 and 23-6).

Is this ventricular tachycardia?

VT is a potentially lethal rhythm requiring rapid identification and intervention. The rate is usually 160 to 200 and regular. The QRS is always greater than 120 msec. The SA node continues to produce independent P waves that may be buried or appear as irregularities on the wide QRS complexes. When sustained VT occurs, evaluate for ischemia and magnesium and potassium disturbances.

How do I evaluate an irregularly irregular rhythm?

Although atrial fibrillation is by far the most likely cause, obtain an ECG to confirm the rhythm. If atrial fibrillation is present, obtain electrolytes, a TSH, and a chest x-ray to look for pulmonary disease or signs of left ventricular (LV) failure. An echocardiogram may be use-

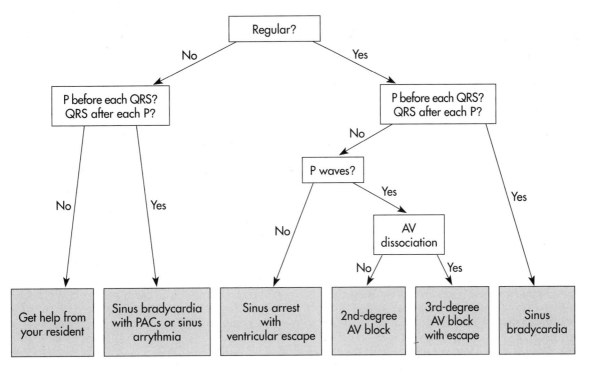

Figure 23-6 Algorithm for identifying bradycardias.

ful to identify valvular heart disease or left ventricular dysfunction. Pulmonary embolism is an unusual but potential cause, so ask about leg swelling, dyspnea, previous clots, and medicines (e.g., oral contraceptives, tamoxifen).

My patient has bradycardia. What evaluation is indicated?

Study the ECG carefully to identify the rhythm. If ischemia is suspected, obtain cardiac enzymes. A list of medications may identify possible precipitants (digoxin, diltiazem, verapamil, β-blockers). Hospitalize symptomatic patients for cardiac monitoring and, possibly, pacing.

How do I evaluate a patient with palpitations?

Get a clear description of what the patient is sensing. Often, it is helpful to have patients tap out the rhythm of abnormal beats with their finger. Ask about prescription and nonprescription medications, caffeine, and substance abuse. Occasional "extra beats" without associated symptoms are almost always PACs or PVCs. An ECG alone is usually adequate evaluation. A history of associated dizziness, syncope, chest pain, or shortness of breath is concerning for supraventricular tachycardia (SVT), VT, ischemia, or structural problems and requires an ECG, electrolytes, a TSH, and ambulatory or inpatient monitoring.

TREATMENT

My patient has atrial fibrillation. What should I do now?

The three main treatment goals are cardioversion, rate control, and anticoagulation. Unstable patients should be cardioverted immediately. Stable patients are treated initially with β-blockers or diltiazem to bring the ventricular rate to less than 100. Digoxin may be used but not as the sole agent because it does not maintain rate control with exercise. If the onset is clearly within the past 48 hours, cardioversion using electricity or medications may be indicated. Because patients with atrial fibrillation for longer than 48 hours have a significant risk of atrial clot and embolism, they should receive anticoagulation for 3 weeks before cardioversion. Patients with persistent atrial fibrillation require anticoagulation to reduce embolic events. If there are no signs of heart failure, cardiac ischemia, or pulmonary emboli, hospitalization is not required.

How do I treat ventricular tachycardia?

VT should be immediately electrically cardioverted to prevent deterioration into ventricular fibrillation. Supraventricular tachycardias (atrial flutter, AVNRT) with aberrancy may look like VT. In the setting of hypotension or chest pain, assume the rhythm is VT and cardiovert immediately.

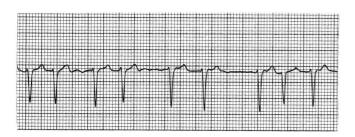

Figure 23-7 Electrocardiogram for patient in Case 23-1.

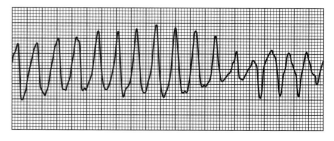

Figure 23-8 Electrocardiogram for patient in Case 23-2.

CASE 23-1

A 67-year-old man reports increasing shortness of breath and fatigue on exertion. He denies associated chest pain, diaphoresis, or nausea. He has noted an intermittently rapid heart rate. He has a history of MI and mild compensated CHF. Examination is significant for a fast, irregular heart rate but is otherwise normal. His rhythm strip is as shown (Figure 23-7).

A. What is the rhythm?

B. How will you treat this patient?

CASE 23-2

A 52-year-old man is admitted to the hospital for an acute MI. He is treated with aspirin, thrombolytics, and heparin. On hospital day 2, he suddenly becomes short of breath and then loses consciousness. His rhythm strip is as shown (Figure 23-8).

A. What is the rhythm?

B. How should this patient be treated?

How do I treat AVNRT?

Hemodynamically unstable patients require immediate electrical cardioversion to restore sinus rhythm. In clinically stable patients, adenosine is the agent of choice to terminate AVNRT. β-Blockers or calcium channel blockers may decrease recurrence. Refer patients with refractory AVNRT to a cardiologist for catheter-directed ablation of abnormal conduction pathways.

How do I treat bradycardias?

In patients without symptoms, intervention is not necessary. Associated dizziness or syncope usually requires hospitalization to initiate cardiac pacing. Stop medications likely to slow the rate. Unstable patients should be given atropine and considered for cardiac pacing.

Key Points

- When reading ECGs, look systematically at the rate, QRS width, RR interval, P waves, and PR intervals to determine the rhythm.
- An irregularly irregular rhythm is almost always atrial fibrillation.
- Electrically cardiovert any patient who has an unstable arrhythmia.
- Assume any wide-complex tachycardia is ventricular in origin, and treat as VT.

CONGESTIVE HEART FAILURE

ETIOLOGY

What are the common causes of heart failure?

CHF affects 1% of all people in the United States and 10% of those over 75 years of age. Hypertension and coronary artery disease account for 50% to 75% of left ventricular (LV) failure. Right ventricular (RV) failure is usually due to LV failure (Table 23-2).

How do I classify a patient's heart failure?

CHF is classified as right or left ventricular failure, with systolic or diastolic dysfunction. In systolic dysfunction, ejection fraction is low because of poor ventricular contraction. In diastolic dysfunction, ejection fraction is normal, but cardiac output is low because of poor filling of a stiff ventricle during diastole. Functional status is classified as I through IV (Table 23-3). These functional categories guide treatment and prognosis.

EVALUATION

What are classic findings in LV failure?

LV failure increases pulmonary venous pressure and causes pulmonary manifestations (Table 23-4): decreased exercise tolerance (dyspnea on exertion), diffi-

TABLE 23-2
Causes of Systolic Dysfunction in Left and Right Heart Failure

	COMMON CAUSES	LESS COMMON CAUSES	RARE CAUSES
LV failure	Ischemia Hypertension Chronic alcohol use	Valvular disease Thyroid disease	Viral myocarditis Hemochromatosis Amyloidosis
RV failure	LV failure COPD RV ischemia	Sleep apnea Pulmonary hypertension	Rare pulmonary diseases

TABLE 23-3
New York Heart Association (NYHA)
Functional Classification

FUNCTIONAL CLASS	SYMPTOMS
I	No limitation with ordinary physical activity
II	Mild symptoms, mild limitation with ordinary activity
III	Marked symptoms of fatigue, dyspnea, palpitations, or angina with minimal activity
IV	Symptoms at rest; symptoms increase with any activity

culty breathing while supine (orthopnea), and episodic severe breathing impairment awakening the patient from sleep (paroxysmal nocturnal dyspnea). You may hear an S_3, an early diastolic filling sound, over the left ventricle. Also look for characteristic chest x-ray findings: enlarged heart, pulmonary edema, pleural effusion, Kerley B lines, or redistribution of pulmonary blood flow against gravity to upper lung zones. LV failure can overload the RV and create signs of RV failure.

What are classic findings in RV failure?

RV failure increases systemic venous pressure. RV failure, in contrast to LV failure, does not cause lung symptoms, although underlying lung disease may complicate the presentation. Pertinent findings are listed (see Table 23-4). To evaluate jugular venous pressure (JVP), place the head of the bed at 30 to 45 degrees and observe for venous pulsations in the neck. Measure the height of the pulsations vertically up from the angle of Louis (where the second rib meets the sternum). Add 5 cm to your measurement to estimate the vertical height in cm of water above the right atrium. To evaluate for abdominojugular reflux, apply pressure to the abdomen for 10 seconds while you watch the JVP. If JVP rises more than 4 cm for the duration of pressure, this implies high right heart filling pressures. Chest films may reveal the underlying lung disease or signs of LV failure.

What diagnostic tests should I do in a patient with new left-sided systolic heart failure?

Standard workup includes CBC, chemistry panel, cholesterol, ECG, chest x-ray, and echocardiogram. Echo estimates ejection fraction (EF) and evaluates ventricular wall motion and valve function. An EF less than 40% is considered systolic dysfunction. A normal EF of greater than 40% does not rule out CHF. LV diastolic dysfunction, seen in up to one third of patients with clinical CHF, presents with normal EF. Focal wall motion abnormalities suggest ischemic injury. If standard workup does not reveal a diagnosis, review the history for alcohol use, then consider further testing for ischemia, thyroid disease, hemochromatosis, amyloidosis, or HIV.

TREATMENT

What are the treatment goals in CHF patients?

Management goals are to reduce symptoms, prevent complications, and improve survival.

What can patients do to improve symptoms?

Patients can restrict salt intake to 3 to 4 g/day, stay as active as possible, and avoid cigarettes and alcohol. They can follow home blood pressures and daily weights and notify their physician of major changes so that medications can be adjusted. Recognize that nonadherence with medications is common in CHF patients (20% to 60%), so counsel patients to take medications as prescribed.

What medicine do I start for LV systolic failure?

Angiotensin-converting enzyme inhibitors (ACEIs) are the first-line agents for LV systolic dysfunction. They reduce LV afterload and decrease morbidity and mortality,

TABLE 23-4
Symptoms and Signs of Left and Right Ventricular Failure

	HISTORY	EXAMINATION
LV failure	Orthopnea Paroxysmal nocturnal dyspnea Dypsnea on exertion Cough Hemoptysis	Rales (crackles) S_3 over left ventricle PMI diffuse and displaced laterally Poor perfusion with cool, mottled extremities Leg edema
RV failure	Exercise intolerance Dyspnea Increasing abdominal girth or pain Leg swelling	Elevated JVP Right ventricular parasternal heave S_3 over right ventricle Abnormal hepatojugular reflux Ascites Leg edema

PMI, Point of maximal impulse.

particularly in patients with decreased ejection fraction from recent myocardial infarction. Increase the ACEI dose as tolerated to decrease systolic blood pressure to 85 to 90 mm Hg. Monitor the serum creatinine and the potassium frequently because both may rise with initiation of ACEI. Common side effects include hypotension, worsening renal function, hyperkalemia, cough, rash, and taste disturbance. The side effect of angioedema is an absolute contraindication to continuing ACEIs. About 10% of patients develop intolerable ACEI cough. Cough is common from CHF itself, but if it is clearly due to ACEI, consider changing to angiotensin II receptor blockers. These new agents also may decrease afterload and mortality but cause less cough than ACEIs. The combination of hydralazine and isosorbide, also used to decrease afterload, is less effective in reducing mortality but should be used when angiotensin-blocking agents are not tolerated.

When do patients need diuretics?

Most patients with CHF have sodium and water overload. Start a diuretic if an ACEI alone does not resolve volume overload. Titrate diuretics to achieve a JVP less than 8 cm H_2O. Dose diuretics once a day unless high doses are required (e.g., furosemide greater than 160 mg/day). Hypokalemia requires replacement if the potassium level is below 4.0 mEq/L; use potassium cautiously in patients on ACEIs. Add digoxin when patients remain symptomatic on full-dose ACEI and diuretics. Digoxin is the drug of choice for patients with atrial fibrillation and CHF. Digoxin increases exercise tolerance and improves functional class; withdrawal of digoxin results in worsening CHF and increased risk for hospitalization. However, digoxin has not been shown to alter the progression of CHF or decrease mortality. Digoxin toxicity causes arrhythmias, confusion, visual disturbances, anorexia, nausea, and vomiting. Levels do not reflect clinical digoxin toxicity, so follow symptoms and ECG changes. Renal in-

sufficiency, hypokalemia, hypothyroidism, and drug interactions increase the risk of digoxin toxicity.

When should I use β-blockers for CHF?

Increased plasma norepinephrine levels in patients with CHF are strongly associated with increased mortality and worsening disease. β-Blockers may block this effect. Use β-blockers in post-MI patients because these agents decrease mortality in these patients, as well as decreasing sudden death in post-MI patients with CHF. Routine use in CHF patients is not yet standard, although recent data suggest that carvedilol (an α-blocker and β-blocker with antioxidant properties) and metoprolol improve LV function, decrease hospitalization, and delay need for heart transplant in CHF patients. Because of negative inotropy with these agents, symptoms may worsen initially; short-acting agents may be preferable to use at first.

How is treatment for diastolic dysfunction different?

Instead of ACEIs and diuretics, use β-blockers or verapamil. These agents increase cardiac output by increasing diastolic filling time for patients with diastolic dysfunction.

What are the major prognostic indicators in patients with CHF?

Poor prognostic signs include symptoms at rest, poor EF, hyponatremia, and ventricular arrhythmias. Major causes of death include progressive CHF (40%) and sudden death (40%). One-year mortality for patients with class IV CHF exceeds 50%.

How do I prevent complications?

Up to 90% of CHF patients demonstrate complex ventricular ectopy. Amiodarone suppresses ventricular arrhythmias. Automatic implantable cardiac defibrillating devices (AICDs) can resuscitate patients with frequent ventricular fibrillation. Thromboembolism is more common when LV EF is less than or equal to 25%, so warfarin is often used. Depression decreases medication adherence. Because tricyclic antidepressants increase the risk of arrhythmias, use a serotonin reuptake inhibitor.

When should I hospitalize patients with CHF?

Hospitalize patients with newly diagnosed CHF of unclear cause to rule out ischemic disease and begin workup and treatment. Admit patients for clinical exacerbations with hypoxia or hypotension or if ECG suggests new ischemic injury. Admit orders should include strict daily weights, records of fluid intake and output, and a low-salt (2-4 g) diet. Monitor clinical volume status daily with examination, serum chemistries, and renal function. Daily examination should include vital signs (including orthostatics), weight, height of the JVP, cardiovascular examination for S_3, lung examination for crackles or effusions, and extremity examination for edema. For significant volume overload, give oxygen, intravenous diuretics, or even a furosemide drip if necessary. Swan-Ganz catheters are used in refractory CHF for careful volume management or when inotropic agents are used. Intravenous dobutamine, an inotropic agent, may be used to increase cardiac output and lower afterload. Some patients require intermittent hospitalization for intravenous dobutamine therapy while they await cardiac transplant.

Key Points

- Patients presenting with CHF should be classified by type of heart dysfunction and by functional class to guide treatment strategies.
- All patients with systolic dysfunction should be treated with ACEIs.
- Treat volume overload with diuretics.
- Consider digoxin or β-blockers in patients who remain symptomatic on ACEIs and diuretics.

CASE 23-3

A 60-year-old man who has had classic angina for years wishes to establish care. After a particularly bad episode of chest pain 2 weeks ago, he began having ankle swelling and more shortness of breath during his daily walks.

A. For what symptoms and signs of heart failure should you seek?
B. What tests do you want to order?
C. What treatment is indicated if he has an EF of 30% and mild volume overload?

CASE 23-4

A 50-year-old truck driver reports morning headaches and increasing difficulty staying awake while driving his truck. On examination, his BP is 185/100, pulse is 82, weight is 297 lb, and height is 6 feet. He has a JVP of 11 cm H_2O, right-sided S_3 with parasternal heave, positive abdominojugular reflux, clear lungs, and 2+ pedal edema.

A. Does he have heart failure, and, if so, why are his lungs clear?
B. What is the cause of his symptoms?

ISCHEMIC HEART DISEASE

ETIOLOGY

What is ischemic heart disease?

Ischemic heart disease is the leading cause of death and disability in the United States and is a spectrum of illness caused by coronary artery atherosclerosis. At the chronic end of the spectrum is stable angina pectoris; at the acute end are unstable angina and acute MI.

What causes chronic stable angina?

Angina is chest pain resulting from inadequate myocardial oxygen supply (Figure 23-9). Most patients with angina have coronary plaque causing focal, fixed vessel narrowing. Blood supply may be adequate at rest but not with the increased demand of exertion.

What causes the acute coronary syndromes?

Acute coronary syndromes are more dynamic and begin with plaque rupture, an event that may be precipitated by inflammation within the plaque. Younger, lipid-laden plaques rich in inflammatory cells are probably more susceptible than older, fibromuscular plaques. With plaque rupture, tissue factor is exposed and stimulates thrombosis. The end result depends on the balance between clot formation and lysis. If clot lysis occurs, patients present with unstable angina. If clot propagation continues, complete coronary occlusion occurs, leading to infarction.

What are the risk factors for coronary artery disease?

Independent risk factors for CAD have been identified (Box 23-1). Several differences in risk for women are worth mentioning. Postmenopausal estrogen replacement may decrease risk by up to 40%. Diabetes is a more powerful predictor of CAD in women than in men. Hypertension in elderly women is also a stronger predictor than in men of similar age. Although high LDL is the best lipid predictor in men, low HDL is a better predictor in women.

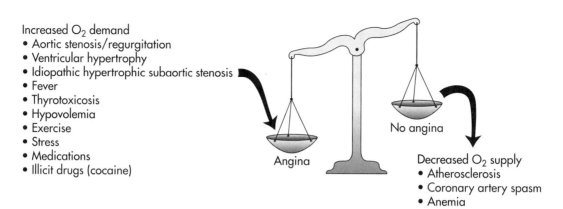

Increased O₂ demand
- Aortic stenosis/regurgitation
- Ventricular hypertrophy
- Idiopathic hypertrophic subaortic stenosis
- Fever
- Thyrotoxicosis
- Hypovolemia
- Exercise
- Stress
- Medications
- Illicit drugs (cocaine)

No angina

Angina

Decreased O₂ supply
- Atherosclerosis
- Coronary artery spasm
- Anemia

Figure 23-9 Myocardial oxygen supply and demand in angina.

| **BOX 23-1** | Risk Factors for Coronary Artery Disease |

Hypercholesterolemia
Smoking
Diabetes
Family history early CAD, first-degree relative younger than 55 years (men) or younger than 65 years (women)
Hypertension

EVALUATION

How do I diagnose chronic stable angina and unstable angina?

Chronic stable angina usually presents as exertional chest pain relieved by rest. Presence of risk factors raises the likelihood of ischemia. Confirm the diagnosis with stress testing (see below). Unstable angina is angina that (1) is new, (2) occurs at rest, or (3) occurs with increased frequency or severity. Although ECG changes may be present, their absence does not rule out the diagnosis.

How do I diagnose acute MI?

Time to reperfusion is critical to outcome in acute MI, so obtain history and ECG expeditiously in those with acute chest pain. Diagnosis of MI requires at least two of the following: (1) typical cardiac chest pain, (2) typical ECG changes (see Figure 6-2, *B*), or (3) rise in cardiac-specific enzymes. CPK with MB bands and troponin I are the enzymes used in most "rule-out MI" protocols. CPK-MB levels rise within 4 to 6 hours of onset of pain, peak in 12 to 20 hours, and return to baseline within 36 to 48 hours. False positives can be seen in some muscle disorders because muscle CPK is approximately

9% MB. LDH peaks later than CPK, at 24 to 48 hours, and remains elevated for 14 days. LDH1/ LDH2 greater than 1 is diagnostic of infarction. Troponin I is a cardiac-specific contractile protein that rises early and remains elevated for longer than 7 days.

What noninvasive stress tests are available for diagnosis and risk stratification?

For *exercise tolerance testing* (ETT), patients walk on a treadmill with continuous ECG monitoring while work is progressively increased. Horizontal or down-sloping ST segment depression of at least 1 mm lasting at least 0.08 seconds is diagnostic of ischemia. False-positive and false-negative rates are both about 15%. The positive predictive value (PPV) is highest in men over age 50 with typical angina. PPV falls progressively with age less than 50 years, atypical symptoms, in premenopausal women, and in those with baseline conduction delay or ST abnormalities on resting ECG. Options when PPV with ETT is low are *exercise-thallium* (radiolabeled thallium identifies myocardial perfusion defects) or *exercise echocardiography* (focal wall motion abnormality localizes areas of ischemia). For patients unable to ambulate, use a pharmacologic stress test, such as *dipyridamole (Persantine) thallium* or *dobutamine echocardiography*.

When is a stress test indicated?

This is a diagnostic tool in patients with typical angina or unexplained chest pain. In addition, it can be used in patients with known CAD to "risk-stratify" and guide subsequent management. For example, ST depression greater than 2 mm, involving greater than 4 leads, or persisting longer than 5 minutes into recovery is associated with multivessel CAD and poor outcome; such patients require catheterization and probable revascularization rather than medical therapy alone. Similarly, after MI, if a low-level ETT shows persistent ischemic changes, revascularization is indicated.

When should patients be referred for coronary angiography?

Most patients with *stable angina* are managed medically. However, angiography is reasonable when medical therapy fails to control symptoms or when noninvasive tests reveal poor prognostic findings: ischemic ST segment depression on ETT, multiple large perfusion defects on thallium imaging, or reduced LV function (EF <40%). In *unstable angina*, angiography is appropriate with severe, recurrent rest angina; hemodynamic instability; or severe ECG abnormalities suggesting large areas of myocardium at risk. Patients with minor ECG changes and pain that responds quickly to medical therapy may safely undergo noninvasive risk stratification. In *acute MI*, angiography and revascularization are appropriate with hemodynamic instability or contraindications to thrombolysis. In addition, primary angiography and angioplasty may be an appropriate alternative to thrombolysis in centers with experienced personnel and an appropriately staffed cardiac catheterization laboratory. Finally, *after MI*, angiography is only indicated if there is recurrent ischemia either spontaneously or with noninvasive testing.

TREATMENT

How do I treat chronic stable angina?

β-blockers and nitrates are first-line agents; long-acting calcium channel blockers may be used when first-line agents are not tolerated. β-*blockers* reduce myocardial oxygen demand by decreasing heart rate, contractility, and blood pressure. β_1-selective agents (metoprolol, atenolol) cause less bronchospasm. Other side effects include bradycardia, AV blockade, fatigue, erectile dysfunction, and CHF. Start at a low dose and titrate up to a resting heart rate of 50 to 60/min. *Nitrates* reduce preload by venodilation; dilate coronary arteries; and, at higher doses, reduce afterload by generalized arterial dilation. Prescribe a long-acting preparation (e.g., isosorbide dinitrate, nitroglycerin patch) plus a short-acting sublingual nitroglycerin for "breakthrough" symptoms. If breakthrough symptoms do not respond to 3 sublingual tablets, advise patients to seek medical attention immediately. With all nitrates, a drug-free interval (usually at night) is necessary to prevent tolerance. Side effects include hypotension and headache, usually responsive to acetaminophen. Nitrates should never be used with sildenafil (Viagra), a drug for erectile dysfunction, because the combination can cause life-threatening hypotension. Recent questions about *calcium channel blocker* safety have relegated them to a second-line role. Do not use short-acting dihydropyridines (short-acting nifedipine). Long-acting preparations are reasonable for those failing, or intolerant of, nitrates and/or β-blockers. Because verapamil and diltiazem both have negative chronotropic and inotropic effects, avoid them in patients with CHF or bradyarrhythmias, or those already receiving β-blockers (pulse in the 50s). The long-acting dihydropyridine amlodipine has been shown to be safe in patients with CHF. Finally, recommend aggressive *risk-factor modification* with smoking cessation, treatment of hyperlipidemia, hypertension, and diabetes for all patients with CAD. Discuss the risks and benefits of estrogen replacement with postmenopausal women.

How should I manage a patient with unstable angina?

Admit for continuous monitoring. Give both aspirin and heparin because the combination of the two has been shown to be superior to heparin alone for preventing further clot formation at unstable plaques. Low-molecular-weight heparin may be more effective than standard unfractionated heparin with similar rates of major bleeding, although its use is not yet widely accepted. Give IV or topical nitrates and β-blockers to improve coronary flow and decrease myocardial work. Once patients with unstable angina are pain-free, risk-stratify by exercise testing.

How do I manage patients with MI?

See Tables 23-5 through 23-7 for management of acute MI and its complications. After patients recover, they should be risk-stratified with a low-level stress test to guide further management.

What are the options for revascularization, and when are they appropriate?

Options for revascularization include percutaneous transluminal coronary angioplasty (PTCA) and coronary artery bypass grafting (CABG). In patients with single-vessel CAD, neither PTCA nor CABG have a proven impact on mortality over medical therapy, although both have been shown to provide greater symptom relief. In contrast, in patients with three-vessel CAD, both PTCA and CABG improve survival over medical therapy. CABG is the preferred intervention in patients with diabetes, reduced LV function, or disease in the left main coronary artery.

What medicines are standard for the post–MI patient?

Give aspirin (81-325 mg), a β-blocker, and a lipid-lowering agent (usually HMGCoA reductase inhibitor) if LDL is greater than 130. LDL goal with CAD is less than 100. Vitamin E (400-800 IU) may help decrease risk of reinfarction. ACEIs are beneficial when EF is less than 40%.

TABLE 23-5
Management of Acute MI

INTERVENTION	INDICATIONS	WHEN	FOR HOW LONG
Bed rest	All patients	Immediately	12-24 hrs
Oxygen	All patients	Immediately	12-24 hrs
Aspirin	All patients	Immediately	Indefinitely
Morphine	All patients	Immediately	prn
Nitrate	Most patients	Immediately	24-48 hrs
β-blocker	Most patients	First 24 hrs	Indefinitely
ACEI	Most patients	First 24 hrs	Indefinitely if EF <40%, 6 wks in others
Thrombolysis: Streptokinase Urokinase TPA	Within 12 hrs of onset ST elevation ≥1 mm in 2 or more contiguous leads New left bundle branch block No contraindications	Immediately	One-time dose
Heparin	TPA Large anterior MI Mural thrombus Prior recent embolic event	Immediately (after TPA when TPA used)	48 hrs
PTCA	Cardiogenic shock Spontaneous or provoked ischemia during recovery An alternative to thrombolysis in experienced centers	Immediately or prn	Repeat if needed

Key Points

- Stable angina is due to fixed arterial narrowing by atherosclerotic plaque; unstable angina and MI occur when atherosclerotic plaques rupture.
- Treat chronic stable angina with aspirin, lipid-lowering agents, nitrates, and β-blockers.
- Treat unstable angina with heparin, aspirin, and nitrates.
- Treat acute MI with thrombolytics or angioplasty, β-blockers, nitrates, aspirin, and heparin.
- Use noninvasive stress tests to risk-stratify patients with angina, unstable angina, and MI.
- Obtain angiography when patients fail medical therapy or are at high risk by stress testing.

CASE 23-5

A 55-year-old man reports several months of intermittent exertional chest pain lasting 1 to 2 minutes and relieved by rest. He has a history of hypertension, 50 pack-years of smoking, and a cholesterol level of 260. He takes one aspirin per day. A recent treadmill test showed a normal resting ECG with chest pressure after 8 minutes of exercise and the ECG shown (Figure 23-10). In your office, BP is 148/103 and P is 90.

A. What is the most likely cause for his chest pain, and what evidence supports this?
B. Would you order any additional diagnostic tests at this time?
C. What medications, if any, would you suggest?
D. What other therapeutic interventions, if any, would you suggest?

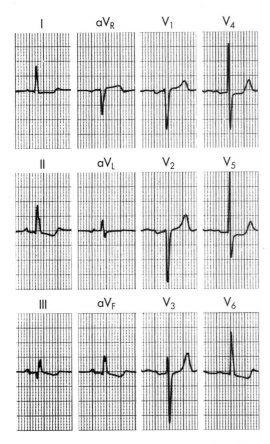

Figure 23-10 Electrocardiogram for patient in Case 23-6. *(From Davison R: Electrocardiography in acute care medicine, St Louis, 1995, Mosby.)*

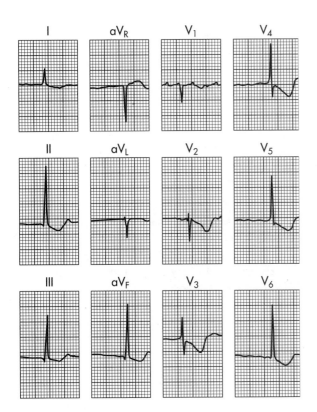

Figure 23-11 Electrocardiogram for patient in Case 23-6.

TABLE 23-6

Contraindications of Key Medications
Used to Treat Acute MI

INTERVENTION	CONTRAINDICATIONS
Nitrates	Systolic BP <90 Pulse >100 and <50
β-blockers	Bronchospasm, COPD Hypotension Bradycardia AV block
ACEIs	Hypotension Renal failure, renal artery stenosis

Thrombolysis:
  Streptokinase
  Urokinase
  TPA (tissue
    plasminogen
    activator)
	Absolute contraindications:
	Active internal bleeding
	Suspected aortic dissection
	Known intracranial tumor
	Hemorrhagic stroke anytime
	  or other CNS event within
	  1 year
	Relative contraindications:
	Severe hypertension (>180/110)
	Chronic severe hypertension
	Prior stroke
	Recent trauma, surgery (<3 wks)
	Prolonged CPR (>10 min)
	Noncompressible vascular
	  punctures
	Recent bleeding (2-4 wks)
	Known bleeding diathesis
	Pregnancy
	Active peptic ulcer

Heparin	Streptokinase Active life-threatening bleed

CASE 23-6

A 65-year-old woman reports chest pain that awoke her from sleep. She has a history of CAD, documented by a Persantine thallium test 4 years ago showing reversible inferior-wall decreased perfusion. She has been treated with a nitroglycerin patch and aspirin. Her pain, which usually occurs with exertion or emotional stress, woke her up from sleep last night and was more severe than usual. It initially responded to 2 sublingual nitroglycerin tablets but recurred several hours later. She received 3 nitroglycerin tablets en route. Her pain is currently mild (2/10) but still present. ECG is shown (Figure 23-11). A prior ECG was normal.

A. What is the most likely diagnosis?
B. What interventions are indicated?
C. The patient rules out for MI, and her pain resolves. What additional tests does she need?

TABLE 23-7
Complicacions of Acute MI

COMPLICATION	PRESENTATION	TREATMENT
Ventricular arrhythmias (VT, VF)	Hypotension, cardiac arrest	Cardioversion Lidocaine
Sinus bradycardia or 2nd-degree AV block type I	Asymptomatic or hypotension, common with inferior MI	Atropine, dopamine Transvenous pacemaker No treatment if no symptoms
1st-degree AV block	Asymptomatic	No treatment required
2nd-degree AV block type II or 3rd-degree AV block	Asymptomatic or hypotension	Transvenous pacemaker Observation is appropriate in stable patients with inferior MI
Congestive left heart failure	Dyspnea, cough, edema, orthopnea, paroxysmal nocturnal dyspnea	Oxygen Furosemide Nitrates ACEIs
Cardiogenic shock	Hypotension, dyspnea, altered mental status, oliguria	Oxygen Furosemide Dopamine, dobutamine Intraaortic balloon pump Angioplasty
RV infarction	Hypotension, JVD	Saline (volume-loading) Dobutamine
Acute mitral regurgitation (papillary muscle rupture)	Dyspnea, hypotension, rales, acute CHF, new apical murmur	IV nitrates, nitroprusside Surgery Intraaortic balloon pump Angioplasty
Acute ventricular septal defect	Dyspnea, hypotension, acute CHF, new murmur	IV nitrates, nitroprusside Surgery
Cardiac wall rupture	Cardiac arrest, hypotension	Surgery; usually fatal

VF, Ventricular fibrillation.

CASE 23-7

A 61-year-old healthy man presents to a rural emergency room with acute onset of crushing, substernal chest pain associated with dyspnea and diaphoresis. On examination, BP is 110/70, P is 104, RR is 24, and he is diaphoretic with a few crackles at both lung bases and an intermittent S_3 on cardiac examination. Chest x-ray reveals a normal cardiac silhouette with mild central vascular prominence and cephalization, suggesting early pulmonary edema. ECG is shown (Figure 23-12).

   A. What is his diagnosis?
   B. What therapies are indicated at this time?

Four days later, he develops acute onset of dyspnea, and his oxygen saturation falls to 80%. On examination, he has crackles involving both lung fields two thirds of the way up the posterior chest and a new systolic murmur at the apex. ECG reveals evolutionary changes of acute MI.

   C. What is your differential diagnosis?
   D. What diagnostic tests are indicated?
   E. How should the patient be treated?

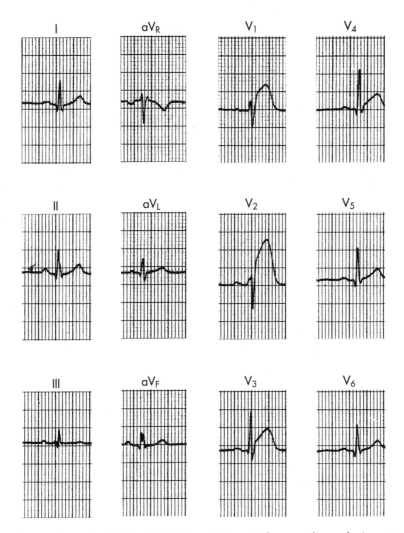

Figure 23-12 Electrocardiogram for patient in Case 23-7. *(From Davison R:* Electrocardiography in acute care medicine, *St Louis, 1995, Mosby.)*

VALVULAR HEART DISEASE

ETIOLOGY

Are all murmurs pathologic?

No. Many murmurs are flow murmurs without valvular pathology. These are benign systolic murmurs, which tend to be less than 2/6 in intensity, are loudest at the upper sternal border, do not radiate to the neck, and do not cause symptoms. Athletes and patients with anemia, fever, or hyperthyroidism often have flow murmurs. Systolic murmurs are more likely pathologic if they are greater than 2/6, radiate to the carotids, are present in older people (older than 55 years), or are accompanied by cardiac or pulmonary symptoms. A diastolic murmur, in contrast, is always pathologic.

What are common causes of systolic murmurs?

Flow murmurs, aortic stenosis (AS), and mitral regurgitation (MR) are common causes of systolic murmurs (Box 23-2). AS is most commonly due to congenital bicuspid aortic valve in adults younger than 55 years and degenerative valve change in adults older than 55 years. Rheumatic AS occurs in people 40 to 60 years old, about 15 years after acute rheumatic fever. Aortic sclerosis is benign calcification of the aortic valve that can cause a systolic murmur and is frequently reported on echocardiograms of older individuals. Causes of MR are listed (see Box 23-2).

What are the key causes of diastolic murmurs?

Aortic regurgitation (AR) and mitral stenosis (MS) are the most common causes. AR can occur with congenital bicuspid valves, rheumatic heart disease, endocarditis,

---

BOX 23-2 Common Causes of Murmurs

SYSTOLIC MURMURS

Flow murmur
Normal turbulence
Anemia, fever, hyperthyroidism

Aortic stenosis
Congenital bicuspid valve (age <55 years)
Degenerative valvular disease (age >55 years)

Mitral regurgitation
Rheumatic heart disease
Mitral prolapse
Ischemic papillary muscle dysfunction

DIASTOLIC MURMURS

Aortic regurgitation
Congenital bicuspid valve
Rheumatic heart disease
Endocarditis
Aortic root dissection
  Marfan syndrome
  Aortitis (syphilis, vasculitis)

Mitral stenosis
Rheumatic heart disease

TABLE 23-8
Grading Cardiac Murmurs

GRADE	DESCRIPTION
I	Cannot hear at first
II	Hear right away, not too loud
III	Loud but no palpable thrill
IV	Loud and associated with palpable thrill
V	Heard with stethoscope angled on chest
VI	Heard with stethoscope off chest

TABLE 23-9
Characteristics of Some Common Valvular Abnormalities

LESION	TIMING	LOUDEST LOCATION	RADIATION
AS	Systolic crescendo-decrescendo	Base	Carotid
MR	Pansystolic	Apex	Axilla, back
AR	Early diastole	Base	Left sternal border
MS	Opening snap in early diastole, murmur in mid-diastole, with crescendo in late diastole	Apex, best to listen with bell, left lateral decubitus position	None

---

ankylosing spondylitis, rheumatoid arthritis, and aortic root dilation/dissection (as with Marfan syndrome, vasculitis, or syphilitic aortitis). The predominant cause of MS is rheumatic heart disease.

EVALUATION

My patient has a murmur. How should I proceed?

Place in systole or diastole by palpating pulse; grade on a scale of I to VI (Table 23-8); and describe pitch, location, and sites of radiation (carotids, chest wall sites). Then find someone to confirm your examination. For example, AR is described as an early diastolic, II/VI, high-pitched decrescendo murmur heard best radiating down the left sternal border.

How do I distinguish between the systolic murmurs of AS and MR?

Specific valvular abnormalities are often identifiable by the location and character of the murmur (Table 23-9, Figures 23-13 and 23-14). AS is heard best at the base (second intercostal space), MR at the apex. Severe AS dampens and delays the carotid pulse (pulsus parvus et tardus). With mild AS, S_2 is clearly heard because the

murmur tapers off before aortic valve closure, whereas with MR, S_2 may be obscured because the regurgitant mitral flow continues after the aortic valve closes.

How do the clinical presentations of the systolic murmur conditions differ?

For both conditions, a long asymptomatic period precedes symptoms of LV failure (fatigue, dyspnea on exertion, orthopnea). AS typically also causes syncope and chest pain resulting from poor coronary artery perfusion in diastole. MR may present acutely if an MI ruptures papillary muscle.

How can I differentiate between the diastolic murmurs of AR and MS?

The early diastolic high-pitched decrescendo murmur of AR is heard maximally at the base with radiation down the left sternal border. It almost mimics a breath

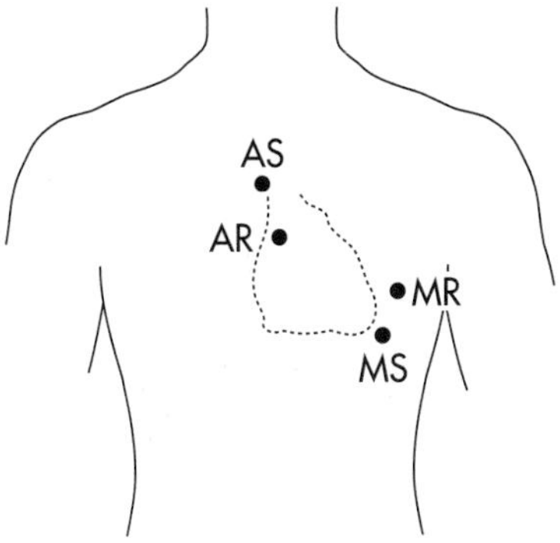

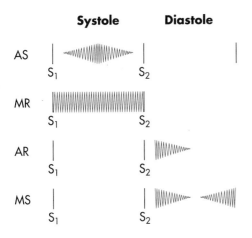

Figure 23-13 Location of murmurs from common valvular disorders.

Figure 23-14 Visual representation of the sounds produced by common murmurs.

sound. A wide pulse pressure often accompanies a bounding, collapsing Corrigan's pulse. MS, in contrast, is low pitched, mid-diastolic, and heard at the apex. A presystolic crescendo is often heard as the atrial kick sends blood across the stenotic mitral valve. Use a lightly placed bell and ask the patient to lie in the left lateral decubitus position to best hear the murmur of MS.

How do the clinical presentations of diastolic murmurs differ?

Both AR and MS can have long asymptomatic periods and both lead to LV failure. AR increases left ventricular work. Mitral stenosis increases left atrial pressure, causing left atrial dilation, atrial fibrillation, pulmonary hypertension and congestion, dyspnea, orthopnea, hemoptysis, and right heart failure. Atrial fibrillation further compromises LV filling and worsens pulmonary congestion.

Which patients need an echocardiogram or ECG?

Obtain both for murmurs with pathologic features: any diastolic murmur, grade greater than II/VI, age greater than 55 years, or concurrent cardiopulmonary symptoms.

TREATMENT

How should I manage a patient with pathologic valvular disease?

All patients with pathologic valvular disease need close follow-up to detect onset of heart failure early. Annual history and physical with particular attention to cardiopulmonary review is key. Obtain echocardiogram every 1 to 3 years in asymptomatic patients and sooner if symptoms of chest pain or dyspnea develop. Patients with AR and MR benefit from afterload-reducing agents (e.g., ACEIs, hydralazine) to increase forward flow through the aortic valve. These drugs can also postpone onset of symptoms and the need for surgery. Diuretics can be added for pulmonary edema refractory to afterload reduction. Atrial fibrillation is a common complication for patients with atrial enlargement from MS or MR. Atrial fibrillation requires anticoagulation (warfarin or aspirin), cardioversion, and/or heart rate control (digoxin, calcium channel blocker). Refer asymptomatic patients for valve replacement when EF is reduced or LV end-systolic measurement is greater than 45 mm for MR and greater than 55 mm for AR. Refer all patients with cardiopulmonary symptoms. Acute AR resulting from endocarditis or aortic dissection requires urgent valve replacement to avoid LV failure.

Are there any special issues in managing patients with AS?

Avoid afterload reduction with ACEIs or hydralazine in patients with AS because these agents worsen coronary artery perfusion. Worsening pressure gradient greater than 80 mm Hg across the valve or valve area less than 0.7 cm² are additional indications for valve replacement.

Are there any special issues in managing patients with MS?

Diuretics are the main treatment for pulmonary congestion. Patients with MS and atrial fibrillation may particularly benefit from cardioversion because the atrial diastolic kick markedly assists LV filling. Systemic emboli can be a problem with MS, and lifelong warfarin is begun after any atrial fibrillation. Consider surgery for limiting dyspnea, uncontrollable pulmonary edema, recurrent systemic emboli on anticoagulation, and severe pulmonary hypertension with RV hypertrophy and hemoptysis. Open mitral commissurotomy and percutaneous balloon valvuloplasty can be considered for non-regurgitant valves or for temporary repair (as in pregnant women). Regurgitant valves require replacement.

How can I prevent endocarditis?

Give high-risk patients (e.g., those with prosthetic valves or prior endocarditis) a single 2-g dose of amoxicillin before dental, respiratory tract, or esophageal procedures, and ampicillin plus gentamicin for genitourinary or gastrointestinal procedures. For moderate-risk patients (e.g., rheumatic or congenital valve dysfunction or significant mitral valve prolapse) amoxicillin alone is sufficient.

Key Points

- All diastolic murmurs are pathologic.
- Monitor significant valvular disease by serial echo, and refer for valve replacement with symptoms or LV dysfunction.
- Acute valvular regurgitation, such as MR with papillary muscle rupture and AR with endocarditis, requires urgent echocardiography and rapid intervention.
- Give endocarditis prophylaxis to all valvular disease patients undergoing dental, respiratory, GI, or GU endoscopic procedures.

CASE 23-8

A 60-year-old woman who recently emigrated from China reports orthopnea for the past 3 months. She has an irregular rhythm and a crescendo-decrescendo systolic murmur loudest at the base. Two diastolic murmurs are heard, a high-pitched decrescendo murmur that radiates down the left sternal border and a low-pitched apical murmur that radiates to the axilla. Her carotid pulse upstroke is blunted.

A. What is the most likely cause of her valvular disease?
B. List the diagnostic studies that you would obtain.
C. Outline your management.
D. She is undergoing a tooth extraction in 2 weeks. How will you prepare her for this?

CASE 23-9

A 65-year-old man reports 6 hours of squeezing throat pain. He is in obvious discomfort. The nurse gets an ECG because his heart rate is 40. You notice a diastolic basal murmur as the ECG is obtained. The strip reads ***ACUTE MI*** and you see 1-mm ST elevations inferiorly. The nurse hangs a bag of streptokinase and asks if he can infuse it.

A. How do you answer?
B. Outline your management in terms of diagnostic tests and treatment.

24

Dermatology

ITCHING

ETIOLOGY

What are common causes of itching?

Xerosis (dry skin), scabies, and eczema are common causes of pruritus (itching). Less common causes include systemic diseases, such as renal failure, cholestasis, polycythemia vera, or lymphoma.

EVALUATION

How do I determine what is causing itching?

Xerosis usually causes diffuse pruritus and is common in the elderly and in patients who bathe frequently. The skin appears dry and may be cracked, although there is usually no erythema. Scabies may be associated with burrows in the interdigital web spaces and a papular rash, especially in the axillae, around the waistline, on the male genitals, or on the buttocks. The organism may be found by collecting scrapings from the white, linear, 1-mm wide burrows less than ½ inch long, often found at the wrists or in the web spaces between the fingers. Patients with scabies often have affected family members and almost always suffer from intense pruritus, often worse at night. If a therapeutic trial for xerosis fails and scabies is not identified, consider workup for a systemic illness with complete blood count, chemistry panel, and liver function tests.

TREATMENT

What treatments are useful?

For dry skin, use moisturizers, minimize bathing, and avoid hot water and deodorant soaps (Ivory is often a culprit). Use moisturizing soap sparingly in essential areas only. Treat scabies with permethrin or lindane cream overnight to the whole body below the neck. Prescribe enough for the simultaneous treatment of all intimate contacts (do not use lindane in children), even if they are asymptomatic. In the morning, patients should wash their bedding and any clothes worn the previous 2 days. Itching may occur for 1 to 2 weeks after treatment but does not indicate treatment failure. A short course of oral prednisone may be indicated if the itching is severe.

MACULOPAPULAR RASHES

ETIOLOGY

What are the most common causes of erythematous macules or papules in adults?

Drug reactions and viral infections cause diffuse maculopapular rashes. Scabies may cause more localized papular eruptions.

EVALUATION

How are the common maculopapular rashes distinguished?

New medications suggest drug reactions, especially common with antibiotics (sulfas and penicillins). Viral prodrome suggests a viral exanthem. Both cause a diffuse, truncal rash. Infestation with *Sarcoptes scabiei* causes papules with their tops scratched off and crusted resulting from itching. Scabies is often localized to the wrists, axillae, waist, or male genitals, although occasionally it is more widespread.

TREATMENT

Viral exanthems resolve spontaneously. Drug reactions often resolve with removal of the offending agent. See previous section for the treatment of scabies.

SCALING RASHES

ETIOLOGY

What are the most common scaling rashes in adults?

Psoriasis, eczema, pityriasis rosea, seborrheic dermatitis, and tinea infection are common causes.

EVALUATION

What helps me tell these conditions apart?

The pattern of body sites involved is helpful (Figure 24-1). Besides distribution, the appearance of the border and scale are also useful. Psoriasis causes well-circumscribed, raised, salmon-colored plaques with adherent silvery scales. Eczema is seen in "atopic" individuals who are prone to allergies and asthma and usually begins with erythema, often with intensely pruritic small vesicles or pustules. If eczema is long-standing, diffuse scaling and thickening (lichenification) can occur. Seborrhea is nonpruritic and has indistinct margins with greasy, fine, yellowish scales and underlying mild erythema. Pityriasis rosea is a mysterious, self-limited rash with distinct, oval-shaped, hyperpigmented lesions, each with an inner scaling ring. These lesions are distributed in an evergreen tree pattern over the trunk. Tinea causes distinct erythematous lesions with scaly borders. Hyphae on potassium hydroxide (KOH) preparations of skin scrapings are diagnostic.

TREATMENT

What treatments are useful for the scaling rashes?

Treat the underlying cause (Table 24-1). Preventive measures can minimize suffering from eczema: Avoid skin irritants, such as wool and household chemicals; minimize scratching with antihistamines; keep fingernails short; prevent skin dryness with moisturizers (avoid lanolin); minimize bathing; and avoid hot water and deodorant soaps. Treat secondary infection of eczematous lesions with antibiotics before initiating steroid treatment.

TABLE 24-1
Treatments for Scaling Rashes

CAUSE OF SCALING RASH	TREATMENT
Psoriasis	Coal tar lotion or shampoo, topical steroids (high to very high potency), sun exposure, UV light, methotrexate
Pityriasis rosea	Resolves without treatment after 2-8 wks, antihistamines decrease itching
Seborrheic dermatitis	Selenium sulfide shampoo, steroid lotion (scalp), ketoconazole shampoo
Eczema	Topical steroids, moisturizer, irritant avoidance
Tinea	Antifungal cream

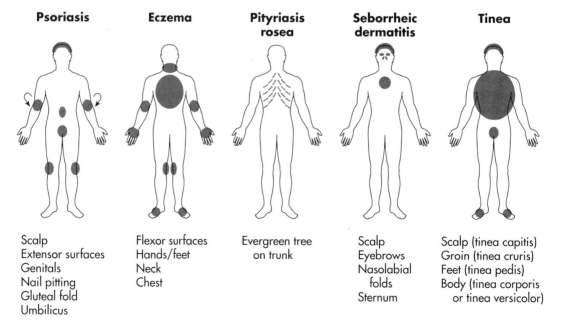

Psoriasis	**Eczema**	**Pityriasis rosea**	**Seborrheic dermatitis**	**Tinea**
Scalp	Flexor surfaces	Evergreen tree	Scalp	Scalp (tinea capitis)
Extensor surfaces	Hands/feet	on trunk	Eyebrows	Groin (tinea cruris)
Genitals	Neck		Nasolabial	Feet (tinea pedis)
Nail pitting	Chest		folds	Body (tinea corporis
Gluteal fold			Sternum	or tinea versicolor)
Umbilicus				

Figure 24-1 Classic sites involved with common scaling rashes.

SKIN CANCERS

ETIOLOGY

What are the different types of skin cancer?

Malignant melanoma is the most aggressive skin cancer. Associated with prior history of blistering sunburns, it grows rapidly, metastasizes early, and can be deadly. Tissue depth of melanoma at the time of diagnosis determines prognosis. Basal and squamous cell skin cancers are slow-growing tumors associated with a large cumulative sun exposure. Although they do not usually metastasize, they can invade local tissues if left untreated. Actinic keratoses are areas of mild atypia of the epidermis from chronic sun damage that may progress to squamous cell carcinoma, but the overall risk of progression is very small—less than 0.1% per year.

EVALUATION

How do I recognize skin cancers?

Features concerning for melanoma are listed in Box 24-1. Basal cell carcinomas (BCCs) appear as shiny pink or pearly papules with telangiectasias. Squamous cell carcinoma (SCC) is an indurated, yellowish plaque, often with scaling, erosions, or ulcerations. Actinic keratoses are usually more easily felt than seen, with patients complaining of a small patch of recurrent, rough, adherent scale. All three of these lesions occur on sun-exposed areas, especially the upper cheeks, below the eyes, on the ears, and around the nose in immunocompetent hosts.

How should a suspicious mole be evaluated?

Remove small lesions with low suspicion for melanoma with a simple punch biopsy. If there is concern for melanoma, refer the patient for definitive excision. Never perform a shave biopsy on a pigmented lesion; the depth of involvement is critical if the lesion is a melanoma.

BOX 24-1	Features Concerning for Malignant Melanoma
A	Asymmetry, especially a notched border
B	Bleeding
C	Color variation
D	Diameter growing or >6 mm
E	Elevation irregularity, e.g., a raised area within a macule
F	Feeling changes, e.g., new itching or burning

TREATMENT

Freeze actinic keratoses with liquid nitrogen, but be aware that the lesions are so superficial that a single 10-second freeze is usually sufficient. Refer to dermatology for wider excision and further treatment of any malignant lesion.

VESICULAR LESIONS

ETIOLOGY

What are common causes of vesicles?

Common causes include herpes zoster reactivation as shingles, as well as herpes simplex infection. Contact allergies also cause vesicles, usually in a limited distribution.

EVALUATION

How do I tell shingles from herpes simplex?

Shingles is reactivation of dormant varicella-zoster virus (chickenpox); the dermatomal distribution clinches the diagnosis. It often starts with painful burning along a dermatome, which is followed by an outbreak of vesicles on an erythematous base. Zoster occurs most commonly in elderly or immunocompromised patients. Herpes simplex is usually sexually transmitted and causes vesicles and ulceration on the lips, in the mouth, or on the genitals. To confirm diagnosis of herpes simplex, obtain a sample of cells for viral culture from the base of an unroofed vesicle (rub firmly for an adequate sample).

What is postherpetic neuralgia?

Postherpetic neuralgia (PHN) is pain occurring after shingles resolves and may continue for months. The incidence increases with age, from 10% at age 40 years to 70% after age 65 years. It typically lasts 1 to 2 months in young patients and 6 to 9 months in elderly patients.

TREATMENT

How do I treat herpes zoster and postherpetic neuralgia?

Treat with either 7 days of acyclovir, famciclovir, or valacyclovir. These drugs are effective at shortening the time to healing of the rash and cutting the average length of PHN, but they do not affect the incidence of PHN. Prednisone may speed the healing of the rash but has little to no effect on PHN and so should only be used when the acute rash is severe. All patients with active zoster should avoid pregnant women and adults who do not have a history of chickenpox. Patients who have lesions on the forehead, the nose, or around the eye should have urgent ophthalmologic evaluation to rule out corneal involvement. PHN may respond to amitriptyline 25 mg or more at bedtime or topical capsaicin, the active ingredient of hot peppers, or the antiseizure drug gabapentin.

How do I treat herpes simplex?

Outbreaks are self-limited but may be shortened by acyclovir, famciclovir, or valacyclovir. Patients with frequent, severe attacks can be given prophylactic acyclovir 400 mg bid. Prevent transmission by avoiding intimate contact with the involved area during outbreaks. Viral shedding occurs even without presence of sores, although the clinical impact of this is unclear.

Key Points

- Psoriasis responds to topical steroids, but if severe, it may require referral for nontopical therapy.
- Pityriasis rosea is a benign, self-limited rash that has a characteristic evergreen-tree pattern.
- Seborrhea is a common scaling rash on the face that responds to low-potency steroids.
- Therapy for eczema consists primarily of skin moisturizing and topical steroids.
- Zoster should be treated with antivirals to speed rash healing and shorten the course of PHN.
- It is very rare for BCCs or SCCs to metastasize; excision halts local spread.

CASE 24-1

A 28-year-old woman with allergic rhinitis and a history of childhood asthma reports an itchy rash on the flexor surfaces of her arms for 4 weeks. On examination, she has symmetric erythema on both antecubital fossae with significant excoriation, and one area of associated yellowish crust.
- A. What is the most likely diagnosis?
- B. What do you make of the yellowish crusting?
- C. What would you recommend for treatment?

CASE 24-2

A 62-year-old man has acute onset of facial pain followed by appearance of a rash on his forehead. His vision is normal. On examination, he has small red vesicles on his left forehead.
- A. What is the most likely diagnosis?
- B. What would you recommend for acute treatment?
- C. Is any other evaluation needed?

CASE 24-3

A 52-year-old woman comes to clinic because her husband has noticed a mole on her back that has grown recently. On examination, there is a 5-mm pigmented macular lesion just below the right scapula with a slightly irregular border.
- A. What other historical and physical examination features should be noted?
- B. What is the main diagnostic concern?
- C. What should be the next diagnostic step?

25

Endocrinology

ADRENAL DISORDERS

ETIOLOGY

What causes adrenal insufficiency?

The most common cause of adrenal insufficiency is exogenous steroid use. Primary adrenal gland destruction worldwide is usually due to TB. In the United States, autoimmune destruction is more common and is often part of a polyglandular deficiency syndrome type 1 (hypoparathyroidism and mucocutaneous candidiasis) or type 2 (autoimmune thyroiditis and type I diabetes). Secondary adrenal insufficiency occurs with decreased adrenocorticotropic hormone (ACTH) production due to disrupted pituitary function.

What are the types of adrenal excess?

Adrenal hypertrophy, adenoma, and carcinoma can all produce excess aldosterone, cortisol (Cushing's syndrome), or catecholamines (pheochromocytoma). Cushing's syndrome is a state of chronic glucocorticoid excess from any source. Long-term steroid use is the most common cause. Cushing's disease is due to a pituitary adenoma secreting ACTH and is the second most common cause of Cushing's syndrome. Less common are adrenal hyperplasia, adrenal adenoma, and ectopic ACTH, usually from small-cell lung cancer.

EVALUATION

How does adrenal insufficiency present?

Adrenal insufficiency may present with acute cardiovascular collapse mimicking sepsis, or more gradually with nonspecific fatigue and abdominal pain (Table 25-1). Assume adrenal insufficiency in any patient on long-term steroids. Diffuse hyperpigmentation, including in the palmar creases and gums, is seen with adrenal gland failure because the compensating pituitary overproduces melanocyte-stimulating hormone, a by-product. Secondary adrenal failure is usually part of panhypopituitarism with hypothyroidism and hypogonadism. Laboratory abnormalities suggesting adrenal insufficiency include hyperkalemia, hyponatremia, hypoglycemia, and eosinophilia.

How do I diagnose adrenal insufficiency?

Random cortisol greater than 20 μg/dl rules out adrenal insufficiency. Gold standard screening is with an ACTH stimulation test: a plasma cortisol of less than 18 μg/dl measured 30 to 60 minutes after 250 μg synthetic ACTH (cosyntropin, given IV or IM) indicates insufficiency. An ACTH level greater than 250 pg/ml then distinguishes adrenal from pituitary (ACTH <50 pg/ml) causes. Small adrenal glands on CT scan suggest autoimmune destruction; large adrenals suggest metastasis or early TB.

When should I suspect adrenal excess?

Aldosterone, cortisol, and catecholamine excess all cause hypertension. Aldosterone and cortisol excess also cause hypokalemia, hypernatremia, and metabolic alkalosis. Screen for adrenal excess with careful history, examination, and electrolytes in very young hypertensive patients and in those with difficult-to-control hypertension. Clues include a cushingoid appearance. Pheochromocytoma causes episodic severe hypertension, with associated sweating or flushing. Some pheochromocytomas are associated with neurofibromatosis or medullary thyroid cancer.

How does Cushing's syndrome present?

Patients rarely complain of symptoms that will suggest this diagnosis; it is diagnosed by an astute physician who thinks to look for it. Consider the diagnosis in

TABLE 25-1

Presenting Signs and Symptoms of Adrenal Insufficiency and Cortisol Excess

ADRENAL DISORDER	SYMPTOMS	SIGNS	LABORATORY TEST RESULTS
Adrenal insufficiency	Weakness Fatigue GI symptoms: anorexia, nausea, vomiting, abdominal pain	Hypotension/orthostasis Weight loss Hyperpigmentation (with adrenal cause only)	Hyperkalemia Non-gap metabolic acidosis Hyponatremia Hypoglycemia Eosinophilia
Cortisol excess (Cushing's syndrome)	Proximal muscle wasting, weakness Easy bruising Acne Hirsuitism	Hypertension Central obesity with thin extremities Facial plethora, moon facies Abdominal striae	Hypokalemia Metabolic alkalosis Hypernatremia Hyperglycemia

patients who look cushingoid, who present with hypertension and central obesity, or with unexplained metabolic alkalosis. If one feature is present, look for others to confirm your suspicion (see Table 25-1).

How do I diagnose Cushing's syndrome?

Screen for cortisol excess by a 24-hour urine cortisol (normal <100 μg/24 hours). Levels greater than 250 μg/day diagnose Cushing's syndrome, whereas levels less than 65 exclude the diagnosis. False-positive tests occur with depression, anorexia, stress, alcoholism, and oral contraceptives.

How do I work-up patients for hyperaldosteronism or pheochromocytoma?

When you suspect hyperaldosteronism, obtain a serum aldosterone-to-renin ratio. When aldosterone is greater than 20 ng/dl, a ratio greater than 100 (with renin units in ng/ml/3 hours) is highly specific for the diagnosis. Suspect pheochromocytoma with presence of the 5 "H"s (each usually episodic): hypertension, headache, hyperhidrosis (sweating), hypotension (orthostatic), and hyperglycemia. Screen for pheochromocytoma by 24-hour urine catecholamines, metanephrines, or vanillylmandelic acid. If screening is positive, obtain abdominal MRI to look for the source.

TREATMENT

How do I treat adrenal insufficiency?

Replace with hydrocortisone for pituitary insufficiency, with the addition of aldosterone (fludrocortisone) for primary adrenal disease. During surgery or infection, pa-

Key Points

- Adrenal insufficiency is most commonly due to steroid use.
- Patients who look septic might have adrenal insufficiency.
- Recognize adrenal insufficiency early, and if the patient is in crisis, do not wait for test results—give hydrocortisone immediately.

CASE 25-1

A 55-year-old man with severe COPD is markedly confused immediately after an elective cholecystectomy. Temperature is 101.5° F, pulse is 130, BP is 76/42, and respiratory rate is 20. Staples are intact, and abdomen is not distended but is tender without guarding or rebound. Blood loss was minimal during the surgery, and 2 L of fluid were administered.

A. What is your differential diagnosis for his confusion and hypotension?

B. What further workup should be done?

C. What treatment does he need?

tients need stress-dose steroids (hydrocortisone 100 mg IV on call to the OR, or 50-100 mg IV q6h).

How do I treat adrenal excess syndromes?

Remove the tumor. This must be done carefully with pheochromocytoma—prepare preoperatively with αblockade and β-blockade to avoid life-threatening catecholamine bolus.

DIABETES

ETIOLOGY

What is the difference between type 1 and type 2 diabetes?

Diabetes occurs when inadequate insulin results in a high blood sugar. Patients with type 1 diabetes stop making insulin. A combination of genetic predisposition and environmental trigger (possibly viral infection) causes autoimmune destruction of pancreatic islet β-cells. These patients are generally young and slender. In type 2 diabetes, insulin resistance is combined with insufficient, but not absent, insulin secretion. Onset is usually after age 30, and patients are often obese.

What are the risk factors for diabetes?

The major risk factor for type 1 diabetes is an identical twin with type 1 diabetes. Risk factors for type 2 diabetes are obesity; prior gestational diabetes; Native American, Hispanic, or African-American race; prior impaired glucose tolerance; hypertension; family history of type 2 diabetes; and dyslipidemia. Many drugs can exacerbate glucose intolerance, including steroids, thiazide diuretics, niacin, and β-blockers.

What is diabetic ketoacidosis?

Diabetic ketoacidosis (DKA) occurs in type 1 diabetes when lack of insulin forces the body to burn ketones for fuel and causes accelerated starvation. Key features include hyperglycemia, elevated ketones, and anion-gap acidosis. Common precipitants include infection (50%), lack of insulin, and new diabetes.

What is hyperglycemic hyperosmolar nonketotic coma?

When patients with type 2 diabetes get extremely hyperglycemic, they become hyperosmolar. Ketoacidosis is uncommon because patients have enough insulin to prevent ketone production. High glucose draws free water out of cells and creates an osmotic diuresis, leading to dehydration and altered mental status. Coma is present in 10%; mortality is 10% to 17%. Many patients with hyperglycemic hyperosmolar nonketotic coma (HHNC) are elderly and unable to drink enough fluids to compensate. Common precipitants include infection, heart attack, stroke, uremia, pancreatitis, and parenteral nutrition.

EVALUATION

How do I diagnose diabetes?

Diagnose diabetes by a single plasma glucose greater than or equal to 200 mg/dl with symptoms such as polydipsia, polyuria, polyphagia, and weight loss, or a fasting plasma glucose greater than or equal to 126 mg/dl on two occasions. Glycosylated hemoglobin ($HgbA_{1c}$) is too insensitive to use for diagnosis. Oral glucose tolerance testing is only used as screening for gestational diabetes.

Who should be screened for diabetes?

Patients have type 2 diabetes on average 10 to 12 years before diagnosis. To diagnose these patients earlier, the American Diabetes Association recommends screening those with more than 1 risk factor every 3 years. Screening includes risk factor evaluation and fasting plasma glucose.

How do patients with diabetes present?

Patients under 20 years old with type 1 diabetes usually present abruptly, often in ketoacidosis precipitated by an acute stressor, such as a bacterial infection. Ketoacidosis may be accompanied by coma (in 10%), Kussmaul's breathing (rapid, deep breaths in response to acidosis), fruity breath from elevated acetone, dehydration, hypotension, and tachycardia. Some patients with type 1 diabetes present with more gradual-onset malaise, weight loss, polydipsia, polyuria, or blurred vision. Patients with type 2 diabetes more commonly present either without obvious symptoms or with weeks to months of polyuria; polydipsia; weight loss; or symptoms of end-organ complications, such as altered vision (retinopathy), peripheral edema (nephropathy), or sensory changes in the distal extremities (neuropathy). Diabetes can also present with recurrent infections, such as boils, carbuncles, and vaginal yeast infections in women. Elderly patients with type 2 diabetes may present with life-threatening hyperosmolar coma.

Once I have made the diagnosis, what other evaluation is important?

Among patients with type 2 diabetes, 10% to 15% have neuropathy, 37% have retinopathy, and 50% have coronary artery disease at diagnosis. Pertinent history and examination (Table 25-2), as well as laboratory monitoring, should be aimed to detect these complications (Table 25-3). Additionally, order TSH because many patients with type I diabetes will have autoimmune destruction of other endocrine glands. $HgbA_{1c}$ estimates average blood glucose over the prior 3 months. Obtain a baseline $HgbA_{1c}$ and repeat every 6 months in patients who are stable on oral agents, and every 3 months in

TABLE 25-2
Pertinent History and Physical in Patients with Diabetes

	HISTORY	EXAMINATION
New diagnosis of diabetes	Duration of symptoms Polyuria, polydipsia Cardiovascular risk factors or symptoms (cigarette use, cholesterol, hypertension, family history of CV disease) Family history of diabetes Vision disturbance Sensory changes in the extremities Medications	Blood pressure (assess CV risk) Weight and height for body mass index Funduscopic exam (for retinopathy) Thyroid exam (concurrent autoimmune disease) Carotid, femoral, abdominal renal artery bruits (for atherosclerotic disease) Sensory exam with monofilament (neuropathy) Extremities for edema, ulcers Skin (acanthosis nigricans, fungal infections may provide portal of entry for cellulitis)
Periodic follow-up	Hyperglycemia or hypoglycemia symptoms Glucose-monitoring results Changes in vision Changes in foot sensation Daily self-exam of feet Medication tolerance Diet and exercise habits Brief review of systems (cardiac, GI, infections)	Same as above

TABLE 25-3
Screening and Treatment for Complications of Diabetes

COMPLICATION	SCREENING TEST	RECOMMENDATION	TREATMENT
Retinopathy	Ophthalmology referral	Type 1: yearly beginning 5 yrs after diagnosis; at diagnosis if age >30 Type 2: yearly	Laser therapy
Nephropathy	Urine protein/creatinine ratio or 24-hr urine (microalbuminuria = 30-300 mg/24 hrs)	Type 1: yearly beginning 5 yrs after diagnosis Type 2: yearly	ACEI Angiotensin receptor blocker BP control
Neuropathy	Foot exam: deformity, lesions, and sensory testing with a 5.0 monofilament	Daily patient foot checks Foot exam at every visit Yearly sensory testing	Capsaicin cream Tricyclic anti-depressants Carbamazepine
Heart disease	ECG at diagnosis in patients with type 2; pursue testing with chest or respiratory complaints.	Type 1: fasting lipids at diagnosis, then follow lipid screening guidelines Type 2: fasting lipids yearly	Lower lipids with "statin" to LDL <100 β-blockers post-MI
Gastroparesis	Ask about symptoms of early satiety, nausea, emesis	Upper GI series or nuclear medicine gastric emptying study	Erythromycin* Metoclopramide Cisapride*

*Do not use concurrently due to risk of cardiac arrhythmia.

TABLE 25-4
Human Insulin Formulations and Pharmacokinetics

INSULIN	ACTION	ONSET (LAG TIME*)	PEAK (HOURS)	DURATION (HOURS)
Lispro (Humalog)	Immediate	5-15 min	0.5-1.5	≤5
Regular (Humulin R)	Rapid	30-60 min	1-5	5-7
NPH (Humulin N)	Intermediate	3-4 hrs	6-12	18-28
Ultralente (Humulin U)	Prolonged	4-6 hrs	12-24	36
70/30 (Humulin, 70%N/30%R)	Mix of intermediate and rapid	30-60 min 3-4 hrs (N)	6-15	22-28

*Lag time refers to the amount of time between an insulin injection and when a patient should eat. Lag time is approximately equal to onset of action (e.g., 30 minutes for regular insulin; little or no lag time with Lispro).

those taking insulin. Refer to ophthalmology for annual retinopathy screening.

What tests are appropriate for patients with DKA or hyperosmolar coma?

Obtain chemistry panel, ABG, CBC, and urinalysis. Look for a precipitating infection with blood and urine cultures, as well as a chest x-ray, even if the patient is afebrile. An elevated WBC count (12-15), glucose greater than 250 mg/dl, elevated potassium resulting from cellular shifts, and an anion gap acidosis with compensatory respiratory alkalosis are expected. Serum osmolarity greater than 330 can cause altered mental status. If the serum osmolarity is less than 330 with altered mental status, or if mental status does not reverse after several hours of treatment, consider head CT and lumbar puncture.

TREATMENT

What are the goals of treatment?

In the Diabetes Control and Complications Trial (DCCT), type 1 patients treated with intensive therapy were 50% to 75% less likely to have progression of retinopathy, nephropathy, and neuropathy than those receiving conventional therapy. The goal of such intensive treatment for type 1 diabetes is a HgbA$_{1c}$ less than or equal to 7% (normal 4% to 6%), equivalent to an average plasma glucose of 150 mg/dl. Similar goals are reasonable for type 2 diabetes, though less outcome data exist.

How do I start treatment in patients with newly diagnosed diabetes?

Diet, exercise, and self-monitoring of blood glucose are the foundation of treatment. Aggressively lower coronary artery disease risk with smoking cessation and treatment for elevated blood pressure and cholesterol. Glucose is best checked 2 to 4 times daily, before meals or before bed. Type 1 patients require insulin. Type 2 patients may require oral medications or insulin. When starting medications, educate patients about sweating, shaking, hunger, or confusion as signs of hypoglycemia, and averting a reaction with candy or juice. Careful glucose monitoring should accompany any change in regimen.

How do I choose a starting dose of insulin?

Patients with type 1 diabetes need multiple daily subcutaneous insulin injections: short-acting to cover meals and long-acting for basal requirements. A number of preparations are available (Table 25-4). Estimate insulin dose by weight, starting at 0.5 to 1.0 U/kg/day. Give two thirds of this dose in the morning (two-thirds NPH, one-third regular), and one third in the evening (split one-half NPH, one-half regular). NPH at bedtime instead of with dinner may prevent nighttime hypoglycemia because its peak effect occurs later when early-morning growth hormone and cortisol levels naturally increase blood sugar. A single dose of bedtime NPH can be added to oral agents in patients with type 2 diabetes. Intensive therapy in type 1 patients adds daily injections of short-acting insulin with each meal or snack. Because type 1 patients are more insulin-sensitive than those with insulin-resistant (type 2) diabetes, you will need to adjust these guidelines to fit individual patients.

When are medications necessary in patients with type 2 diabetes?

Asymptomatic patients near ideal body weight, with no complications, or with a fasting glucose level less than 200 mg/dl may do well with diet and exercise alone. For patients who are symptomatic, have complications, or have a fasting glucose greater than 300 mg/dl, diet and oral agents are usually not enough, so insulin is appropriate initial therapy. Most patients with type 2 diabetes require diet and an oral agent. About one third of type 2 patients initially need insulin; many patients feel better and achieve better glycemic control on insulin.

TABLE 25-5
Common Oral Agents Used to Treat Patients with Type 2 Diabetes

DRUG	PRIMARY ACTION	MAJOR SIDE EFFECTS	DOSE
Sulfonylureas glyburide	Increases pancreatic insulin secretion	Hypoglycemia Weight gain	1.25-20 mg/day
Biguanides metformin	Decreases gluconeogenesis	GI intolerance, lactic acidosis	1000-2550 mg/day divide bid-tid

Which oral agent should I use?

Multiple oral agents are available (Table 25-5). Nonobese patients who need more than dietary treatment should start a sulfonylurea to stimulate pancreatic insulin secretion and decrease insulin resistance. Patients who are overweight or have high triglycerides do well on metformin, which lowers lipids and does not cause the weight gain common with sulfonylureas and insulin. Metformin is contraindicated in patients with CHF or creatinine greater than 1.4 mg/dl because of the risk of lactic acidosis. Increase doses of oral medications weekly as needed. Oral agents generally lower the HgbA$_{1c}$ 1% to 2%, except acarbose, which only achieves a 0.5% reduction.

What should I do if one oral agent is not enough?

Many patients require combination therapy, either with a sulfonylurea plus metformin, or with an oral agent plus insulin. 0.1 U/kg of intermediate or long-acting insulin can be added at bedtime. Bedtime insulin decreases fasting glucose and causes less weight gain. Acute illness or medications such as prednisone can exacerbate hyperglycemia, necessitating short-term insulin use.

How can I prevent nephropathy and renal failure?

Slow the progression of nephropathy by controlling hypertension aggressively to a goal systolic blood pressure less than 135 and diastolic less than 85. Use ACEIs when urine microalbumin is greater than 30 mg/L (or per gram of creatinine or per 24 hours). ACEIs cannot be used in pregnancy, or when they cause hyperkalemia or angioedema. Elevated creatinine alone should not prevent ACEI use because even patients with creatinines of 4 to 5 may benefit. β-Blockers and thiazide diuretics are second choices for hypertension because of adverse effects on glycemic control and lipids, although patients with concurrent coronary artery disease gain greater benefit than harm from β-blockers.

How do I adjust therapy when patients cannot eat?

When patients are ill or fasting for a procedure, adjust therapy to avoid hypoglycemia. Patients with type I diabetes always need insulin, regardless of food intake, to prevent ketoacidosis. Because hepatic production accounts for about half of the serum glucose, give patients half their usual insulin in long-acting form and monitor frequently. Alternatively, you may use an insulin drip. Patients with type 2 diabetes can hold or decrease sulfonylurea doses and monitor chemsticks. Patients on metformin should stop this medication before procedures or surgery because of the small risk of lactic acidosis; restart after 48 hours if creatinine is stable.

How do I treat hypoglycemia?

Hypoglycemia is the most common endocrine emergency. Intensive therapy and decreased renal clearance of insulin or sulfonylureas are risk factors. Low serum glucose alters mental status and induces a catecholamine response (sweating, shakiness, weakness, nausea, and anxiety). β-Blockers blunt hypoglycemic symptoms except for sweating. Give oral glucose to conscious patients and intravenous glucose and glucagon to unconscious patients. Hospitalize if the patient does not respond rapidly or if decreased renal clearance may cause recurrent symptoms.

When do I need to hospitalize patients with diabetes?

DKA, hyperosmolar coma, severe infections, severe nausea and vomiting, and cardiac ischemia are common reasons to hospitalize patients with diabetes. Cellulitis and foot ulcers often require intravenous antibiotics. Malignant otitis externa is an uncommon but life-threatening external ear canal pseudomonal infection that requires intravenous antibiotics. Other life-threatening infections seen with diabetes include rhinocerebral mucormycosis, emphysematous cholecystitis (*Escherichia coli* or *Clostridium*), emphysematous pyelonephritis (*E. coli* or other gram-negative rods), and necrotizing fasciitis (mixed anaerobes and aerobes).

A patient with diabetes is hospitalized for cellulitis. How should I manage the glucose?

Patients can be given their usual regimen if glucose is less than 250 mg/dl. "Supplemental" insulin (additional insulin before meals for high glucose measurements) may be appropriate. However, "sliding scale" insulin given for a high glucose without anticipating caloric intake is unacceptable because of the risk of hypoglycemia. If the patient's glucose cannot be easily controlled by insulin injections, use a continuous insulin drip, and add glucose if the patient is not eating.

How do I treat patients with DKA?

Patients with DKA usually require intensive care for aggressive hydration with normal saline, intravenous insulin, and electrolyte monitoring and replacement. Give regular insulin, 10-U IV bolus, followed by an insulin drip for at least 12 to 24 hours, with hourly glucose checks; adjust as needed. Check potassium and phosphate because these are often depleted. Serum potassium levels may not reflect total body depletion because acidosis causes shift from cells to plasma. When the serum glucose drops to 250, intravenous fluid can be changed to D5½NS to prevent hypoglycemia and provide calories and free water. Insulin can be changed to the outpatient regimen when bicarbonate normalizes and patients can eat. Continue the insulin drip at least 1 hour after the first subcutaneous injection to prevent recurrent ketone production. Give DVT prophylaxis to comatose patients. Use antibiotics when indicated.

How do I treat patients with hyperosmolar coma?

Hydration with isotonic saline is the mainstay of therapy. Insulin may be needed in lower doses than for DKA (5- to 10-U bolus and 0.1 U/kg/hr). Give antibiotics as indicated.

Key Points

- Type 1 diabetes is caused by lack of insulin. Type 2 diabetes results from insulin resistance.
- Diagnose diabetes by 2 fasting glucoses greater than 126 or a random glucose greater than 200 plus symptoms.
- Patients with type 1 require insulin to avoid DKA; intensive therapy reduces complications.
- Therapy for type 2 diabetes begins with diet and exercise; oral agents or insulin may be required to optimize glucose levels and prevent complications.

CASE 25-2

A 27-year-old man complains of thirst, frequent urination, and a 20-pound weight loss over 4 weeks. He has no significant past medical history and takes no medications. He does recall a viral illness approximately 3 months before admission, during which he missed a week of work. His maternal grandmother has type II diabetes, and his mother is obese. He is a bicycle delivery person. His weight is 150 pounds, and his height is 6 feet 1 inch. Vital signs and examination are normal. His glucose is 360 and his urine is positive for glucose, ketones, and protein.

A. Does he have type I or type II diabetes, and what evidence do you need to decide?
B. Assuming he needs insulin, calculate a starting dose for a twice-daily injection regimen using intermediate and short-acting insulin.
C. What screening does he need now?

CASE 25-3

A 45-year-old overweight Hispanic man comes to your office at the request of his wife for a "check-up." His father had a heart attack at age 50, and his mother has diabetes. He has no complaints, but on review of systems he notes fatigue, nocturia, and occasional paresthesias. His weight is 210 pounds; height is 6 feet. His blood pressure is 150/90; other vital signs are normal. He has dark pigmentation at the collar line and under his arms. Prostate examination is normal. He has hammer toes and decreased sensation at 4/10 points on monofilament testing. Chemstick is 240.

A. What is his diagnosis?
B. Outline your treatment and screening plan.
C. Which oral agent would you choose for this patient and why?

HYPERLIPIDEMIA

ETIOLOGY

Why is cholesterol important?

Elevated cholesterol is clearly associated with an increased risk for coronary artery disease (CAD). Lowering cholesterol reduces the risk of CAD, slows progression of existing CAD, may cause regression of atherosclerotic plaques, and may reduce stroke risk.

What causes hypercholesterolemia?

The great majority of cases are primary disorders of lipid metabolism or production. Secondary causes may contribute to elevated cholesterol (Box 25-1). Note that the medications listed are not contraindicated if otherwise medically important.

Do triglycerides have an effect on the heart?

There is a positive correlation between elevated triglycerides and risk for CAD. However, isolated hypertriglyceridemia is not a clear risk factor for CAD. One theory is that elevated triglyceride levels are not directly atherogenic but instead reflect abnormalities in HDL or LDL. When triglyceride levels are greater than 1000 mg/dl, there is an increased risk for pancreatitis.

EVALUATION

Whom should I screen for high cholesterol?

Controversy exists about when to start cholesterol screening because agencies that establish standards vary in their approach and recommendations. The National Cholesterol Education Program (NCEP) currently recommends screening cholesterol every 5 years in all adults over the age of 20. However, the U.S. Preventive Services Task Force, which uses stricter requirements for evidence-based benefits, recommends screening men ages 35 to 65 and women ages 45 to 65. One approach is to begin screening for cholesterol at age 35, and earlier

---

BOX 25-1   Secondary Causes of Hyperlipidemia

Poorly controlled blood glucose
Hypothyroidism
Nephrotic syndrome
Drugs:
    Progestins
    Steroids
    High-dose thiazide diuretics
    High-dose β-blocker
    Protease inhibitors
Smoking

BOX 25-2   Cardiovascular Risk Factors Applied in Cholesterol Management

Male gender
HDL <35 mg/dl
Family history of an MI or sudden cardiac death in a parent or sibling <55 years old
History of cerebrovascular or peripheral vascular disease
Hypertension
Diabetes mellitus
Cigarette smoking (>10 per day)

NOTE: HDL >65 counts as a negative risk factor.

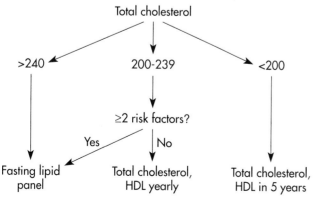

Figure 25-1 Follow-up testing recommendations for total cholesterol.

---

if the patient has cardiovascular risk factors (Box 25-2). Whether to screen after the age of 65 is debated.

What test should I use to screen?

In any patient with known coronary disease, go directly to the fasting lipid panel. Otherwise, start with a nonfasting total cholesterol and HDL. Whether to test further depends on total cholesterol and risk of CAD (Figure 25-1).

What is a fasting lipid panel, and what do I do with the results?

The fasting lipid panel is drawn after a 12-hour fast. In this test the total cholesterol, HDL, and triglycerides are all measured. LDL is estimated by the following calculation: $LDL = $ total cholesterol $-$ (HDL $+$ triglycerides/5). If the patient's triglycerides are too high (>400), the LDL cannot be accurately calculated.

TREATMENT

What modifiable cardiovascular risk factors should I treat?

Diabetes, smoking, and hypertension are each independent cardiovascular risk factors. In fact, their role in cardiovascular and cerebrovascular disease is so strong that it makes little sense to work on controlling a patient's cholesterol without managing these risk factors aggressively. Patients with diabetes have an especially high risk of CAD.

How does LDL guide cholesterol management?

LDL levels predict adverse events. Cardiovascular risk determines specific treatment goals for LDL levels. Whether to start with diet or medications depends on the measured LDL level (Table 25-6). For patients with diabetes, the goal LDL is 100, regardless of whether other risk factors are present.

What treatment plan do I follow, and how closely do I monitor treatment?

For all patients with high cholesterol (even those starting medications), the NCEP recommends dietary intervention with a Step 1 Diet, which limits daily intake of total fat to 30% of total calories and dietary cholesterol to 300 mg/day. If the goal LDL is not achieved after 6 months, advance to a nutritionist-guided Step 2 Diet, which further limits fat and cholesterol intake. Because compliance is difficult on the more stringent diet, many physicians begin medications at this point. Regardless of the treatment plan, measure the LDL at 6 weeks and 3 months until goal LDL is reached, then every 6 months thereafter.

What other alternatives are there to cholesterol-lowering medications?

Regular exercise lowers triglycerides, raises HDL, and can lower LDL levels. In postmenopausal women, estrogen replacement therapy is an important intervention. The onset of CAD occurs 10 years later in women than men, a fact attributed to the cardioprotective effects of estrogen. Estrogen reduces LDL and triglycerides and increases HDL. However, these benefits have to be weighed against the increased risk of endometrial

and possibly breast cancers in patients taking unopposed estrogen therapy. Concomitant progestins reduce the risk of endometrial cancer but may offset the benefits of estrogen on the lipid profile.

What about other dietary interventions?

Increasing dietary omega-3 fatty acids by consuming fish and fish oil (30 g/day or 2 fish meals weekly) has been shown to reduce total cholesterol, reduce triglycerides, raise HDL, and lower cardiovascular mortality. Dietary fiber (e.g., legumes, oat bran, fruit, and psyllium) has also been associated with significant lowering of cholesterol levels. Mild-to-moderate consumption of alcohol (2 oz whiskey, 8 oz wine, or 24 oz of beer per day) is associated with reduced incidence of CAD. HDL is increased in patients with moderate alcohol intake. However, the potential harmful effects of excess alcohol ingestion preclude routine recommendations for its use in preventing CAD. Vitamin E and β-carotene are antioxidants that have been shown to reduce the oxidation of lipids, but clinical benefits are not yet clear.

What are the cholesterol-lowering medications, and how should I use them?

Factors to be considered are efficacy with certain lipid profiles, side effects, and convenience (Table 25-7). For patients with elevated LDL and known coronary artery

TABLE 25-6
Coronary Artery Disease Risk Determines Treatment Goal for LDL

PATIENT'S CARDIOVASCULAR RISK	GOAL LDL*	THRESHOLD LDL FOR STARTING DRUG THERAPY*
≤2 risk factors	<160	>190
≥2 risk factors	<130	>160
Known CAD or diabetes	≤100	≥130

*In mg/dl.

TABLE 25-7
Lipid-Lowering Medications

DRUG	COST	ACTION	SIDE EFFECTS
HMG CoA Reductase inhibitors "Statins" Simvastatin Atorvastatin	$$$	LDL ↓↓ TG* ↓ HDL ↑	Rhabdomyolysis, slightly increased risk with fibric acid Hepatotoxicity GI distress Headache, insomnia
Nicotinic acid Niacin	$	LDL ↓ TG ↓↓ HDL ↑	Flushing, headache, tachycardia, pruritus Hyperuricemia Hyperglycemia Hepatotoxicity
Fibric acid Gemfibrozil Clofibrate	$	LDL ↓ TG ↓↓ HDL ↑↑	Rhabdomyolysis, slightly increased risk with statins, greatly increased with cyclosporine, erythromycin, and ketoconazole Gallstones Hepatotoxicity GI malignancy Nausea
Bile-acid sequestrants Colestipol Cholestyramine	$$	LDL ↓ TG ↑ HDL —	Decreased absorption of many other medications GI distress, constipation

TG, Triglycerides.
*High-dose simvastatin (80 mg/d) and atorvastatin at regular doses lower triglycerides.

disease, HMG CoA reductase inhibitors are first choice because clinical benefits beyond simple cholesterol lowering have been demonstrated with these drugs. At high doses, or with higher potency formulations (e.g., atorvastatin), HDL is increased and triglycerides are lowered. For primary prevention, niacin and bile-acid sequestrants are quite effective; niacin is the cheapest cholesterol-lowering drug available. Gradually increase niacin to minimize the immediate flushing/headache reaction that many patients experience; pretreating with aspirin can also help. For low HDL, treat with niacin, gemfibrozil, atorvastatin, or estrogen in women. Because of side effects of gastrointestinal distress and constipation, bile-acid sequestrants are generally only added as a second- or third-line agent when other drugs are not adequate for control.

When do I treat hypertriglyceridemia?

If your patient has mild elevation (up to 400 or so) and is otherwise healthy, treatment is not indicated. On the other hand, if your patient has known vascular disease, treat triglycerides aggressively, even though the association with CAD is not clearly causative. If the triglycerides are markedly elevated (>1000), treatment will decrease the risk of pancreatitis.

What is the best treatment for high triglycerides?

Begin with nonpharmacologic management (unless TG >1000): weight loss, alcohol restriction, exercise, and dietary change. Treat secondary causes when they are found. Nicotinic (niacin) and fibric (gemfibrozil) acids are the drugs of choice for lowering elevated triglycerides.

Key Points

- Screen otherwise healthy patients with nonfasting total cholesterol and HDL.
- Goal LDL for patients with coronary artery disease or diabetes is 100.
- Treat accompanying risk factors, such as smoking, diabetes, and hypertension, aggressively.

CASE 25-4

A 57-year-old postmenopausal woman has persistent hypercholesterolemia after 6 months of diet therapy. Her only other risk factor is hypertension. Laboratory test values are as follows: total cholesterol 293, TG 159, LDL 215, HDL 46, glucose 90, and TSH 9.3 (this is high).

A. What is her goal cholesterol?
B. Would you start a medication now, and if so, which medication would you choose?

CASE 25-5

A 69-year-old woman with a history of myocardial infarction comes to you on pravastatin 20 mg in the morning. Her total cholesterol is 284, triglycerides are 146, LDL is 228, and HDL is 72. She recently had a stress thallium study that demonstrated no ischemic changes.

What treatment changes, if any, do you advise?

CASE 25-6

A 64-year-old man comes to your clinic for follow-up after being hospitalized 4 weeks ago for a "small heart attack." He has stopped smoking. He says he feels "terrific" and is walking 2 miles daily. He is taking atenolol 25 mg and an aspirin daily. He asks you if he should do anything else. Laboratory test values are: total cholesterol 198, TG 95, LDL 132, and HDL 45.

Does he need any further treatment at this time?

THYROID DISEASE

ETIOLOGY

What are the most likely causes of hyperthyroidism?

Graves' disease is commonly seen in young women and is due to an antibody that turns on the TSH receptor. *Toxic multinodular goiter* is seen in the elderly and occurs when one or more clones of cells grow into nontender, autonomous nodules. *Subacute thyroiditis* follows viral respiratory infection, causing painful, transient hyperthyroidism and elevated ESR. *Silent thyroiditis* may be a nonpainful variant of subacute thyroiditis occurring postpartum and is less clearly associated with viral infection or elevated ESR.

What causes hypothyroidism?

In more than 95% of cases, hypothyroidism is due to thyroid gland failure. *Iatrogenic* hypothyroidism from ablation or removal of the thyroid gland is the most common cause in developed nations. Worldwide, *iodine insufficiency* is most common, causing diffuse thyroid enlargement, or goiter. Where iodine is plentiful and the thyroid is intact, *Hashimoto's thyroiditis* is most common, an autoimmune disease associated with antimicrosomal antibodies against thyroid peroxidase. Hashimoto's may coexist with other autoimmune disorders, including

Sjögren's syndrome, diabetes, pernicious anemia, and lupus, and it can be complicated by lymphoma, especially in the few men with Hashimoto's. Less than 5% of hypothyroidism is secondary, usually resulting from *pituitary failure*. This diagnosis is important to make because thyroid replacement in panhypopituitarism can precipitate fatal adrenal insufficiency if no steroids are given.

What causes thyroid nodules?

Although thyroid nodules are recognized in about 5% of patients, autopsies show 50% prevalence. Approximately 5% to 10% of solitary thyroid nodules are malignant, most of which are papillary or follicular carcinomas—well-differentiated, slow-growing, and curable by resection when found early. Medullary thyroid carcinoma is uncommon and may be sporadic or inherited as part of a multiple endocrine neoplasia type II (MEN II) syndrome. Lymphoma rarely complicates Hashimoto's thyroiditis. Anaplastic carcinoma is rare but aggressive, with less than 1-year survival.

EVALUATION

What questions are pertinent if I suspect hyperthyroidism?

Ask about weight loss despite a healthy appetite, nervousness, emotional lability, sweating, tremor, palpitations, heat intolerance, frequent bowel movements, amenorrhea, and insomnia. Elderly patients may present less typically with "apathetic" hyperthyroidism with anorexia, weakness, blunted affect, depression, or slowed mentation. CHF, angina, or arrhythmias often dominate the clinical picture in the elderly, so ask a good cardiopulmonary review of systems.

How does thyroid storm present?

Thyroid storm is a life-threatening extreme presentation of hyperthyroidism. Decompensation in one or more organ systems occurs with fever as high as 106° F, delirium or even frank psychosis, seizures, tachyarrhythmia, angina, high-output cardiac failure, or cardiogenic shock. Precipitants include infection, surgery, iodine in contrast dyes or ablative therapy, amiodarone, and trauma.

What should I look for on examination when I suspect hyperthyroidism?

Observe for sweating, agitation, fine tremor, nail clubbing, and onycholysis (fingernail separation from the nail bed). Pretibial myxedema is seen rarely in Graves' disease. Palpate the thyroid: multiple nodules suggest multinodular goiter; diffuse enlargement is seen in more than 95% of those with Graves' disease; a tender,

hard gland suggests viral thyroiditis. Check pulse for tachycardia and arrhythmias. Ask patients to rise from a chair with arms crossed to detect proximal muscle weakness. Check for hyperreflexia, lid lag on oculomotor testing (white sclera visible above the iris with downward gaze), and widened palpebral fissures causing a frightened stare; these are all signs of sympathetic overstimulation that reverse with therapy for the hyperthyroid state. Check for exophthalmos (protrusion of the eyeballs) resulting from infiltration of eye muscles in Graves' disease. Unlike lid lag, exophthalmos does not reverse with treatment.

What history and examination suggest hypothyroidism?

Onset is often insidious and may be overlooked by patients and physicians because hypothyroidism can mimic normal aging. Hypothyroid patients are often fatigued (although most fatigued patients do not have hypothyroidism). Also ask about dry skin, menorrhagia, hoarseness, cold intolerance, muscle stiffness, weakness and cramping, depression, constipation, and weight gain. Anorexia and poor bowel motility may actually lead to weight loss, especially in the elderly. On examination, look for hypothermia; bradycardia; pale, cool, doughy skin; nonpitting diffuse myxedema; periorbital edema; coarse skin and hair; macroglossia; peripheral edema; bradycardia; or distant heart sounds, suggesting a pericardial effusion. Neurologic manifestations can include impaired mentation, dementia, ataxia, psychosis, carpal tunnel syndrome, "hung-up" reflexes with a delayed relaxation phase, and bradykinesia. Severe hypothyroidism may cause cardiac failure or coma.

What studies do I order if I suspect thyroid disease?

Order a TSH and free T_4. Other laboratory abnormalities that may accompany hypothyroidism include anemia, hypercholesterolemia, hyponatremia, elevated liver enzymes (e.g., SGOT), LDH, and CPK. Chest film may reveal cardiomegaly in hypothyroid patients caused by pericardial effusion. ECG may show bradycardia or decreased voltage (if pericardial effusion is present) with hypothyroidism; sinus tachycardia or possibly atrial fibrillation may accompany hyperthyroidism.

What does it mean if my patient has a high TSH?

TSH cannot be interpreted alone. The most common cause of a high TSH is an underactive thyroid gland (primary hypothyroidism). A concomitant low free T_4 confirms this. Because TSH is very sensitive to small changes in T_4, it may rise before a drop in T_4 is detected. This situation is called *subclinical hypothyroidism* because patients are usually asymptomatic. In rare cases, both free T_4 index and TSH will be high, implicating a TSH-producing pituitary or gynecologic tumor. TSH takes 4 to 6 weeks to reflect changes in thyroid hormone replacement.

Does a low TSH imply primary hyperthyroidism?

Yes, usually. This is confirmed by a high free T_4. In the rare instance in which both TSH and free T_4 are low with hypothyroid symptoms, secondary hypothyroidism from pituitary failure is likely.

When do I need to check a free T_3?

T_4 is the inactive form of hormone produced in the thyroid and converted to active T_3 in the periphery. Elevated T_3 can be missed if not specifically measured. If TSH is low in the setting of hyperthyroid symptoms but free T_4 is normal or low, obtain free T_3 to look for T_3 toxicosis.

When do I need to check antithyroid antibodies?

Most Hashimoto's and many Graves' disease patients have antimicrosomal and/or antithyroglobulin antibodies. Graves' patients may also have antithyroid receptor antibodies. Occasionally Graves' ophthalmopathy causes proptosis without hyperthyroidism; the presence of thyroid antibodies avoids further workup for retroorbital mass or vascular lesion. Patients with other autoimmune disorders can be checked for antithyroid antibodies to determine if frequent TSH monitoring is warranted.

How do I tell the difference between a malignant and benign thyroid nodule?

The strongest risk factor for thyroid malignancy is prior head and neck irradiation—one third of nodules in these high-risk patients are malignant. Other risk factors include male gender; family history; onset in childhood; rapid growth; hard, fixed, nontender nodule larger than 4 cm; hoarseness; local compressive symptoms; ipsilateral adenopathy; and a Delphian node in the midline just above the thyroid isthmus. *Fine-needle aspiration* (FNA) is the initial procedure of choice, with 90% sensitivity and 70% specificity. FNA yields a benign diagnosis in 70% to 80% of patients and a malignant diagnosis in 5%. The remaining 10% to 20% are nondiagnostic and require further workup, usually by surgical removal. Although ultrasound distinguishes solid from cystic lesions, this is not that useful because either could be malignant. Radioactive iodine scan identifies "hot" nodules (take up radiolabeled iodine) that are unlikely to be malignant. Unfortunately, only 10% of nodules are "hot," so this test avoids exploratory surgery in only 1 out of 10 patients with nondiagnostic FNA. Of the 90% of nodules (with nondiagnostic FNA) that are cold by scan,

20% are malignant, making surgical exploration mandatory in all cold nodules.

TREATMENT

What are the options for treatment of hyperthyroid patients?

Propranolol blocks sympathetic stimulation and decreases adrenergic and cardiac symptoms, although it may worsen CHF. Glucocorticoids shorten the course and decrease the pain of acute thyroiditis, although these are rarely needed. Correction of sustained hyperthyroidism is important to avoid the long-term sequelae of osteoporosis, cardiac arrhythmias, and CHF. For this, use *propylthiouracil* (PTU) or *methimazole* to decrease thyroid hormone production and release. PTU also blocks peripheral conversion of T_4 to active T_3. These antithyroid drugs can rarely cause agranulocytosis, especially in older patients. *Radioiodine ablation* is effective for both Graves' disease and multinodular goiter and leads to iatrogenic hypothyroidism 75% of the time. Check TSH periodically after ablation. *Surgical removal* of the thyroid gland is reserved for local compressive symptoms, failure to respond to other therapies, or possible malignancy.

How do I treat hypothyroid patients?

Asymptomatic subclinical hypothyroidism can be followed without therapy, although patients may feel better if it is treated. Start symptomatic patients on oral *thyroxine* at around 100 μg/day. Start more gingerly in the elderly (25 μg) to avoid precipitating angina or MI. Intravenous thyroxine is reserved for life-threatening myxedema coma.

When should I hospitalize a patient for thyroid disease?

Hypothyroid myxedema coma is an endocrine emergency presenting with stupor, hypothermia, bradycardia, and hypoventilation and may be associated with hypoglycemia, anemia, and hyponatremia. Treat in the hospital with parenteral levothyroxine, high-dose glucocorticoids to prevent adrenal crisis, and intensive supportive therapy. It may develop insidiously or be precipitated by infection, cold exposure, sedative drugs, or failure to take thyroid replacement. Life-threatening hyperthyroidism, or thyroid storm, also requires hospitalization for monitoring and initiation of antithyroid drugs, iodine to inhibit hormone release, glucocorticoids to decrease peripheral T_4 levels, and propranolol to decrease adrenergic effects and block peripheral conversion of T_4 to T_3. Iopanoic acid or ipodate (radiographic contrast agents) can be added to block hormone release and decrease peripheral T_4-to-T_3 conversion.

Key Points

- TSH is very sensitive: small changes in T_4 cause large changes in TSH.
- When TSH and free T_4 are abnormal in opposite directions, there is a primary thyroid problem.
- TSH levels take about 4 to 6 weeks to adjust to changes in therapy.
- The procedure of choice for the initial workup of a thyroid nodule is FNA.

CASE 25-7

A 75-year-old man is brought to your office by his daughter because he seems depressed and weak. He has been losing weight with a poor appetite, has become much less interactive, and is now unable to climb the 3 stairs to his room without assistance. On examination, he is a slender elderly man in no acute distress with a mild tremor; an irregular pulse of 100; a lumpy, nontender thyroid; and clear lung sounds.

A. What is your differential diagnosis?
B. TSH is less than 0.1, free T_4 is elevated. What thyroid condition is most likely?
C. What treatment do you want to offer him?

CASE 25-8

A 63-year-old woman is brought in to the ER. She was found slumped in her easy chair by her landlord after he noticed she had not paid her rent. On examination, she moans to painful stimuli, temperature is 34° F, pulse is 45, BP is 110/80, and RR is 6. Skin is cool, dry, and doughy; tongue is large; heart sounds are inaudible; lungs reveal diffuse rales; rectal vault contains hardened pellets of stool; and chest x-ray reveals a massive heart, pleural fluid, and pulmonary vascular cephalization.

A. What is your differential diagnosis for her altered mental status?
B. TSH is 95, and free T_4 is low. Name your diagnosis and seven features of her presentation to support it.
C. How will you manage this patient?
D. What other laboratory tests are likely to be abnormal?
E. What are likely causes of her hypothyroidism?

Gastroenterology

BILIARY TRACT DISEASE

ETIOLOGY

What are causes of biliary tract disease?

Blockage of the bile ducts leads to cholecystitis or cholangitis. Blockage is usually due to gallstones. Rarer causes include extrinsic compression by tumor or adenopathy, cholangiocarcinoma, or primary sclerosing cholangitis (PSC). Cholecystitis is inflammation or infection of the gallbladder from obstruction of the cystic duct, usually by a gallstone. Cholangitis is a deadly infection arising in the common bile duct resulting from ductal obstruction; the gall bladder is uninvolved. PSC causes inflammation and scarring from unclear cause. PSC leaves the biliary ducts thickened and irregularly narrowed and eventually causes cirrhosis and hepatic failure. Patients with ulcerative colitis are at risk for PSC.

EVALUATION

What is a pertinent history?

The classic patient with gallstones is "fat, fertile, 40, and female," a derogatory but accurate characterization. Cholecystitis starts with postprandial right upper quadrant pain, which is worse with fatty food ingestion, as much as 3 to 4 hours after eating. As the condition worsens, pain becomes steady, often radiating to the right shoulder. High fever is rare. In contrast, cholangitis is a gastrointestinal emergency, presenting with a triad of high spiking fevers with rigors, jaundice, and right upper quadrant pain. If tumor is obstructing the common bile duct, painless jaundice may develop gradually over weeks before onset of infection. When bile flow to the intestine is completely obstructed, urine is dark (bilirubinuria) and stools are light. More than 30% of patients have concomitant pancreatitis with pain radiating to the back. With PSC, patients have intermit-

tent flares of jaundice, pruritus, right upper quadrant pain, and, sometimes, frank cholangitis.

What do I look for on physical examination?

Fever, tachycardia, hypotension, right upper quadrant pain, and guarding can occur with both cholecystitis and cholangitis. Peritoneal signs are usually absent. Jaundice is a feature of cholangitis but is absent in cholecystitis. Approximately 50% of patients with cholecystitis have a palpably enlarged gallbladder. The classic examination finding is Murphy's sign: Palpate the liver edge deeply at the midclavicular line and ask patient to inhale. When the inflamed gallbladder meets the hand, the patient abruptly stops breathing in. Sensitivity and specificity are low for this maneuver.

What laboratory tests and studies should I order?

The hallmark of ductal blockage is elevated alkaline phosphatase, GGT, and bilirubin. When either cholecystitis or cholangitis is suspected, order CBC, blood cultures, LFTs, amylase, and an imaging test. Common bile duct dilation on ultrasound or CT suggests cholangitis; a thickened, edematous gallbladder wall suggests cholecystitis. If cholecystitis is suspected but ultrasound is normal, a radionuclide scan can confirm cholecystitis by absence of uptake in the gallbladder. Endoscopic retrograde cholangiopancreatography (ERCP) confirms PSC by the beaded appearance of the bile ducts, or cholangiocarcinoma by biopsy.

TREATMENT

What treatment steps are appropriate for patients with cholecystitis or cholangitis?

For cholecystitis or cholangitis, start broad-spectrum IV antibiotics to cover gram-negative enterics, gram-positives *(Clostridium, Enterococcus)*, and anaerobes *(Bacteroides)*. Perform volume resuscitation as needed. Cholecystis may respond to antibiotics alone and warrants later elective cholecystectomy; asymptomatic gallstones do not require removal. Worsening fever or leukocytosis warrants urgent cholecystectomy. For cholangitis, consult GI immediately for emergent ERCP with sphincterotomy to decompress the common bile duct.

Do most patients get better from cholecystitis and cholangitis?

Cholangitis is fatal if untreated. Approximately 25% of cholecystitis requires urgent surgery. Complications of cholecystitis include empyema, gangrene, and gallbladder perforation (mortality 30%). Suspect coexisting pancreatitis with pleural effusion or pain left of the midline or radiating to the back.

Key Points

- Right upper quadrant pain, high fever, and jaundice indicate cholangitis until proven otherwise.
- Cholangitis is a GI emergency and warrants urgent imaging and GI consultation.

CASE 26-1

A 49-year-old woman with obesity, diabetes, and hypertension has had several hours of severe, steady abdominal pain with an episode of emesis. Temperature is 102° F, pulse is 120, BP is 100/80, and RR is 28. Her abdomen is obese with right upper quadrant tenderness.

A. *What information do you need to narrow your differential diagnosis (history, examination, laboratory tests)?*

B. *Which of the diseases on your list of possibilities is most worrisome? Which is most likely?*

C. *Where do you want to take care of her?*

D. *What intervention is most important right now?*

LIVER DISEASE

ETIOLOGY

How is liver disease categorized?

Liver disease is categorized by whether it affects the biliary tree or the cells of the liver parenchyma. Biliary tree disorders generally elevate alkaline phosphatase and bilirubin. Hepatocellular injury elevates liver transaminases (ALT, AST) more dramatically than bilirubin or alkaline phosphatase. This chapter focuses on causes of hepatocellular and parenchymal injury.

What are the causes of elevated transaminases?

Transaminases greater than 1000 are caused by viral hepatitis, drug-induced hepatitis, or ischemic hepatitis. Other causes of hepatocellular injury raising transaminases more modestly include alcohol, autoimmune disorders, inherited storage disorders, tumors, and nonalcoholic steatohepatitis.

What epidemiologic features distinguish the major causes of viral hepatitis?

Viral hepatitis epidemiology is summarized in Table 26-1. Hepatitis A and E are passed by the fecal-oral route, whereas hepatitis B, C, and D are acquired parenterally, usually through sexual contact, transfusion, or injection drug use. *Hepatitis A virus* (HAV) is endemic in developing countries, where it causes approximately 35% of cases of acute viral hepatitis. Infection with *hepatitis B virus* (HBV) is often asymptomatic. Few infected individuals develop chronic infection unless infection was acquired perinatally. *Hepatitis C virus* (HCV) is the most common chronic bloodborne infection in the United States, with 60% of transmission resulting from IV drug use. Unlike hepatitis B, most individuals with hepatitis C develop chronic infection. The course of infection is insidious,

---

TABLE 26-1

Epidemiologic Features of Viral Hepatitis

VIRUS	TRANSMISSION	RISK FACTORS	% WHO BECOME CHRONIC CARRIERS	INCUBATION PERIOD (DAYS)
A	Fecal-oral	Travel in developing countries	None	15-60
B	Parenteral	IV drug use, male-male sex, health care worker, unprotected sex	10% (80% if perinatal)	45-160
C	Parenteral	Same as HBV, but sexual transmission much less	80%	14-180
D	Parenteral	IV drug use, coinfection with HBV, unprotected sex	2%-70%	42-180
E	Fecal-oral	No cases seen in U.S.	None	15-60

and most patients do not notice any symptoms during the first two decades of infection. *Hepatitis D virus* (HDV) requires coinfection with HBV to replicate. Seroprevalence is low in the United States except in IV drug users and recipients of multiple transfusions. *Hepatitis E virus* (HEV) infection is usually inconsequential and self-limited, although mortality rates greater than 30% have been seen in women infected during the third trimester of pregnancy.

What are the most important causes of chronic liver disease?

Chronic liver disease is any condition that causes hepatic inflammation for longer than 6 months and is the tenth-leading cause of death among adults in the United States. The most common causes include chronic viral hepatitis from HBV and HCV. Other causes include alcohol, autoimmune disease, drugs, hemochromatosis, Wilson's disease, and α_1-antitrypsin deficiency. Each of these disorders can lead to cirrhosis, with alcohol abuse as the leading cause.

How does alcohol cause liver damage?

The pathogenesis is unknown. The spectrum of disease includes fatty liver infiltration, alcoholic hepatitis, and cirrhosis. Cirrhosis occurs more frequently in individuals who have a history of alcoholic hepatitis and continue to drink.

What drugs cause hepatocellular injury?

Methyldopa, acetaminophen, NSAIDs, trazodone, phenytoin, nitrofurantoin, isoniazid, antilipid agents (statins and fibrates), and sulfonamides are associated with drug-induced hepatitis.

What is autoimmune hepatitis?

Autoimmune hepatitis causes liver inflammation. Although autoantibodies are often found, they do not directly cause the hepatitis. Types 1 is responsible for 80% of adult cases in the United States. Most of type 1 occurs in young women, whereas type 2 is more common in children.

What are some of the inherited causes of liver disease?

Autosomal recessive causes of liver disease include α_1-antitrypsin deficiency, hemochromatosis, and Wilson's disease. α_1-Antitrypsin deficiency causes emphysema, chronic hepatitis, and eventual cirrhosis. Hemochromatosis is caused by abnormally increased intestinal iron absorption with resulting iron deposition in a variety of organs (liver, heart, pancreas, and pituitary). In Wilson's disease, impaired copper excretion into the bile results in accumulation of copper in the liver and other tissues, resulting in cirrhosis and/or neuropsychiatric abnormalities. A new diagnosis of Wilson's disease is extremely rare in patients older than 35 years of age.

What are the complications of cirrhosis?

Cirrhosis leads to fibrosis of the liver parenchyma with increased vascular resistance in the hepatic sinusoids, resulting in increased resistance to portal blood flow. This is referred to as *portal hypertension*. Associated clinical features may include esophageal varices as blood detours around the liver through small vessels in the esophagus, massive GI bleeding if these varices rupture, ascites resulting from leakage of fluid from the portal system, spontaneous bacterial peritonitis, hepatic encephalopathy, hepatorenal syndrome, and hepatocellular cancer.

EVALUATION

When should I suspect chronic liver disease?

Presentation is often insidious and nonspecific with fatigue, anorexia, and/or pruritus.

What components of the clinical history are pertinent?

Assess risk factors for viral hepatitis (i.e., IV drug use, prior transfusion, occupational exposure, sexual behavior, travel history, and birthplace). Ask about toxin exposure, including alcohol and medications. Family history of liver or autoimmune disease is also pertinent.

What clues to liver disease should I look for on physical examination?

Scleral icterus is visible when bilirubin level is greater than 3 mg/dl. Most patients remain anicteric until acute exacerbation or end-stage disease occurs. Other signs of chronic liver disease result from cirrhosis and include spider angiomata, palmar erythema, Terry's nails (dark red distal nail, pale proximal nail), gynecomastia, and jaundice. Advanced disease with postnecrotic cirrhosis and severe hepatic fibrosis causes portal hypertension and, beyond a critical threshold, results in ascites, caput medusa (engorged vessels around the umbilicus), bleeding esophageal varices, severe hemorrhoids, muscle wasting, encephalopathy, and peripheral edema.

What laboratory tests should I order when I suspect chronic liver disease?

Liver enzymes (also called *liver transaminases* or *aminotransferases*) are sensitive indicators of liver injury. These include alanine aminotransferase (ALT) and aspartate aminotransferase (AST). The ALT is more specific for liver injury, whereas the AST may be elevated because of skeletal, cardiac, and liver muscle injury or injury to the brain and kidney. Transaminases are elevated with all causes of hepatitis. The degree of elevation is usually higher in acute than in chronic injury and does not correlate with the severity of liver injury. Acute viral hepatitis can cause transaminase elevations up to 100 times normal. In contrast, alcohol-induced hepatitis usually elevates transaminases to about 2 to 3 times normal, with a characteristic AST/ALT ratio of 2:1. Once you detect liver disease, continue workup with viral hepatitis antibody screening. If viral serologies are negative, look further for storage or autoimmune disorders (see below). For patients with alcohol use that is mild or who deny a previously applied diagnosis of alcohol-induced liver disease, have a low threshold for ruling out other treatable causes of liver disease.

What laboratory tests can I use to assess the severity of liver disease?

Because aminotransferase levels do not correlate with the degree of injury, use albumin and prothrombin time to assess hepatic biosynthetic function. Albumin less than 3 g/dl or an increased prothrombin time (longer than 11 to 16 seconds) indicate significantly reduced hepatic function.

How do I interpret hepatitis serologic profiles?

Some general rules are helpful: antigen is present with active infection, either acute or chronic; IgM antibodies signal early response to acute infection; and IgG antibodies develop later in infection and persist with chronic infection or resolution (Table 26-2). Because the risk of chronic carrier state is so high with HCV, positive antibody tests are usually presumed to indicate chronic infection. Active HCV infection can be confirmed by testing for HCV RNA viral load, although the test is not currently FDA approved for this use.

When should I screen for hemochromatosis?

Screen all first-degree relatives of affected patients for iron overload with serum iron, ferritin, or transferrin saturation. Also screen patients with chronic liver disease and negative workup for viral cause. Elevated ferritin or a transferrin saturation greater than 55% requires liver biopsy to confirm the diagnosis. Be aware that other causes of chronic liver disease may also elevate these tests,

TABLE 26-2
Interpretation of Serologic Tests for Viral Hepatitis

TEST	INTERPRETATION
HEPATITIS A	
IgM antibody	Acute infection
IgG antibody	Past infection
HEPATITIS B	
Surface antigen (Hb$_s$Ag)	Acute or chronic infection
Envelope antigen (Hb$_e$Ag)	Correlates with higher infectivity
IgM antibody against core protein (Hb$_c$IgM)	Acute infection
IgG antibody against core protein (Hb$_c$IgG)	Prior infection or vaccination
HEPATITIS C	
IgG antibody	Infection, likely chronic
Viral load	Active infection

making interpretation challenging. Some physicians advocate screening the general population given the high prevalence of heterozygotes and the therapeutic efficacy of phlebotomy in preventing cirrhosis. This is currently not an established standard, although it may be soon.

What laboratory tests suggest autoimmune hepatitis?

Type 1 autoimmune hepatitis is characterized by hypergammaglobulinemia, antinuclear antibody (ANA), and anti-smooth muscle antibody (ASMA). Type 2 is characterized by antibody to liver/kidney microsome type 1 (anti-LKM1) without ANA and ASMA. Either type may be accompanied by other autoimmune diseases, although this is more common with type 2.

What laboratory tests do I use to diagnose Wilson's disease?

Wilson's lowers serum ceruloplasmin to less than 20 mg/dl and increases urinary copper excretion, although up to 20% of patients with Wilson's have a normal ceruloplasmin. Kayser-Fleischer rings, a single brownish line on the outer edge of the cornea seen by slit lamp, are pathognomonic.

Should I screen for hepatocellular carcinoma in patients with chronic liver disease?

In areas in which hepatitis B is endemic, one half of hepatocellular carcinoma patients are Hb$_s$Ag-positive. A similar risk pattern is seen with HCV infection. Cirrhosis of any cause is associated with the development of hepatocellular carcinoma. α-Fetoprotein and imaging studies, such as ultrasound or CT, are used to detect hepatocellular carcinoma. However, there is no evidence that screening increases the rate of detecting potentially curable tumors.

When should a patient be referred for liver biopsy?

Use liver biopsy to confirm hemochromatosis and Wilson's disease or to determine eligibility for antiviral therapy in hepatitis B or C. Biopsy is also a prognostic tool: patients with evidence of portal or mild periportal hepatitis tend to have a benign course; those with bridging or multilobular necrosis or cirrhosis are at a high risk of progressive disease.

TREATMENT

What treatments are available for chronic viral hepatitis?

The treatment of chronic viral hepatitis is a rapidly evolving field. α-Interferon is FDA approved for the treatment of both hepatitis B and C. This treatment is expensive and has multiple side effects, including flu-like symptoms, fatigue, bone marrow suppression, and neuropsychiatric effects. With hepatitis B, treatment is reserved for those with active viral replication and elevated aminotransferases. From 30% to 40% of treated individuals respond to therapy, as evidenced by loss of Hb_eAg and a return of the serum ALT to normal. Interferon is recommended for chronic hepatitis C in patients at the greatest risk for the progression to cirrhosis, as evidenced by elevated ALT levels, detectable HCV RNA, and liver biopsy findings of either portal or bridging fibrosis. Approximately 50% of treated individuals have normalization of ALT levels, and 33% have loss of detectable HCV RNA. Unfortunately, 50% relapse when therapy is stopped, and only 15% to 25% have a sustained response. Recent studies show benefit from combination therapy with interferon and ribavirin in patients with chronic hepatitis C and relapse after interferon treatment. Refer patients to a hepatologist for consideration of inclusion in clinical trials. Advise patients with chronic hepatitis of any type to abstain from all alcohol ingestion to prevent accelerated progression to cirrhosis.

What treatments are available for drug-induced or autoimmune hepatitis?

Stop the drug and watch to make sure liver function tests and clinical symptoms improve. For autoimmune disease, steroids prolong survival and may be augmented with azathioprine.

What is the treatment for alcoholic liver disease?

Stop the use of alcohol; there may be reversal of liver damage.

How do I treat the complications of cirrhosis?

Esophageal variceal hemorrhage is treated with endoscopic variceal banding (preferred) or sclerotherapy. Transjugular intrahepatic portal systemic shunt (TIPS) has been used to decompress portal hypertension, which often stops refractory or recurrent variceal bleeding. Treat *ascites* with sodium restriction to less than 2 g per day. A loop diuretic, such as furosemide, and/or an aldosterone antagonist, such as spironolactone, can be added. Use large-volume paracentesis for tense ascites in symptomatic patients in whom diuretics fail or are contraindicated. The mainstay of treatment for *hepatic encephalopathy* is lactulose, which facilitates the removal of ammonium ion. *Hepatorenal syndrome* with oliguria and poor renal perfusion causing a renal sodium concentration less than 10 mEq/L is a grave prognostic sign. There is no treatment other than temporizing with dialysis while awaiting liver transplantation. Hepatocellular tumors can be resected if they involve only one lobe of the liver. Otherwise, elective palliative therapy involves angiographic embolization of affected areas.

How do I treat hemochromatosis?

Treat hemochromatosis with phlebotomy, removing 500 ml 1 to 2 times per month to a goal hemoglobin less than 11 g/dl and ferritin less than 100 ng/ml. This prevents iron overload and cirrhosis.

Who should be referred for liver transplantation?

Patients with end-stage liver disease or fulminant hepatic failure should be referred early to transplant centers for consideration of liver transplantation. Waiting lists are long, and patients must fulfill specific criteria, including mental stability, psychosocial support, probability that they will survive the operation, and funding. Contraindications include alcohol intake over the preceding 6 months, other substance abuse, AIDS, infection outside the hepatobiliary system, metastatic liver disease, hepatic carcinoma, and uncorrectable coagulopathies.

How can I prevent hepatitis?

Vaccines are available for both hepatitis A and B. The hepatitis A vaccine is given in 2 doses 6 to 12 months apart and is recommended for travelers to endemic areas, military personnel, people with chronic liver disease, and persons engaging in high-risk sexual activity. Hepatitis B vaccine is given in 3 doses, spaced by 1 and 6 months. It is recommended in infants, persons at occupational risk, sexually active young adults, IV drug users, inmates of correctional facilities, hemodialysis patients, international travelers, and populations where HBV is endemic.

> ## Key Points
> - The most common presenting symptoms of liver disease are fatigue, anorexia, and pruritus.
> - Hepatitis C is the most common chronic bloodborne infection in the United States, with the majority of patients unaware that they are infected.
> - Prothrombin time, not liver enzymes, reflects the degree of liver injury.
> - Use liver biopsy for diagnosis and prognosis, and to plan and assess treatment.

CASE 26-2

A 70-year-old man comes to clinic reporting that he and his friends have noted that he has looked yellow for the last week. He reports feeling quite tired and is particularly bothered by generalized itching. His stool is light in color, and he thinks that his urine looks brown. He has not been eating because of loss of appetite.
  A. What is your differential diagnosis?
  B. What laboratory tests would be useful in determining the cause of his illness?
  C. What other information would be useful?

CASE 26-3

A 42-year-old woman and former IV drug user reports feeling tired lately. She has been working long hours as a bartender and stays late after work to share a beer with her co-workers. On examination, the right upper quadrant is tender. Liver function tests show a slightly elevated ALT and AST, bilirubin is 1.4 mg/dl, albumin is 3.0 g/dl, and prothrombin INR is 1.8.
  A. What further diagnostic studies are indicated?
  B. Read answer to A for test results and then decide what further studies are indicated.
  C. Read answer to B. What advice do you give this patient regarding her treatment options?

PANCREATITIS

ETIOLOGY

Causes of acute pancreatitis are listed in Table 26-3, with no cause identified in 15% to 20% of cases. Pancreatitis can become chronic if the underlying cause is not treated.

TABLE 26-3
Causes of Pancreatitis

COMMON	UNCOMMON
Alcohol	Drugs (ddI, ddC, d4T, trimethoprim/
Gallstones	sulfamethoxazole, tetracycline,
	thiazides, pentamidine)
	Viral
	Triglycerides >1000
	Idiopathic
	Trauma

EVALUATION

How do patients with pancreatitis present?

Patients report severe, steady epigastric pain, often radiating to the back, worse with lying down, and relieved by sitting up. Nausea and vomiting are common and exacerbated by eating. If pancreatic edema or gallstones occlude the common bile duct, jaundice ensues.

What do I look for on physical examination?

Look for tachycardia, hypotension, volume depletion resulting from third spacing of fluids, or low-grade fever of inflammation or infection. The abdomen is diffusely tender. Retroperitoneal pancreatic hemorrhage manifests as bruising around the umbilicus (Cullen's sign) or flank (Turner's sign).

What tests should I order?

Order CBC, amylase or lipase, chemistry panel, calcium, liver function tests, triglycerides, and x-rays of the abdomen. Pancreatic calcifications on x-ray are pathognomonic for chronic pancreatitis. Ultrasound or CT scan confirms diagnosis (see Figure 6-3, C).

TREATMENT

Use bowel rest (nothing to eat) and IV fluids. Place nasogastric tube to low-intermittent suction if vomiting is present. ERCP will relieve an obstructing gallstone but may worsen pancreatic inflammation. Watch for complications of pseudocyst, abscess, sepsis, and adult respiratory distress syndrome. Severely ill patients may benefit from broad-spectrum antibiotics (imipenem or cefuroxime). Refer for elective cholecystectomy when the pancreatitis resolves if stones were the cause. Mortality is 10% overall in patients hospitalized with pancreatitis. Ranson's criteria have been used to predict mortality rates (Box 26-1).

BOX 26-1   Ranson's Criteria Predict
              Mortality Rates*

INITIAL EVALUATION
Age >55 years
WBC >16,000
SGOT >250
LDH >350
Glucose >200

CHANGES IN THE FIRST 48 HOURS
HCT drop >10%
BUN rise >5 mg/dl
Ca <8
Pao$_2$ <60
Base deficit >4

*Mortality is 2% with 0-2 criteria, 40% with 5-6 criteria, nearly 100% with >7 criteria.

Key Points

- Pancreatitis radiates to the back, whereas cholecystitis radiates to the right shoulder.
- Gallstone disease and alcohol abuse are the two main causes of pancreatitis.

CASE 26-4

A 45-year-old man has several hours of severe abdominal pain radiating to the back with emesis worsened by eating. He smokes half a pack of cigarettes and drinks at least a 6-pack of beer daily. Pulse is 90, BP is 145/90, temperature is 99° F, R is 20. His upper mid-abdomen is very tender, and you cannot find any costovertebral angle or point tenderness on his back.

A. Name three possible causes of abdominal pain that are associated with back pain.
B. Which of the three diagnoses you named is most likely for this patient and why?
C. What will help you confirm your diagnosis and assess his prognosis?
D. His amylase is 500 (normal 20-90), WBC is 19, SGOT is 300, and glucose is 160, and he has several more episodes of emesis. What treatment is warranted now?

27

Geriatrics

BENIGN PROSTATIC HYPERPLASIA

ETIOLOGY

What causes benign prostatic hyperplasia?

Benign prostatic hyperplasia (BPH), a nonmalignant enlargement of the prostate, is caused by excessive cellular growth of both glandular and stromal elements of the prostate. Increasing evidence suggests that BPH is an endocrinopathy related to dihydrotestosterone (DHT, the chief intracellular androgen) and aging.

EVALUATION

How do I make the diagnosis of BPH?

The diagnosis of BPH is suggested by symptoms that reflect bladder irritation (i.e., urinary frequency, urgency, nocturia) and obstruction (i.e., hesitancy, straining, weak stream/dribbling, retention). Rule out other conditions causing these symptoms (e.g., prostatitis, urethral stricture or infection, prostate or bladder cancers) by history, rectal examination, and urinalysis.

How can I gauge the severity of my patient's BPH?

The American Urological Association (AUA) Symptom Index is a valid and reliable indicator of symptom severity using seven questions regarding specific symptoms (Box 27-1). Peak urine flow (normal >15 ml/sec) and postvoid residual can be useful to gauge disease severity. Prostate size does not correlate well with symptom severity or the degree of obstruction.

Besides symptoms, are there any other serious problems associated with BPH?

Long-standing BPH can infrequently cause urinary retention, renal insufficiency, urinary tract infections, gross hematuria, and/or bladder stones. If these occur, surgery is generally indicated.

TREATMENT

How do I decide when and how to treat BPH?

BPH is a disease that primarily affects quality of life, and thus patient perception of symptom severity (AUA Symptom Score) is a major determinant in making treatment decisions. Treatment options range from watchful waiting to surgery (Figure 27-1).

What are the differences between the drugs used in the medical management of BPH?

Two classes of medication can improve symptoms. α-*Adrenergic blockers,* such as doxazosin, terazosin, and tamsulosin, work rapidly over several weeks to block α_1-adrenergic receptors in the bladder neck and prostate that constrict outflow. Side effects in 5% to 10% of patients include orthostatic hypotension and weakness. Tamsulosin selectively blocks prostatic α-receptors and causes less asthenia, dizziness, and hypotension but can cause more retrograde ejaculation. *Finasteride* requires 6 to 12 months for benefit, decreases prostatic DHT, and shrinks prostate size by about 20%. In patients with enlarged prostates, finasteride reduces urinary retention and need for surgery. This medication may be less useful in patients without prostatic enlargement. Finasteride has fewer side effects than α-blockers (decreased libido, impotence in 3% to 4%). *Invasive or surgical interventions* offer benefit for patients in whom medical therapy fails

---

BOX 27-1   The American Urological Association Symptom Index for Patients with BPH

OVER THE PAST MONTH, HOW OFTEN HAVE YOU . . .

1. Had the sensation of not emptying your bladder completely?
2. Had to urinate again within 2 hours of last void (frequency)?
3. Stopped and started again several times while urinating?
4. Found it difficult to postpone urination (urge)?
5. Had a weak urinary stream?
6. Had to push or strain to begin urination?
7. Had to get up to urinate after going to bed?

ANSWER OPTIONS:
0 = Not at all
1 = Less than 1 time in 5
2 = Less than half the time
3 = Half the time
4 = More than half the time
5 = Almost always

SYMPTOM SCORE (SUM OF ANSWERS):
0-7: Mild BPH
8-19: Moderate BPH
20-35: Severe BPH

---

*Adapted from Berry, et al: *J Urol* 148:1541-1547, 1992. Used with permission from the AUA.

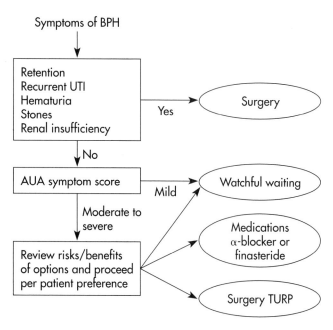

Figure 27-1 Treatment algorithm for benign prostatic hyperplasia.

but entail risks, including impotence, incontinence, blood loss requiring transfusion, and infection. The most common surgical procedure is transurethral resection of the prostate (TURP).

Key Points ··

- Use history and directed examination to detect and assess severity of BPH.
- In the absence of clear surgical indications, patient symptoms and preferences should guide interventions for BPH.

DEMENTIA

ETIOLOGY

What are the three most common causes of dementia in older adults?

Alzheimer's disease accounts for about two thirds of dementia cases. Traditionally, multiinfarct dementia accounts for about 15% to 25%. However, recent studies suggest that vascular dementia may be overdiagnosed and that a previously underdiagnosed entity, Lewy Body disease, may account for up to 15% to 25% of cases. Alcohol, at 10%, is the third most common cause in some studies.

What are the most common causes of "reversible dementia"?

Drugs and depression ("pseudodementia") are by far the most common reversible causes. After drugs and depression, only 5% of remaining cases are potentially treatable; 1% or less are truly fully reversible. The most common potentially reversible causes are vitamin B_{12} deficiency, hypothyroidism, and normal-pressure hydrocephalus. Dementia is often only partially reversed with treatment of these conditions (perhaps because they often coexist with Alzheimer's disease).

EVALUATION

How does one establish the diagnosis of dementia?

Although a hallmark sign, memory deficits alone are not sufficient to diagnose dementia. Impairments must exist in at least one other cognitive area (e.g., language, motor skills, personality), at a level severe enough to interfere with usual function. The mini-mental state examination (MMSE) is one way to objectively measure and document cognitive impairment.

What is the appropriate workup for a patient suspected of having dementia?

Perform a thorough history and examination with focus on neurologic and mental status. Obtain CBC, electrolytes, BUN, creatinine, liver function tests, vitamin B_{12}, thyroid screen, and syphilis serology. Although optional, most experts recommend a noncontrast head CT to rule out tumor, subdural hematoma, or hydrocephalus. Brain imaging is required for patients with focal neurologic signs, headache, or other atypical features. Lumbar puncture and electroencephalogram (EEG) are not routinely required.

What red flags increase the likelihood of a diagnosis other than Alzheimer's disease?

Sudden onset or onset at a younger age (especially age <60), a history of rapid cognitive decline over weeks to months rather than years, or the presence of focal neurologic signs or symptoms increases the chance of a diagnosis other than Alzheimer's disease.

TREATMENT

What are the basic management approaches to patients with dementia?

Review and discontinue drugs likely to impair cognition. Consider depression and a trial of selective serotonin reuptake inhibitor (SSRI) therapy. Diagnose and treat coexisting medical conditions that, although not the cause of cognitive impairment, can affect mood and function. Use nonpharmacologic approaches to improve patient function and behavior, along with caregiver education, support, and respite.

What pharmacologic treatments are available to patients with Alzheimer's dementia?

Primary treatments currently available are the cholinesterase inhibitors, such as donepezil. These agents can improve cognitive function and, in some studies, behavior and overall function. Vitamin E and ginkgo biloba have slowed the rate of decline in Alzheimer's disease in randomized trials. Estrogen and antiinflammatory agents may also delay onset and slow decline of Alzheimer's disease, but confirmatory randomized trials are needed.

How about managing common behavioral problems such as agitation and sleep problems?

Nonpharmacologic strategies may work as well, if not better, than medications. Seek out and address medication side effects, infection, injury or pain, exacerbation of preexisting illness, or inconsistency in the environment that may be causing agitation. Low-dose neuroleptics (haloperidol 0.5 mg, risperidone 0.5 mg, or thioridazine 10 mg at night) may be helpful for persistent hallucinations or delusions. Trazodone may be useful for sleep problems.

Key Points

- Most dementia is not reversible; Alzheimer's disease is the most common cause.
- Drugs and depression are the most common potentially reversible causes of dementia.
- Function and behavior are optimized through excellent general medical care, nonpharmacologic interventions, and the judicious use of drugs.

POLYPHARMACY

ETIOLOGY

Why do older adults have more adverse drug effects than younger patients?

Most studies on the efficacy and safety of medications exclude the very old (age >75) and those with multiple medical problems. As a result, the benefits, risks, and dosages of drugs seen in younger, healthier populations may not apply to older patients. Older adults are at higher risk for adverse effects because they take more medications (30% take at least 4 drugs) and have more underlying disease. Older adults also have altered pharmacokinetics (e.g., reduced renal clearance not accurately reflected by serum creatinine) and pharmacodynamics (e.g., more sensitive to warfarin, psychoactive drugs). Finally, polypharmacy decreases compliance, with its own adverse effects.

EVALUATION

When should I suspect an adverse effect from drugs/polypharmacy?

Always suspect drugs as a cause of new symptoms. Adverse consequences are often nonspecific, such as dizziness, falls, confusion, or altered bowel and bladder function. Particularly scrutinize hospitalized patients because up to 25% of admissions of older adults are for drug-related problems—most often resulting from adverse effects rather than patient errors or noncompliance.

Are particular medications more commonly associated with adverse effects in the elderly?

Problematic drugs include antihypertensives, NSAIDs, H_2-blockers, tricyclic antidepressants, narcotics, and sedatives. These agents are often clearly medically indicated; they are mentioned here to increase vigilance rather than prohibit their use. Review over-the-counter agents, as well.

TREATMENT

How can I best avoid polypharmacy and adverse drug events in elderly patients?

Regardless of age, the risk for adverse reactions increases with each added medication. Thus, be particularly judicious when initiating drugs in the elderly. Try to limit patients to at most four drugs, which is often difficult in patients with multiple chronic conditions. Start at the lowest recommended dose. Carefully assess for drug interactions and for dosage changes necessitated by altered metabolism. Calculate creatinine clearance rather than relying on serum creatinine to assess renal function. Use Medisets, simple regimens, and patient education to reduce patient errors.

How can I safely withdraw medications in older adults?

Although some drugs require slow tapering to avoid physiologic withdrawal (e.g., steroids or drugs that interact with receptors, such as β-blockers, benzodiazepines, antidepressants), do not be reluctant to carefully withdraw drugs whenever problematic polypharmacy is suspected. In one study of drug reduction among older adults, about 1 in 4 medications was stopped and 74% of drug discontinuations occurred without incident; no deaths were associated with the infrequent disease exacerbations that did occur when medications were stopped.

URINARY INCONTINENCE

ETIOLOGY

What are the basic categories of urinary incontinence?

Keeping in mind that mixed etiologies are common, there are four basic categories, each with characteristic symptoms and risk factors (Table 27-1).

What are the common causes of acute (sudden onset, usually reversible) incontinence?

Remember reversible causes with the mnemonic DRIP (Box 27-2). Frequently implicated drugs include diuretics, agents that impair bladder contractility by anticholinergic effects, and narcotics. Isolated nocturnal incontinence is often from volume overload states (CHF, lower extremity edema) resulting from the supine diuresis that occurs when these patients are recumbent.

EVALUATION

What is the best way to discern the cause of my patient's incontinence?

If incontinence is new or suddenly worse, consider DRIP causes. If incontinence persists, inquire about timing and volume of urine loss and about specific symptoms related to urge or stress incontinence, outlet obstruction, and functional problems. Because the bladder control reflex arc is located at S2-S4, focus the examination on relevant neurologic evaluation of sacral dermatomes and lower extremity function. Also perform rectal (impaction, prostate, sphincter tone, anal wink) and pelvic examinations (atrophy, vaginitis, prolapse). Assess for volume-overloaded state, cognitive impairment, and/or physical impairment. Send for urinalysis, glucose, BUN/creatinine, and calcium. Obtain postvoid residual (PVR); greater than 100 ml is likely overflow, whereas less than 100 ml is likely urge or stress incontinence.

Key Points ································
- The biggest risk factor for adverse drug events is number of medications prescribed.
- Compliance decreases with the number of drugs that an individual takes.
- With careful monitoring, many medications can be safely stopped in older adults.

BOX 27-2   Common Reversible Causes of Acute Incontinence, by the Mnemonic "DRIP"

D	Drugs, delirium
R	Restricted mobility, retention
I	Infection, fecal impaction
P	Polyuric states, such as CHF, diabetes

TABLE 27-1
Categorization, Symptoms, and Treatment of Urinary Incontinence

TYPE	MECHANISMS AND RISK FACTORS	SYMPTOMS	TREATMENT
Stress	Weak sphincter, altered pelvic muscle strength from multiple childbirths or vaginal atrophy	Small-volume leakage with cough, laugh, bending	Pelvic muscle exercises Estrogen α-Agonists Refer (periurethral injections, surgery)
Urge	Detrusor hyperreflexia: ↓ CNS inhibitory input to bladder (Parkinson's, stroke) Detrusor instability: ↑ bladder contraction from local causes (UTI, stone, early obstruction)	Sudden urge, large-volume leakage	Scheduled voiding Avoid irritants (caffeine, alcohol) Bladder muscle relaxing agent (e.g., oxybutynin)
Overflow	Poor bladder emptying from obstruction (e.g., BPH, stricture) or poor contractility (e.g., diabetic neuropathy)	Hesitancy, dribbling, small-volume leakage	α-Blockers or finasteride for BPH Refer to urology
Functional	Physical or cognitive impairment	Inability to get to toilet	Scheduled voiding Adapt environment (e.g., commode, urinal)

TREATMENT

What are common treatment approaches, and how successful are they?

Over 50% of patients are cured, and most others are markedly improved with standard therapies. Nonpharmacologic interventions include scheduled voids, bladder training, addressing mobility issues, and adult protective garments. Treatments are guided by etiology (see Table 27-1 and Figure 27-2). Refer to urology for hematuria, PVR greater than 100 ml, prostate nodule, uterine prolapse, or if diagnosis is unclear after initial evaluation and/or empiric therapy fails.

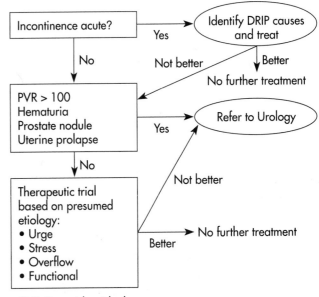

PVR, Postvoid residual.

Figure 27-2 Algorithm for the management of urinary incontinence.

Key Points

- Most urinary incontinence can be cured or markedly improved using combined nonpharmacologic and pharmacologic interventions.
- History and directed examination are the key to determining the causes of incontinence.

CASE 27-1

An 82-year-old woman is brought to see you by family members concerned about her slowly worsening memory and increasing difficulties with shopping and handling her finances. The patient states that she is doing fine and has no physical complaints. She takes clonidine for hypertension, ibuprofen for knee pain, and Tylenol PM to help her sleep at night. Her physical and neurologic examination are notable only for an MMSE score of 23/30.

A. What should you do next in terms of her diagnostic workup?

B. After medications are adjusted—clonidine changed to Dyazide, ibuprofen to plain Tylenol, Tylenol PM eliminated—her MMSE improves to 25/30 but she still has obvious memory and other cognitive deficits. What is the most likely diagnosis, and what tests should be performed?

C. Assuming normal laboratory tests and imaging, what treatments should be offered?

CASE 27-2

A 79-year-old man relates several months of increasing difficulties holding his urine. Occasionally he gets little warning, cannot to make it to the bathroom, and completely soaks himself. He voids frequently, including twice at night, and notes a decrease in the force of his stream, but he denies a sense of incomplete emptying and does not have dysuria. He has diet-controlled diabetes and degenerative joint disease (DJD) in his knees but is otherwise healthy and takes only acetaminophen.

A. What type of incontinence does he have, and how should your workup proceed?

B. On rectal examination, his prostate is soft, enlarged, and nontender. The remainder of his examination is normal, including a nonfocal neurologic examination with intact sacral dermatomes and good sphincter tone. His urinalysis is normal, and his postvoid residual is 40 ml. What is his likely diagnosis?

C. With AUA symptom score of 12, what treatment options should be considered?

Hematology and Oncology

BLEEDING DISORDERS

ETIOLOGY

What general processes cause abnormal hemostasis?

Hemostasis requires a dynamic balance between factors that promote clot formation and factors that promote anticoagulation. The tendency to bleed or to clot can be inherited or acquired. The types of bleeding problems you encounter in the outpatient setting are likely to be quite different from those you might see in hospitalized patients.

What are the most common causes of abnormal bleeding?

Common causes are summarized in Table 28-1. *von Willebrand's disease* (vWD) is the most likely inherited cause, resulting from lack of the protein that links platelets to damaged endothelium. The most common acquired cause is *nonsteroidal antiinflammatory drugs* (NSAIDs and aspirin), with bleeding in up to 10% of patients on these agents. *Immune thrombocytopenic purpura* (ITP) is an acquired disease caused by autoantibodies that bind to the surface of platelets and shorten their life span. These antibodies may be associated with a variety of systemic illnesses, such as lupus, HIV infection, or lymphoproliferative disorders. ITP is usually an outpatient diagnosis. Hospitalized patients with thrombocytopenia should be evaluated for cause.

What are some of the most likely causes of bleeding in a hospitalized patient?

The leading diagnosis depends on how sick your patient is and what underlying medical problems are present. In the ICU setting, for example, *disseminated intravascular coagulopathy* (DIC) is a fairly common cause of abnormal bleeding. This is a final common pathway of many conditions, including sepsis, massive trauma, transfusion, acute head injury, acute promyelocytic leukemia, and adenocarcinoma. *Liver disease* (acute or chronic), with its associated vitamin K–dependent fac-

tor deficiencies (II, VII, IX, X), is common in the patient who is bleeding briskly enough to be hospitalized. Unfortunately, overanticoagulation is a common cause of bleeding necessitating hospitalization. Of the several million patients in the United States on warfarin for CHF or atrial fibrillation, about 1% have significant bleeding complications.

What is hemophilia?

Hemophilia A and B are X-linked deficiencies of factors VIII and IX, respectively (see Table 28-1). Although one would expect a pedigree like that of the royal families of Victorian Europe, about 30% of hemophilia patients have a spontaneous, de novo mutation.

EVALUATION

How do I gauge if prior bleeding is "excessive"?

Although prior excessive bleeding is the clue to a true bleeding disorder, it is often overreported. Quantify the blood loss. Did epistaxis require cautery, packing, or transfusion? Was transfusion required after a minor surgical procedure (e.g., dental extraction, tonsillectomy, circumcision)? Have menses been heavy, for longer than 3 days, or prolonged, for more than 6 to 7 days? Has there been anemia or iron therapy in the past, especially in men who do not have menses or pregnancy to blame?

How do I distinguish between hereditary and acquired disorders?

A careful history reveals helpful clues. Ask about lifelong problems with hemostasis to uncover inherited problems: birth, circumcision, tonsillectomy, tooth extractions (requiring wound packing or suturing), postpartum, and nosebleeds. The one exception to this rule is vWD because severity is variable and may worsen later in life. Ask about medications because recent addition of antiinflammatories or anticoagulants suggest an acquired cause. Acute bleeding in a hospitalized patient who has a history of excellent hemostasis is almost always from an acquired condition.

TABLE 28-1

Prevalence of Common Inherited and Acquired Bleeding Disorders

BLEEDING DISORDER	PREVALENCE	FACTORS INVOLVED
INHERITED DISORDERS		
vWD	1/100	von Willebrand factor deficiency
Hemophilia A	1/5000-10,000*	VIII deficiency
Hemophilia B	1/30,000-50,000*	IX deficiency ("Christmas disease")
ACQUIRED DISORDERS		
NSAIDs/Aspirin	1/10	Platelet dysfunction
ITP	1/10,000	Platelet antibodies
DIC		Platelet and factor consumption
End-stage liver disease		Vitamin K–dependent factor deficiency (II, VII, IX, X)
Warfarin	1/100	Vitamin K–dependent factor deficiency (II, VII, IX, X)

*Prevalence among live male births only because these are X chromosome–linked conditions.

TABLE 28-2

Type of Bleeding Suggested by Particular History and Examination Clues

CLINICAL SYMPTOM	LIKELY BLEEDING PROBLEM
Bruising	Connective tissue disorder (Ehlers-Danlos, scurvy)
Bruises on extremity extensor surfaces	Physical abuse
Delayed (hours to days) postsurgical bleeding	Hemophilia, vitamin K deficiency, factor deficiency (secondary hemostasis problem)
Joint or deep muscle bleed	Hemophilia
Oozing catheter sites in hospitalized patient	DIC
Palpable purpura	Vasculitis, cryoglobulinemia, endocarditis
Petechiae, mucosal hemorrhage, bruises from minor trauma	Decreased or dysfunctional platelets (primary hemostasis problem)

TABLE 28-3

Key Features of Laboratory Abnormalities Seen With Specific Bleeding Disorders

CONDITION	BT	PLTS	PT	PTT	FDP	F
ASA or NSAIDs	↑↑					
vWD	↑	↓*		↑		
Hemophilia A or B				↑		
Warfarin			↑↑↑			
Liver disease		↓	↑↑		↑	
DIC	↑↑	↓↓	↑	↑	↑↑↑	↓↓

BT, Bleeding time; *F,* fibrinogen; *PLTS,* platelets; *PT,* prothrombin time; *PTT,* partial thromboplastin time; *FDP,* fibrin degradation products.
*Decreased in some types.

TABLE 28-4
Use of Blood and Other Products for Bleeding Disorders

PRODUCT	CONTENTS	WHEN TO USE
Fresh frozen plasma (FFP)	All clotting factors, no plts	Multifactor deficiency, vitamin K deficiency, warfarin excess, liver disease with bleeding
Vitamin K		Same as for FFP
Cryoprecipitate (from FFP)	Fibrinogen, VIII, vWF, XIII	Prolonged PTT, heparin excess, severe vWD, fibrinogen depletion, DIC, factor VIII deficiency
Protamine sulfate		Prolonged PTT, from regular heparin (*not* low molecular weight)
Platelets		Prolonged bleeding time, NSAIDs, aspirin, DIC, massive bleeding or transfusion
Specific factor concentrates	VIII or IX	Hemophilia chronic maintenance
Desmopressin (DDAVP)		Preoperatively for mild vWD

Does the type of bleeding help me generate a differential diagnosis?

Yes (Table 28-2). Hematochezia, melena, hematemesis, hemoptysis, and hematuria are almost never the presenting symptom of a bleeding disorder, so evaluate for another cause of blood loss.

What laboratory tests do I order if I suspect a bleeding problem?

Common tests ordered are listed (Table 28-3). CBC determines if bleeding has caused anemia. Platelet count identifies altered platelet numbers but provides no information about platelet function. Bleeding time assesses platelet function (primary hemostasis). Prothrombin time (PT) assesses activity of the extrinsic and common pathways in the coagulation cascade and is elevated with warfarin, vitamin K deficiency, liver disease, and DIC. Partial thromboplastin time (PTT) measures intrinsic pathway activity and is prolonged with DIC and heparin use (but not low-molecular-weight heparin). Prolonged PTT can also occur with deficiency of a clotting factor or presence of a lupus inhibitor. To tell which is true, mix some normal serum with the patient's sample (a "1:1 mix") and repeat the assay: factor deficiencies correct while inhibitors continue to prolong the PTT. Fibrin degradation products appear with thromboembolism or DIC.

TREATMENT

How do I use blood products?

Supply the missing component(s) needed for adequate hemostasis (Table 28-4). If the problem is DIC, the key to your patient's survival is to quickly correct the underlying disorder. Mortality in DIC attributed to shock and sepsis exceeds 50%.

If the diagnosis is most likely ITP, do I give platelets?

No. Transfused platelets will be destroyed about as fast as they are infused. Use high-dose prednisone (1 mg/kg/day) to block the immune process responsible for destroying platelets for 2 to 7 days, or until the platelet count rises sufficiently. Then taper prednisone slowly over 3 to 4 weeks. If bleeding is severe, or if the initial platelet count is below 10,000/μl, give intravenous immunoglobulin (IVIG) 1 g/kg/day IV for 2 days. The response to IVIG is quicker than to prednisone, such that the platelet count usually rises within 24 hours. About two thirds of patients with chronic ITP require splenectomy. Immunize these patients with the hemophilus,

---

Key Points ⋯⋯⋯⋯⋯⋯⋯⋯⋯⋯⋯⋯⋯

- Give FFP to stop bleeding in patients with liver disease or warfarin excess.
- Give prednisone or IVIG but not platelets to patients with ITP.
- Ask about prior dental procedures, surgeries, and menses to uncover excessive bleeding.
- Mucosal and catheter site oozing in hospitalized patients suggests DIC; petechiae suggest a platelet problem; palpable purpura suggests vasculitis or immune complex deposition; and delayed bleeding suggests factor deficiency.
- Bleeding from the bowel, bladder, or lungs is *not* the typical presentation of a bleeding disorder and requires rapid evaluation.

polyvalent pneumococcal, and meningococcal vaccines several weeks before splenectomy. A platelet count as low as 10,000 may be adequate in ITP.

CASE 28-1

A 47-year-old healthy man reports recurrent epistaxis. He has never had a surgical procedure, although he recalls bleeding from the gums for days after he lost a tooth in a soccer game in college. His only medication is occasional ibuprofen for musculoskeletal pain. On examination, he has an eschar in the right nostril. There are no petechiae, bruises, or organomegaly. He has several small, tender lymph nodes in the anterior cervical chain that he had not noticed until you examined them. HCT is 35%, MCV is 82, and platelet count is normal.

A. What are the two most likely diagnoses?
B. Do you want any further laboratory studies, and if so, which ones?
C. How do the results of his CBC help you?
D. What do you recommend for therapy?

CASE 28-2

A 52-year-old homeless alcoholic man is admitted with chronic liver failure and tense ascites. During his first night in the hospital, he begins to pass moderate amounts of guaiac-positive stool. His systolic blood pressure dips into the 80s. Despite intravenous saline, vitamin K, renal-dose dopamine, and 2 units of whole blood, he remains hypotensive.

A. Given the clinical situation, what are your two leading diagnoses at this point?
B. What further physical examination would you perform?
C. What laboratory studies would you order?

CLOTTING DISORDERS

ETIOLOGY

What are heritable causes of hypercoagulability?

The list of possible heritable causes is growing steadily; all listed below are autosomal dominant. Deficiencies of the physiologic anticoagulant proteins C, S, and antithrombin III are detected in 5% to 15% of patients under age 45 with deep venous thrombosis (DVT). Activated protein C resistance (also called *factor V Leiden mutation*) may be diagnosed in up to 50% of patients with DVT. This is extremely common in women who develop blood clots while taking oral contraceptives. The prevalence of this mutation is estimated at 3% to 5% in Caucasians, although it is rarer in Asian-Americans and African-Americans. A new prothrombin variant (G20210A) has been identified recently and is associated with an in-

creased risk of thromboembolism and MI in young patients (3% prevalence in Caucasians). Hyperhomocystinemia is associated with arterial and venous clots. Thromboembolism remains idiopathic in 25% of cases.

What are other risk factors for thrombosis?

Risk factors for arterial thrombosis (MI, stroke) include hypertension, hyperlipidemia, elevated lipoprotein (a), diabetes, smoking, and vasculitis. Risk factors for venous clotting include immobilization, anesthesia, surgery, pregnancy, estrogen use, malignancy (typically mucin-secreting adenocarcinomas), nephrotic syndrome, CHF, age greater than 50 years, and prior thrombosis.

What is a lupus anticoagulant?

Lupus anticoagulants are acquired IgG or IgM antibodies (also called *antiphospholipid* or *anticardiolipin antibodies*) that artifactually prolong the PTT assay. The name is a misnomer because these antibodies are not uniformly associated with lupus and they cause clotting rather than bleeding. Presence of lupus anticoagulant is also called *antiphospholipid antibody syndrome* (APAS) and is an acquired hypercoagulable state associated with lupus and other autoimmune disorders. It is typically seen in young women with recurrent spontaneous abortions and thrombocytopenia. Up to 35% of patients with APAS suffer venous and/or arterial thromboembolism; the risk of clot approaches 70% with concurrent lupus.

EVALUATION

Whom do I screen for the presence of an underlying hypercoagulable state?

The British Society for Hematology has recommended screening in the following situations:

- Thrombosis under the age of 45 without risk factors (even with the first event)
- Recurrent thrombosis or thrombosis at an unusual site
- Arterial thrombosis before the age of 30
- Family history of a heritable clotting disorder
- Recurrent fetal loss

How do I screen for hypercoagulable state?

Obtain protein C and S activity levels before starting warfarin, and antithrombin III activity level before starting heparin. Activated protein C, antiphospholipid antibodies, and homocysteine levels can be assayed while patients are on either anticoagulant. The prothrombin variant can be detected on DNA/PCR screening, although this test may not yet be widely available.

TREATMENT

How do I anticoagulate a patient with a DVT?

Start with an IV heparin bolus of 80 U/kg (ideal body weight) followed by a continuous infusion at 18 U/kg/hr. As this is a rough estimate, adjust infusion rate to maintain PTT at 1.8 to 2.5 times control. PTT can be followed to monitor heparin therapy every 6 hours until stable, then less often. Twice-daily subcutaneous low-molecular-weight heparin can be given instead; although more expensive, LMW heparin does not require PTT monitoring. Begin oral warfarin 24 to 48 hours after initiating heparin. Physicians vary widely in how aggressively they "load" the warfarin therapy, starting with 5 to 10 mg for the first few days, then adjusting based on the PT INR. Continue heparin until PT is therapeutic on warfarin (INR >2). Some hematologists continue heparin 2 days beyond the time a therapeutic INR has been reached to prevent warfarin-associated skin necrosis, especially a risk in patients with protein C or S deficiency. Generally, the target INR is 2 to 3. However, patients with APAS routinely fail less intense therapy and are at high risk of recurrence (>70%), so their target INR is higher at 3 to 4.

My patient with a postsurgical DVT has been therapeutic on heparin for 5 days, but his platelet count is dropping and his DVT is extending. What's going on?

Yours is one of about 2% of patients who develops heparin-induced thrombocytopenia (HIT). HIT is suspected when platelets drop below normal or decline more than 50% from baseline. Unfortunately, extension of the DVT despite adequate anticoagulation means that your patient is also one of the 0.2% to 0.6% who develop HIT-associated thrombosis (HITT). A heparin-dependent antibody (usually IgG) that activates platelet aggregation causes HITT. The clotting events associated with HITT may be venous or arterial and are life threatening. *Stop* all heparin, including catheter flushes. Remove all heparin-bonded catheters. Post a sign above the patient's bed explicitly stating, "NO HEPARIN FLUSHES." Call a hematologist to assist with options for replacing heparin. Danaparoid (a heparinoid) and LMW heparin are *not* options because they worsen the problem 10% and 80% of the time, respectively. If an arterial thrombosis develops, directed thrombolytic therapy may be necessary to save a limb. HIT and HITT are the reason that careful platelet monitoring must accompany all heparin use.

How long do I continue warfarin therapy?

Warfarin is usually given for 3 to 6 months after an initial event when a reversible cause was present, such as surgery or trauma. Consider indefinite warfarin therapy if the hypercoagulable state is a persistent risk (e.g., APAS, CHF with EF less than 25%, paroxysmal nocturnal hemoglobinuria, nephrotic syndrome). Lifelong anticoagulation is also recommended in those with a history of multiple events, multiple genetic risk factors, a strong family history (regardless of the results of the $3,000 workup), or an initial event in an unusual site. Although it is tempting to hinge the length of warfarin therapy on the severity of the initial event, this has no real bearing on the patient's subsequent risk for recurrence. Of patients who develop a lower extremity DVT, 40% to 50% will suffer a pulmonary embolism. Overall, the risk of a significant bleeding complication resulting from warfarin therapy is about 1% per year. Avoid warfarin in women planning pregnancy and through the first trimester in pregnant women.

When should I consider prophylactic anticoagulation?

Any patient with a prior clot (e.g., with surgery) or with an identified genetic risk, even in the absence of a personal history of thrombosis, should receive prophylactic subcutaneous heparin during immobility (e.g., postoperatively).

Is there a role for aspirin in the hypercoagulable patient?

Aspirin and NSAIDs are antiplatelet agents and are useful in preventing arterial thrombosis (such as MI and stroke). A patient with APAS who has a history of predominantly arterial thromboses is often treated with the combination of warfarin and aspirin, with very close monitoring of the INR and clinical status. In all other patients taking warfarin for venous thrombosis, aspirin and NSAIDs are discouraged because the risk of bleeding complications is compounded with the use of these agents.

Key Points

- Monitor platelets in patients on heparin to look for heparin-induced thrombocytopenia.
- Factor V Leiden accounts for up to 50% of identifiable clotting disorders.
- Overlap heparin and warfarin use in patients with DVT to prevent warfarin-induced skin necrosis.
- Screen for hypercoagulable state in patients younger than age 45 with DVT and no risk factors, recurrent thrombosis, unusual or arterial sites of clotting, a family history of a heritable clotting problem, or a history of recurrent fetal loss.

CASE 28-3

A 23-year-old Hispanic woman is admitted to the ICU with sinus vein thrombosis. She is 6 weeks postpartum after delivering her first child. This was her fourth pregnancy, with one of her miscarriages a stillbirth at 20 weeks. She denies any prior thrombosis. Her family history is significant for a maternal aunt with severe arthritis and kidney failure who died at the age of 42. Her musculoskeletal examination shows moderate effusions in both knees and tenderness at the wrists.

A. What laboratory studies would you perform?

B. What do you recommend for therapy?

BREAST CANCER

See the section on Breast Health in Chapter 36.

COLON CANCER

ETIOLOGY

Who gets colon cancer?

In the United States, 47,000 people die from colon cancer each year, making it the second deadliest malignancy. As with breast cancer, most victims have no risk factors other than age. Certain conditions impart a particularly high risk: *familial adenomatosis* (50% by age 40), *ulcerative colitis* (after 10 years the relative risk [RR] is 20), and a *family history* in first-degree relatives (RR = 2-3).

EVALUATION

What screening is recommended?

For people over age 50, screen for polyps or early disease with sigmoidoscopy every 3 to 5 years and annual stool occult blood testing to reduce mortality. People at higher risk need earlier screening. Digital rectal examination may detect rectal cancers but have not been shown to improve outcome.

What symptoms might my patient with colon cancer develop?

Distal colon cancers tend to obstruct, producing cramps, thin stools, bloating, or perforation. Stool in the proximal colon is more liquid, so cancers there cause symptoms by ulcerating and bleeding. Every adult with unexplained iron-deficiency anemia needs a complete colon examination. Dyspnea may be the chief complaint of your patient with a cecal carcinoma and a low hematocrit. Unfortunately, too many patients present with an abdominal mass or liver metastases from advanced disease.

How do I stage colon cancer?

"Duke's classification" is a simple staging system that guides treatment and prognosis (Table 28-5).

TREATMENT

How do I treat colon cancer?

Stage A, B, and C tumors are resected. Stage C tumors are also treated with chemotherapy. Stage D tumors receive chemotherapy or irradiation. Small, isolated liver metastases can be resected. Studies to date have failed to show any benefit of chemotherapy in stage B tumors.

How do I catch recurrences early?

Once treated, perform regular examinations, laboratory tests, and colonoscopy. Measure the carcinoembryonic antigen (CEA) level before excision; a persistently elevated or rising level predicts recurrence.

TABLE 28-5
Duke's Classification of Colon Cancer

STAGE	DEFINITION	TREATMENT	5-YEAR SURVIVAL
A	Limited to mucosa and submucosa	Excision	90%
B	Local extension to subserosa or beyond	Excision	70%
C	Regional lymph node involvement	Excision, plus 5-FU and levamisole	40%
D	Metastases (liver first; then lung, bone, CNS)	Chemotherapy or irradiation, excision of 1-3 liver metastases	7%

LEUKEMIA

ETIOLOGY

What causes leukemia?

Leukemias are the neoplastic, clonal proliferation of blood cells or their precursors. The cause is unknown. Leukemias are classified according to the maturity and type of cell involved. Immature cells, such as blasts, replicate quickly and produce "acute" leukemias. Mature clones are less aggressive and cause "chronic" leukemias that have an indolent course. Any type of cell can cause leukemia: myeloid cells (usually granulocytes), lymphoid cells, and, much less commonly, red blood cell or platelet precursors. Thus there are four common leukemias: chronic lymphocytic leukemia (CLL), chronic myelogenous leukemia (CML), acute lymphocytic leukemia (ALL), and acute myelogenous leukemia (AML). Almost all patients with CML have a translocation between chromosomes 9 and 22, called the Philadelphia chromosome. AML and ALL are associated with myelodysplastic syndromes and certain genetic conditions, as well as exposure to radiation, benzene, and chemotherapy.

EVALUATION

What will I see on a peripheral blood smear?

If you see more than 15,000 mature lymphocytes in the blood of an elderly person, this almost certainly is *CLL*. In *CML*, there are 30,000 to 300,000 WBCs in final stages of maturation (bands). "Leukemoid reactions," caused by certain infections, such as TB, may look similar; in this case a high serum leukocyte alkaline phosphatase rules out CML. Peripheral cells in *AML* may be elevated or reduced. You may see circulating blasts or Auer rods that look like red cigars in the cytoplasm.

What other tests are used to diagnose leukemias?

In CLL, bone marrow shows greater than 40% mature B lymphocytes. Immature cells and blasts predominate in CML and AML, respectively. Membrane antigens differentiate ALL and the seven types of AML (M1-M7). Cytogenetics may identify specific leukemias. The Philadelphia chromosome is pathognomonic for CML.

What are common symptoms of leukemia?

Infiltration may result in enlarged nodes, liver, and spleen, and gingival, skin (leukemia cutis), or soft tissue masses (chloroma). When the WBC is greater than 150,000, vascular sludging, or leukostasis, may result in stroke, headache, tinnitus, blindness, or CHF. Destruction of normal bone marrow causes pancytopenia, resulting in infection, dyspnea, fatigue, bleeding, and bruising.

What complications might occur?

In CLL, clonal lymphocytes produce abnormal immunoglobulins. The resulting hypogammaglobulinemia impairs humoral immunity, causing infections by *Staphylococcus aureus, Pneumococcus,* and *Haemophilus influenzae.* Approximately 15% of patients have antibodies against erythrocytes or platelets, conditions known as autoimmune hemolytic anemia or thrombocytopenia. In AML and ALL, bone marrow failure at presentation is the rule, often with sepsis, DIC, or renal failure. Cranial nerve palsies and leukemic meningitis are common in ALL, especially in children.

TREATMENT

Do I need to treat the chronic leukemias?

CLL may not cause symptoms for many years, and it affects older people, who often die of other diseases first. Late-stage CLL or acute complications of CML respond to oral alkylating agents, such as hydroxyurea. Treatment can cause renal failure or tumor lysis syndrome (purine metabolites released from leukemic cells raise uric acid and potassium). After a few years, patients develop a blast crisis (such as AML), which responds poorly to chemotherapy and is usually lethal.

How do I treat the acute leukemias?

ALL and AML are treated in stages: induction, consolidation, and maintenance. Induction chemotherapy is the initial, often successful, attempt to induce a complete remission (CR). Recurrence within 1 year is the rule. Monthly consolidation chemotherapy ($\times$ 6 months) reduces recurrence. People with ALL may receive low-dose maintenance therapy for years. Long-term disease-free survival is 15% to 20% for AML and up to 40% for ALL (much better in children).

What is the role of bone marrow transplant?

Transplant technology allows you to give otherwise lethal doses of chemotherapy and radiation. AML patients older than age 60, in first remission, and with HLA-matched donors benefit the most from transplant (40% long-term survival). In CML, transplant is the only potentially curative therapy, and only if done under optimum circumstances before the "accelerated" or "blast" phase.

Key Points ··················

- Symptoms of leukemia are caused by infiltration of organs, destruction of bone marrow, alterations in immunity, and the large burden of clones in the blood.
- Diagnose by peripheral smear, bone marrow biopsy, immunologic markers, and cytogenetics.
- CLL may never need treatment; CML always becomes acute over time, and early transplant is the only cure. Acute leukemias must be forced into remission quickly.

LUNG CANCER

ETIOLOGY

Who gets lung cancer?

Lung malignancies killed 160,000 people in the United States in 1997—more than any other cancer. Because of higher smoking rates, women now die more often of lung cancer than of breast cancer. Some 90% of patients who die of lung cancer are smokers, and many of the nonsmokers die from passive exposure. Workers exposed to asbestos (plumbers, ship-builders) have up to 4 times the risk of nonsmokers. Smoking is synergistic with asbestos, and together they increase the risk of lung cancer 100 times. Screening is not recommended because sputum cytology and chest x-rays in smokers do not reveal tumors early enough to decrease mortality.

EVALUATION

What types of lung cancer are there?

Multiple histologic types of lung cancer are classified into one of two groups based on natural history and response to therapy (Table 28-6). *Small-cell lung cancer (SCLC)* is a "systemic" disease—it spreads very early to the mediastinum, nodes, liver, bone, and CNS. Systemic therapy, also called chemotherapy, is relatively effective. Squamous cell carcinoma, adenocarcinoma, and large-cell cancer (subtypes giant-cell and clear-cell) are lumped together as *non–small-cell lung cancer (NSCLC)* because localized disease may be cured surgically.

How might my patient present with lung cancer?

A lung mass may bleed or obstruct an airway, producing hemoptysis, dyspnea, cough, or postobstructive pneumonia. Local extension to the mediastinum, pleura, and chest wall may result in pleural and pericardial effusions, compression of the superior vena cava, or paralysis of mediastinal nerves. Metastases may cause bone pain, liver failure, adrenal insufficiency, or neurologic symptoms. Many paraneoplastic syndromes are associated with particular lung cancers. For example, the syndrome of inappropriate antidiuretic hormone secretion (SIADH) occurs in about 10% of people with SCLC and causes hyponatremia. Humorally mediated hyper-

---

TABLE 28-6
Classification of Lung Cancers

STAGE	INVOLVEMENT	TREATMENT	5-YEAR SURVIVAL
SMALL-CELL LUNG CANCER			
Limited	1 lung, regional nodes (hilum, supraclavicular)	Chemotherapy + radiotherapy +/− prophylactic cranial irradiation rarely, surgical resection	5%-10%
Extensive	More than "limited"	Chemotherapy +/− prophylactic cranial irradiation	<1%
NON–SMALL-CELL LUNG CANCER			
I	No nodes or metastases	Surgical resection	30%
II	Ipsilateral bronchial or hilar nodes only	Surgical resection	30%
III	Distal nodes or local extension	Chemotherapy and/or radiotherapy	<5%
IV	Distant metastases	Palliative radiotherapy or chemotherapy	<1%

calcemia is common in squamous cell carcinoma. These tumors increase serum calcium by secreting parathyroid hormone analogues; bone metastases are rarely a cause of hypercalcemia in lung cancer.

How do I evaluate a single nodule on a chest x-ray?

Many diseases may cause nodules, such as benign tumors (hamartomas, lipomas); AV malformations; infections (TB, abscesses, fungal diseases); rheumatologic diseases (Wegener's granulomatosis, RA); infarction; hemorrhage; or primary lung or metastatic cancers. Thus a complete history and examination is important. Certain features of the nodule suggest cancer, including irregular borders and eccentric calcification. Nodules that are unchanged after 2 years are unlikely to be cancer, so old chest x-rays may be helpful. A CT scan might rule out cancer, but suspicious lesions require biopsy.

TREATMENT

What is the approach to treatment?

Limited SCLC may be cured with chemotherapy. You may need a bone marrow biopsy, brain imaging, and a bone scan to assure that the disease is limited (see Table 28-1). For NSCLC, the essential task is to determine if the tumor can be resected for cure. Imaging, bone scans, and even mediastinoscopy may be necessary. For late-stage SCLC or NSCLC, treatment is palliative.

Key Points ···

- Screening asymptomatic people for lung cancer does not decrease mortality.
- Use chemotherapy for both limited and extensive lung cancer; some limited cancers are curable.
- NSCLC is best treated by surgery, but you must look hard to prove that the tumor is resectable.
- Talk to smokers about quitting every time you see them.

NON-HODGKIN'S LYMPHOMA

ETIOLOGY

What causes non-Hodgkin's lymphoma (NHL)?

Non-Hodgkin's lymphomas are a diverse group of lymphoid tumors of unknown etiology. They cause about 12,000 deaths each year, mostly in middle-aged people. NHL can be a complication of HIV infection. Because of the relatively low prevalence, screening is not recommended.

EVALUATION

How is NHL classified?

There are many histologic types of NHL that are described as low, medium, or high grade based natural history. *Low-grade* lymphomas may exist for years before the patient notices painless lymph nodes. Sometimes, there are complaints of abdominal fullness as a result of massive hepatosplenomegaly. *High-grade* lymphomas usually occur in children and may act like acute leukemias. Any lymphoma may present with generalized "B" symptoms, which are fever, night sweats, and 10% weight loss over the previous 6 months.

What workup is necessary?

Lymphomas can involve any lymphoid tissue and the CNS, so complete review of systems and examination are key. You will also want a lymph node biopsy, bone marrow biopsy, LP, and head and body imaging for diagnosis, grading, and staging of the tumor.

What defines the stages of NHL?

The stages are I to IV, as follows: I—single site, II—several sites on the same side of the diaphragm, III—several sites on both sides of the diaphragm (+/− local organ involvement), and IV—disseminated disease. Each stage is subclassified as "B" for presence of B symptoms as above, and as "A" if B symptoms are absent.

TREATMENT

Which patients with NHL require treatment, and how effective is therapy?

Some asymptomatic indolent lymphomas are not treated. For symptomatic or more aggressive tumors, various combinations of radiation and chemotherapy are used. Overall, 5-year survival is about 50%, but that does not tell the whole story. People with low-grade lymphomas live many years but are rarely cured, whereas aggressive grades are cured about half the time.

Key Points ···

- Non-Hodgkin's lymphoma is a common cause of diffuse lymphadenopathy.
- Non-Hodgkin's lymphoma is a common complication of HIV infection.
- Treatment decisions depend on grade, stage, and the age and condition of the patient.

PROSTATE CANCER

ETIOLOGY

How many men have prostate cancer?

Prostate cancer is the most common newly diagnosed cancer in men. About 40,000 men die of this disease each year. It is unique in its high prevalence of "latent" disease: 70% men in their 80s who die from something else have microscopic foci of prostate cancer. The incidence is highest in African-Americans, less in Caucasians, and least in Asians. Mortality per case is higher in African-Americans. Family history of prostate cancer before age 60 is a risk factor.

EVALUATION

Should I screen my patient for prostate cancer?

There is currently insufficient evidence to recommend screening. Digital rectal examinations, PSA, and transrectal ultrasound can detect tumors that would never cause symptoms or are already incurable. Additionally, treatments may cause incontinence and impotence with unclear long-term benefit. You must help your patient make a personal decision in the face of uncertainty.

What symptoms suggest prostate cancer?

Early cancers often produce no symptoms. Some men report BPH-like symptoms of dysuria, hematuria, or trouble voiding. The first symptom may be metastatic bone pain. Sorting out the few men with treatable prostate cancer from the millions with symptomatic BPH is a clinical dilemma.

TREATMENT

Is treatment based on stages?

Yes. Cancer limited to the gland (stages A and B) may be cured with either radical prostatectomy or radiation therapy. The treatment for stage C tumor extending through the capsule is controversial. Stage D involves lymph nodes, bone, lung, or liver and cannot be cured. In contrast to breast and colon cancer, even a single positive lymph node makes recurrence nearly certain.

Is there a role for palliative therapy?

Palliative treatment is the rule for symptomatic metastatic disease. This tumor is responsive to androgens. Orchiectomy eliminates the body's major source of an-

drogens. Estrogens or luteinizing hormone-releasing hormone (LHRH) analogues suppress LH release and androgen synthesis. All of these treatments are effective in decreasing symptoms, but they may not increase survival.

How long will my patient live?

The 5-year survival for local disease is over 90%. It drops to 80% for locally invasive disease, and 25% for those with metastases (better than for most other metastatic cancers). All of these rates are lower for African-Americans, who may get higher-grade tumors or less timely or aggressive treatment.

> **Key Points**
> - It is not known whether screening for prostate cancer is beneficial or harmful.
> - The treatment tools are surgery and radiation, but some patients may be better off untreated.
> - Metastatic disease cannot be cured, but antiandrogen therapies may reduce symptoms.

TUMORS IN YOUNG ADULTS

What cancers are more likely in young adults?

Hodgkin's disease is a tumor of lymphoid tissue, commonly presenting as painless, rubbery nodes. It is highly curable with radiation and/or chemotherapy, but staging must be done carefully. *Testicular cancer* is the most common cancer in men ages 15 to 35. It is also highly curable and, because the ignorance and embarrassment of patients and physicians, the diagnosis is often made later than necessary. It is more common in Caucasians and 40 times more likely with undescended testes. Your patient may present with a painless testicular mass or supraclavicular nodes. Early stages are usually cured with excision. The cure rate in advanced stages is greater than 60% with chemotherapy and irradiation. Early stages of *ovarian cancer* are asymptomatic. It presents late, often with ascites or pain from peritoneal spread. Most patients die (15,000 each year in the United States), and there is no effective screening. Deaths from *cervical cancer* have dropped to fewer than 5000 per year in the United States, and most of these could be prevented with regular Pap smears. The major risk factor is infection with human papilloma virus, and the disease is particularly aggressive in patients with HIV infection.

CASE 28-4

A 61-year-old, heavy smoker presents with neck and upper back pain. Chest x-ray shows hyperinflation, flattened diaphragms, bullae, and a 2-cm right upper lobe nodule. Calcium 10.5.

A. What is your diagnostic plan?
B. What are the characteristics of a lung nodule that suggest malignancy?
C. What are possible explanations for his abnormal calcium level?

CASE 28-5

A 50-year-old immigrant from Chernobyl comes to your office because she has been feeling very tired. She used to play soccer with her daughters, but now she gets out of breath just unloading the car. She had a prolonged nosebleed yesterday for the first time in years.

A. What diagnoses are you considering, and what questions will you ask?
B. What will you look for on examination? Will this pin down the diagnosis?
C. What complications might occur?

CASE 28-6

A 40-year-old man complains of chills for the last few days. He has smoked 2 packs per day since age 15, and says that he "coughs all the time, but I think it has been worse." His 43-year-old brother had a bleeding adenoma removed from his colon last year. You see that he is tired and thin, and you find a clump of nodes in the left supraclavicular fossa. A chest x-ray shows left hilar enlargement.

A. What is a Virchow's node?
B. What tests do you order?
C. If he is cured by chemotherapy, will there be long-lasting effects?

Infectious Diseases

ENCEPHALITIS

ETIOLOGY

What is encephalitis, and what causes it?

Encephalitis is inflammation of the brain tissue. Viral causes predominate, but fungus, rickettsial infection, toxoplasmosis, and tuberculosis are also important causes. Without question, the most important cause of acute encephalitis in the United States is the herpes virus, especially HSV-1 (note that HSV is also an important cause of meningitis). Rare cases of eastern equine encephalitis, St. Louis encephalitis, and rabies are reported each year. Toxoplasmic encephalitis is common in HIV-infected patients with low CD4 counts (see the HIV Infection Primary Care section in this chapter). The mortality rate of untreated HSV encephalitis is 70%.

EVALUATION

What are the typical clinical features of encephalitis?

The clinical features of herpes encephalitis include nausea, vomiting, headache, and alterations in level of consciousness with lethargy and confusion. HSV can involve the temporal lobe, causing confusion, personality change, and odd behavior. Other symptoms include seizures, ataxia, cranial nerve defects, and visual field loss.

What testing should be done to evaluate suspected encephalitis?

Cerebrospinal fluid (CSF) in patients with HSV encephalitis usually shows a pleocytosis with lymphocytes and polymorphonuclear cells (PMNs). PMNs may predominate early in infection. Red blood cells are fre-

quently present in the CSF. Definitive diagnosis is made by PCR of CSF; culture of HSV from CSF is difficult. CT scan, MRI, or EEG can localize the area of brain involved.

TREATMENT

How do you treat HSV encephalitis?

Treat with high-dose IV acyclovir. Because of high mortality rates, begin therapy as soon as you consider the diagnosis. No treatment is effective for other viral encephalitides.

Key Points ....
- HSV encephalitis may present with personality change, odd behavior, and confusion, as well as fever, headache, and vomiting.
- Early therapy with IV acyclovir is critical to decrease permanent neurologic sequelae and mortality.

ENDOCARDITIS

ETIOLOGY

What causes endocarditis?

Endocarditis is an infection of one or more heart valves. Endocarditis usually begins with seeding of a preexisting valve abnormality during a period of transient bacteremia. Native and prosthetic valve infections are caused by different organisms. Native valve disease is usually caused by *Staphylococcus aureus* in IV drug users and by streptococcal species in other patients. Prosthetic valve disease is more likely a result of *S. epidermidis, S. aureus,* or a gram-negative organism within 2 months of valve placement, or streptococcal species or *S. aureus* if more than 2 months have passed. *Streptococcus bovis* endocarditis is associated with colon cancer and so should prompt colonoscopy.

EVALUATION

How do I recognize the clinical presentation of endocarditis?

Endocarditis can be subtle or acutely obvious. Consider it in any patient with unexplained fever. Other symptoms include signs of LV dysfunction (dyspnea, orthopnea, PND), chest pain from septic infarcts, or neurologic compromise. In IV drug users, the tricuspid valve is most frequently involved; fever and pulmonary symptoms are the usual presentation. Ask about risk factors, including drug use, prior valve abnormality, or recent invasive procedures (e.g., dental, endoscopic) likely to cause transient bacteremic episodes. On examination, look for septic emboli in the fundi (Roth's spots), the palms and finger pads (tender Osler's nodes, red nontender Janeway lesions), and nail beds (splinter hemorrhages). Listen for a new murmur or abnormal lung sounds. Document a thorough neurologic examination as a baseline for potential future embolic events. Chest x-ray may show multiple peripheral patchy infiltrates with tricuspid valve endocarditis.

How do I diagnose endocarditis?

Diagnose with three sets of blood cultures over a 24-hour period, best drawn before starting antibiotics (do not withhold antibiotics in the acutely ill). Echo can confirm the diagnosis by showing a valvular vegetation, but it cannot rule it out because small vegetations may be missed.

TREATMENT

What antibiotics are appropriate for endocarditis?

Treat with empiric bactericidal antibiotics based on your best guess at the organism. For patients using IV drugs, start gentamicin and nafcillin to cover presumptive *S. aureus* (substitute vancomycin for nafcillin if the patient is penicillin allergic). Most native valve streptococcal infections can be covered with penicillin and gentamicin. Prosthetic valve infections should be covered empirically with vancomycin and an aminoglycoside.

Narrow therapy when culture results are available and treat for 6 weeks with IV antibiotics.

Key Points
- Endocarditis in IV drug users most frequently infects the tricuspid valve with *S. aureus.*
- Prosthetic valve endocarditis is caused by different organisms, depending on when it occurs after valve placement.
- Obtain colonoscopy in patients with *Streptococcus bovis* endocarditis to rule out colon cancer.

GENITAL INFECTIONS

ETIOLOGY

What are the common causes of genital discharge?

In women, normal physiologic vaginal discharge varies in amount and quality. Other causes to consider in women are *cervicitis* (gonorrhea, chlamydia) and *vaginitis* (candidal, trichomonal, bacterial vaginosis, estrogen deficiency atrophic vaginitis). Discharge is never normal in men. Male *urethritis* is caused by gonorrhea, chlamydia, and, occasionally, Reiter's syndrome. In men and women, discharge may be absent despite infection. Chlamydia is often clinically silent and has been implicated as a cause of infertility.

What is bacterial vaginosis?

This condition is an overgrowth of normal vaginal flora. There is no true infection or inflammation, hence the term *vaginosis* rather than *vaginitis*. The copious discharge is bothersome to patients, as is the postcoital fishy odor, but it is not a dangerous or sexually transmitted condition. However, bacterial vaginosis in pregnancy may be associated with preterm labor.

What causes genital ulcers?

HSV infection can be silent or can cause a syndrome of fevers, myalgias, and painful genital ulcers. Painless ulcers occur with chancroid and primary syphilis. Toxic epidermal necrolysis is a potentially fatal drug reaction causing painful oral and genital ulcers.

What causes genital growths?

HPV causes genital warts, which are broad-based and verrucous. These can appear at any location in the perineum, including perirectally. Condom use does not prevent the spread of this highly infectious virus, which is easily transmitted by skin-to-skin contact. More than half of the general population has serologic evidence of exposure. Patients are distressed at this common malady; some strains are associated with cervical and vulvar cancer. The differential for genital growths also includes skin tags, molluscum contagiosum, and skin cancer.

My patient reports pelvic pain. What are common genitourinary causes?

Deep pelvic or perineal pain in men can be a manifestation of prostatitis or, less commonly, urinary tract infection. In women, think of urinary tract infection, menstrual pain, ovarian cyst rupture, endometriosis, and PID. The latter is usually due to chlamydia or gonorrhea but may be cervical culture-negative. PID is diagnosed based on a symptom complex of fever, elevated WBC, and cervical motion or adnexal tenderness. Do not miss ectopic pregnancy or tuboovarian abscess. Chronic pelvic pain is closely associated with a history of sexual abuse.

EVALUATION

What historical points are important in evaluating genital infections?

Ask about new sexual partners; condom usage; previous infections; last menstrual period; and current symptoms including discharge, pain with intercourse, fevers, and skin lesions.

What examination is important for men and women reporting genital symptoms?

Examine the external genitalia for dermal or mucosal ulceration, redness, or discharge. Include testicular and prostate examinations in men, pelvic bimanual and speculum examinations in women, and inguinal lymph nodes in both genders. For adnexal tenderness, obtain CBC and pregnancy test, and screen for chlamydia and gonorrhea.

What is an appropriate evaluation for a woman reporting discharge?

Examine the external genitalia for ulceration or erythema. Take cervical swabs for gonorrhoeae culture and chlamydia LCR (ligase chain reaction, a DNA test) or culture. Obtain discharge from the vaginal wall and place on one slide with normal saline and a second slide with KOH. First, view the saline slide ("wet mount") under the microscope for WBCs, clue cells suggesting bacterial vaginosis (squamous cells covered in bacteria, giving them a granular appearance), or twitching trichomonads

slightly larger than WBCs. For the KOH slide, sniff above the slide for the characteristic strong fishy odor of bacterial vaginosis. Viewed under the microscope, the KOH will have lysed all cells, leaving yeast hyphae. Because yeast is a common colonizer of the vagina, WBCs should also be present to make this diagnosis.

Should I perform routine screening for any of these infections?

Studies show benefit in prevention of PID (and by extension, perhaps long-term infertility) with screening for chlamydia in high-risk populations: women younger than age 25 and those with two or more new sexual partners per year. Annual Pap smears in young, sexually active women screens for atypia from HPV. There are no current recommendations for screening in men. Always offer HIV and RPR testing to high-risk individuals.

When is vaginal pH helpful?

Normal vaginal pH is acidic at 4.5. pH is increased during menses, with atrophic vaginitis from estrogen deficiency, and in all vaginal infections except *Candida*.

TREATMENT

Can I treat empirically for discharge?

Studies show that both patients and physicians are unable to diagnose the cause of vaginal discharge by history and gross examination alone, without microscopic or culture evaluation. This includes vaginal candidiasis, although women frequently treat presumptively with over-the-counter topical antifungals. One exception is when pruritus and discharge follow antibiotic therapy; these patients may be empirically treated for vaginal candidiasis. Treat vaginal candidiasis with either topical or oral antifungals. A single oral 150-mg dose of fluconazole treats 90% of cases, but 15% relapse. Prescribe a second dose to be taken after 4 days for persistent symptoms. Topical therapy with vaginal creams alleviate the perineal irritation and itching more rapidly but are messy. All other causes of genital symptoms should be carefully evaluated and treated according to accurate diagnosis (Table 29-1).

Key Points ··
- Screen high-risk patients for chlamydia with LCR.
- Accurate diagnosis of most genital infections requires microscopic examination and culture.
- HPV exposure is common, and certain subtypes correlate with cervical cancer.

TABLE 29-1
Evaluation and Treatment of Genital Infections

PATHOGEN	EVALUATION	TREATMENT (ORAL UNLESS OTHERWISE NOTED)
CERVIX/URETHRA		
Chlamydia	LCR* or Culture	Azithromycin 1000 mg × 1
Gonorrhea	Culture	Ceftriaxone 125 mg IM or cefixime 400 mg × 1
VAGINA		
Candida	pH <4.5 +KOH WBC	Fluconazole 150 mg × 1, may repeat ×1 Topical antifungal
Trichomonas	pH >4.5 Flagellates	Metronidazole 2 g × 1
Bacterial vaginosis	Clue cells pH >4.5 +whiff test	Metronidazole 500 mg bid × 7 d Topical metronidazole gel 0.75% bid × 5d
GENITAL MUCOSA OR SKIN		
Herpes simplex	Tzanck prep Serology	Suppressive: Acyclovir 400 mg bid or valacyclovir 500 mg qd Acute: Acyclovir 400 mg tid × 5-10d or valacyclovir 500-1000 mg bid × 5-10 d
Human papilloma virus	Exam Biopsy Routine Paps	Topical imiquimod or podophyllum Cryotherapy Laser therapy for cervical atypia

*LCR is a DNA-based assay that can be performed on cervical/urethral secretions or on first-void urine. It is greater than 98% sensitive and specific. Culture is slightly less sensitive.

CASE 29-1

An 18-year-old woman comes to clinic for routine care. She has had two partners in the last year with whom she used condoms 90% of the time. She has no history of sexually transmitted diseases. She reports mild vaginal discharge, pruritus, and mild dyspareunia. Focused examination reveals white flocculent discharge in vaginal vault, normal cervix, and normal bimanual examination.
A. What further history would you obtain?
B. What examination would you perform?
C. She reports that her partner has warts. What do you advise?

CASE 29-2

A 45-year-old woman presents with low-grade fever, vaginal pain, and dysuria after unprotected sex several weeks ago. Last menstrual period was 3 months ago. She was diagnosed with a UTI a few days ago by urine dipstick and received 3 days of trimethoprim/sulfamethoxazole. On genital examination, mucosa is erythematous and tender to palpation. Cervix is normal, and bimanual examination reveals no adnexal or cervical motion tenderness.
A. What is in the differential to explain her symptoms?
B. What, if any, further evaluation would you pursue?
C. KOH shows occasional hyphae without white cells. How do you interpret this result?

HIV INFECTION PRIMARY CARE

ETIOLOGY

What terminology is useful in categorizing HIV infection?

HIV infection is classified by numbers 1, 2, or 3, depending on the CD4 count, and by letters A, B, or C, depending on the occurrence of specific conditions (Table 29-2). AIDS is defined as category C disease or a CD4 count less than 200 (A3, B3). Begin your oral presentation of any HIV-infected patient by giving the classification, last CD4 count, and viral load.

Why are CD4 cell counts and HIV viral load important?

CD4 count indicates the severity of immune suppression and is used to determine (1) disease classification, (2) when to start or change antiretroviral therapy; (3) when certain opportunistic infections are likely; and (4) when to start opportunistic infection prophylaxis. Specific opportunistic infections are more likely

TABLE 29-2

Classification of HIV Infection

CD4 COUNT (PER MM³)	A*	B†	C‡
500	A₁	B₁	C₁
200-499	A₂	B₂	C₂
<200	A₃	B₃	C₃

Grey shading = diagnosis of AIDS.
*A-asymptomatic, or persistent generalized lymphadenopathy.
†B-symptomatic, not category C diseases, can include bacillary angiomatosis, oral thrush, cervical dysplasia/carcinoma, oral hairy leukoplakia, herpes zoster (recurrent or multidermatomal), and ITP.
‡C-AIDS indicator conditions, including PCP, cryptococcal meningitis, toxoplasmosis, CMV retinitis, AIDS dementia complex, tuberculosis, recurrent bacterial pneumonias, Kaposi's sarcoma, CNS lymphoma, and other non-Hodgkin's lymphomas.

TABLE 29-3

Occurrence of AIDS-Indicating Conditions in the Natural History of HIV Infection, According to CD4+ Cell Count

CONDITION	CD4 COUNT
Bacterial pneumonia/sinusitis	500
Typical presentation of tuberculosis	500
Herpes zoster	400
Herpes simplex ulcers	300
PCP	200
Atypical presentation of tuberculosis	200
Esophageal candidiasis	100
Cryptococcus	100
Toxoplasmosis	100
Disseminated MAC	75
CMV retinitis	50

to occur below specific CD4 counts (Table 29-3). Quantitative HIV viral load gives prognostic information beyond that provided by the CD4 count. The higher the viral load, the more rapidly the patient is becoming immune-suppressed. In addition, viral load is used to assess efficacy of antiretroviral therapy within weeks of any change.

What is the risk of acquiring HIV infection from a needle–stick injury?

Fear of contracting HIV in the health care setting through needle-stick or mucosal splash accidents is a significant stress for all health professionals. The risk of infection is low, estimated in a Centers for Disease Control and Prevention (CDC) study to be 0.5% for percutaneous exposure (3/860). Based on other data, the risk is probably somewhat less (~0.2%) than that reported by the CDC. The risk for HIV transmission is greater if blood is seen on needle, the needle stick is a deep wound

from a hollow-bore needle, gloves were not worn, or the source patient has advanced HIV disease.

EVALUATION

How do I diagnose HIV infection?

Screen for HIV infection with an enzyme-linked immunosorbent assay (ELISA) test. This detects HIV antibodies with sensitivity and specificity of greater than 99%. The positive predictive value of the ELISA (i.e., the likelihood that a patient with a positive test actually has HIV infection) ranges from 20% in very low-risk populations to greater than 95% in patients with strong risk factors. Because the ELISA is not 100% specific, use a Western blot to confirm any positive ELISA. This test detects serum antibodies directed against specific HIV-1 proteins of various molecular weights and is defined as positive when two or more of the following antibody bands are present: p24, gp41, or gp120/160. Indeterminate Western blots can occur; without p24, gp41, or gp120/160 bands, the patient does not need further evaluation and does not have HIV infection.

What is the window period?

This is the time between acquiring infection and development of antibodies. Antibody-based tests remain negative in this window period. Over 90% of patients seroconvert within 4 weeks of infection. Three tests can detect HIV infection before the appearance of antibody: viral p24 antigen, nucleic acid polymerase chain reaction (PCR) testing, and branch chain DNA assays. The p24 antigen is transiently positive and less sensitive for acute HIV infection than are the viral load tests (PCR or branch chain DNA assay).

What key questions should I ask of patients with HIV infection at clinic visits?

Your main goal is to assess the immune status of your patient. In patients with high CD4 counts, focus on skin or mouth symptoms, side effects from any medications, general health (weight loss, fatigue, itching, loss of appetite), and any patient concerns. In patients with low CD4 counts (<300) the risk of opportunistic infection is much greater. Mean CD4 count is less than 100 for most common opportunistic infections. Ask these patients about diarrhea, dysphagia, thrush, headache, fever, or changes in vision (Table 29-4).

What are the important parts of the physical examination to include in all visits?

Perform skin and oral examinations at each visit in all patients. Look for any of the three forms of candidiasis: pseudomembranous candidiasis is classic, well-recognized

TABLE 29-4

History Questions to Ask HIV-Infected Patients at Routine Clinic Visits

Patient with high CD4 count (>300)	Diseases concerned about
Medication side effects	Pancreatitis: ddI, d4T, ddC
	Neuropathy: ddI, ddC, d4T
	Myositis: AZT
	Kidney stones: indinavir
	Diarrhea: nelfinavir, ritonavir
	Hepatitis: all protease inhibitors
Skin changes	Seborrheic dermatitis, generalized pruritus
General health (fatigue, weight change, anorexia)	Medication side effects, depression, TB
Patient with low CD4 count (<300)	
Headache, seizure, weakness, general fever, weight loss, night sweats	MAC, AIDS wasting syndrome, toxoplasmosis, cryptococcus
Dysphagia	Candidal esophagitis (CMV/HSV esophagitis less commonly)
Diarrhea	*Clostridium difficile*, cryptosporidia, MAC
Abdominal pain	MAC, lymphoma, acalculous cholecystitis
Cough, dyspnea	Pneumonia, especially PCP
Visual changes	CMV
Skin changes	Kaposi's sarcoma, molluscum

thick white plaques on the tongue and palate; atrophic candidiasis causes a painful red shiny tongue or hard palate; and angular cheilitis causes cracking and fissuring at the corners of the mouth. Look for hairy leukoplakia, aphthous ulcers, Kaposi's sarcoma, and gingivitis, as well. Perform a careful skin examination. Test for peripheral neuropathy in patients on didanosine (ddI), zalcitabine (ddC), or stavudine (d4T). This can be done easily by breaking a cotton-tipped applicator and using the sharp wooden end versus the soft cotton end.

When should I obtain HIV RNA viral load and CD4 counts?

Current recommendations for obtaining quantitative measurement of HIV RNA are (1) before starting antiretroviral therapy, (2) 4 weeks after starting a new antiretroviral regimen, and (3) every 3 to 4 months during antiretroviral therapy to assess whether modifications are needed. Check CD4 counts every 6 months when CD4 is greater than 500 and every 3 months when CD4 is less than 500.

TREATMENT

When should I start antiretroviral therapy?

Patients with acute HIV infection should be enrolled in trials looking at the efficacy of aggressive antiretroviral therapy in early infection. Some providers treat acute infection with triple drug combinations, including protease inhibitors, although long-term outcomes are not known. In patients with CD4 counts greater than 500

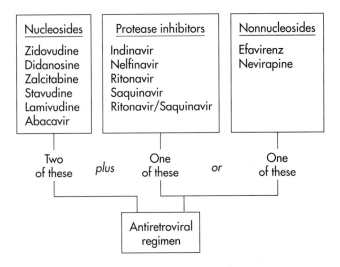

Figure 29-1 Designing antiretroviral therapy for HIV-infected patients.

and an undetectable viral load, monitoring without antiretroviral therapy is appropriate. A high viral load (>10,000) is reason to start antiretroviral therapy regardless of CD4 count. When the CD4 count is less than 500, antiretroviral therapy is appropriate regardless of the viral load. Only start antiretroviral therapy in patients committed to medication compliance.

What antiretroviral drug should I use?

Combination therapy is the rule. The most potent combination is two nucleoside reverse transcriptase inhibitors (zidovudine [AZT], ddI, ddC, d4T, lamivudine [3TC], or abacavir) with a protease inhibitor (Figure 29-1). Another

---

TABLE 29-5

Antiretroviral Medications, Dose and Side Effects

DRUGS	TYPICAL DOSE	SIDE EFFECTS
NUCLEOSIDE REVERSE TRANSCRIPTASE INHIBITORS		
Zidovudine (AZT)	300 mg bid	Nausea, headache, myopathy, anemia, neutropenia
Didanosine (ddI)	400 mg qd	Neuropathy, pancreatitis
Zalcitabine (ddC)	0.75 mg tid	Neuropathy, pancreatitis, mucosal ulcer
Stavudine (d4T)	40 mg bid	Neuropathy, pancreatitis
Lamivudine (3TC)	150 mg bid	Minimal
Abacavir	300 mg bid	Rash, life-threatening hypersensitivity
NONNUCLEOSIDE REVERSE TRANSCRIPTASE INHIBITORS		
Nevirapine	200 mg bid	Rash
Efavirenz	600 mg qd	Rash, agitation, confusion
PROTEASE INHIBITORS*		
Indinavir	800 mg q8h	Kidney stones, elevated bilirubin
Nelfinavir	750 mg tid	Diarrhea
Ritonavir	400 mg bid with saquinavir	Nausea, vomiting, perioral paresthesias
Saquinavir	400 mg bid with ritonavir	Nausea, diarrhea

*All can raise cholesterol, triglycerides, and transaminases.

option is two reverse transcriptase inhibitors with the nonnucleoside drug efavirenz, a combination that appears to equal protease inhibitor combinations in efficacy (Table 29-5).

What are the side effects of antiretroviral agents (Table 29-5)?

Zidovudine can cause headaches, nausea, and vomiting when first started. Anemia and neutropenia occur with longer-term use and are more common in patients who have lower CD4 counts. Patients on the drug for more than 6 months can develop myopathy. All the drugs that begin with "d" (ddI, d4T, ddC) can cause peripheral neuropathy and pancreatitis. In addition, ddC can also cause mucosal ulceration. The nonnucleoside drugs efavirenz and nevirapine can cause rash in 10% of patients. All the protease inhibitors (indinavir, ritonavir, nelfinavir, saquinavir) can cause transaminase elevations. Indinavir is known for its propensity to cause kidney stones. All protease inhibitors can raise triglyceride and cholesterol levels.

When should I start prophylaxis against *Pneumocystis carinii* pneumonia?

Patients who have any of the following conditions should receive *Pneumocystis carinii* pneumonia (PCP) prophylaxis: CD4 count less than 200, previous PCP, oral candidiasis, or unexplained fever greater than 100° F for longer than 2 weeks. Trimethoprim/sulfamethoxazole is

by far the most effective agent. It also provides prophylaxis against toxoplasmosis and may prevent bacterial sinusitis and bacterial pneumonias. For patients who cannot tolerate trimethoprim/sulfamethoxazole, dapsone is a reasonable option. Aerosolized pentamidine is a third option but is less effective than trimethoprim/sulfamethoxazole or dapsone. Because aerosolized pentamidine is not a systemic therapy, patients may develop *Pneumocystis* at sites other than their lungs.

When should patients receive *Mycobacterium avium complex* prophylaxis?

Current recommendations start *Mycobacterium avium complex* (MAC) prophylaxis when CD4 count is less than 50, although some experts suggest a higher cutoff at CD4 less than 100. Favored regimens are azithromycin 1200 mg/wk or clarithromycin 500 mg bid.

What do I do if I get a needle stick from an HIV–infected patient?

First of all, try to prevent this by wearing gloves whenever you draw blood, manipulate intravenous lines, or examine a mucosal surface. Wear eye protection for any procedure (e.g., endoscopy, bronchoscopy, surgery). *Never* recap needles; this is the most common cause of needle-stick injury. Use of AZT after needle-stick injury appears to decrease the risk of transmission. Current practice is to give AZT + 3TC ± protease inhibitor for high-risk exposures.

Key Points

- Perform skin and oral cavity examinations at all visits.
- Use HIV viral load to decide when to start antiretrovirals, and to assess response to treatment.
- Use combination therapy, beginning with two nucleoside reverse transcriptase inhibitors and a protease inhibitor; alternately, a nonnucleoside reverse transcriptase inhibitor can be substituted for a protease inhibitor.
- Prevent needle sticks: never recap needles, wear gloves, and discard all sharps appropriately.

CASE 29-3

A 27-year-old HIV-infected man with A2 HIV disease comes to establish primary care. He was diagnosed with HIV 3 years ago and believes he was infected about 6 years ago. His CD4 count 2 months ago was 405, and viral load was 30,000. He has no complaints. He has had only sporadic, routine care in the past and was previously on AZT + ddI for about 6 months.

A. Would you start antiretroviral therapy? If so, what combination would you use?

B. What tests would you want to obtain?

HIV INFECTION COMPLICATIONS

ETIOLOGY

What types of skin problems affect patients with HIV infection?

Skin findings that occur at higher CD4 counts include *seborrheic dermatitis, allergic reactions* (medication, insect bites), and exacerbations of *psoriasis*. Later in the course of HIV infection, patients can develop *Kaposi's sarcoma* (KS) and *molluscum contagiosum.* In patients with HIV infection, molluscum bodies can cluster together to form giant molluscum up to 1 to 2 centimeters across; this is an indication of a markedly depleted immune system. Patients with very low CD4 counts (<50) can develop large cutaneous ulcers, often in the perirectal region, which should be considered *herpes simplex virus* until proven otherwise.

My patient with HIV infection has a mouth lesion. What could this be?

Possibilities include hairy leukoplakia, candidal infection, aphthous ulcers, gingivitis, and KS. Hairy leukoplakia (HL) appears as white plaques on the side of the tongue and is caused by Epstein-Barr virus. HL is specific for HIV infection and indicates a higher risk for disease progression to AIDS. In one study of CD4 count-matched patients, 22% of patients with HL progressed to AIDS within 2 years compared with 9% of patients without HL. Candidiasis ("thrush") occurs generally when the CD4 count is less than 300 and is a marker of immune deficiency. Patients with oral candidiasis are at higher risk for developing other opportunistic infections and should therefore receive *Pneumocystis* prophylaxis. Some 30% of patients with KS have mouth involvement.

My patient is short of breath. What diseases do I need to consider?

Some 95% of cases of *Pneumocystis carinii* occur with CD4 counts less than 200, with a mean CD4 count less than 100. *Tuberculosis* is more common in patients with HIV, especially in the presence of IV drug use, homelessness, or origin from an endemic area (Africa, Latin America, and Southeast Asia). The yearly rate of developing TB with HIV infection and a positive PPD is 7%. This compares with a lifetime risk of less than 10% with positive PPD but no HIV infection. *Bacterial pneumonia* is also more common. It occurs at high CD4 counts and may be the first hint to the presence of HIV disease. *Pneumococcus* and *Haemophilus influenzae* are the most common organisms involved. Estimated annual rates of pneumococcal pneumonia in HIV-infected individuals are as high as 10%. *Pseudomonas aeruginosa* is another important cause of community-acquired pneumonia when the CD4 count is less than 50. Bacteremia and recurrent pneumonias are more likely in the setting of HIV infection. HIV infection also causes *cardiomyopathy,* which may present as dyspnea.

What causes headaches in HIV-infected patients?

Headache is common. If the CD4 count is greater than 500, nonopportunistic infections are more likely (*sinusitis, HIV meningitis*). When the CD4 count is less than 200, consider the big three opportunistic diseases: *cryptococcosis, toxoplasmosis,* and *lymphoma.* Sinusitis, HIV meningitis, or *tuberculous meningitis* can also occur at these lower CD4 counts.

My patient has diarrhea. What causes do I need to consider?

Approximately 50% of AIDS patients have GI problems, with diarrhea from infectious cause being the most common complaint. Common pathogens include CMV, *Cryptosporidia, Giardia, M. avium,* and *Clostridium difficile. Cryptosporidia* is a small, noninvasive parasite of animals and was a rare cause of self-limited diarrhea in immunocompetent patients before the AIDS epidemic.

Cryptosporidiosis is characterized by a persistent watery diarrhea, cramping abdominal pain, anorexia, and weight loss. *Giardia* is the most common nonopportunistic protozoan parasite in AIDS patients. It is seen in up to 15% of AIDS patients with symptomatic diarrhea. *C. difficile* is extremely common in patients with HIV disease because frequent hospitalizations allow for colonization and frequent antibiotic use leads to overgrowth. HIV infection itself can also cause diarrhea but is a diagnosis of exclusion.

What are the causes of esophagitis?

Dysphagia (difficulty swallowing) and odynophagia (painful swallowing) are symptoms suggesting esophagitis in AIDS patients. These symptoms can significantly decrease food intake and worsen nutritional status. *Candida* esophagitis is the most frequent cause, especially when oral candidiasis is present. *CMV, Herpes simplex,* and the drug *ddC* can also cause symptomatic esophageal ulcerations.

What can cause fever in HIV infected patients?

When CD4 count is greater than 500, nonopportunistic causes are more common: bacterial pneumonia, pulmonary TB, or sinusitis, an almost universal problem in patients with HIV. In patients with lower CD4 counts, especially less than 200, opportunistic infections are more likely. With diarrhea, consider the pathogens *C. difficile, Salmonella,* and MAC. For fever with pulmonary symptoms, consider bacterial pneumonia, TB, or *Pneumocystis.* If no focal signs accompany fever, think of cryptococcal meningitis (10% to 20% of patients do not have headache). Other poorly localized conditions include extrapulmonary TB, common with low CD4 counts; MAC, which can cause night sweats and anemia; hepatitis, either resulting from hepatitis B or C or toxin effect (e.g. from trimethoprim/sulfamethoxazole); CMV infection; or sinusitis.

EVALUATION

When should I suspect pneumonia in an HIV-infected patient?

The symptoms of bacterial pneumonia in HIV-infected patients are similar to those in non–HIV-infected individuals: dyspnea, productive cough, high fever, and fatigue. In patients with *Pseudomonas* and CD4 counts less than 100, x-ray may show cavitary lesions.

Does TB present differently in HIV-infected patients?

Clinical manifestations of TB vary by the CD4 count. At CD4 counts greater than 300, symptoms and x-ray findings are more typical: weight loss, night sweats, fevers, and productive cough, with upper lobe infiltrates, pleural effusions or cavitary lesions on x-ray. At CD4 counts less than 200, clinical manifestations are less typical, extrapulmonary TB becomes common (in two thirds of cases), and chest x-ray findings are atypical with bilateral hilar adenopathy and lower lobe disease. Upper lobe infiltrates and pulmonary cavities are rare in patients with low CD4 counts.

How does PCP present?

PCP usually presents with progressive dyspnea over 2 to 3 weeks, dry nonproductive cough, and fever. Examination is often unrevealing except for an increased respiratory rate. ABG often shows a decreased Po_2 and a widened A-a gradient. LDH is commonly elevated and is a prognostic factor for severity of illness. Bilateral interstitial infiltrates are typical on x-ray, but in severe cases, alveolar/lobar infiltrates occur, as well. In up to 20% of cases, the chest x-ray is normal. Spontaneous pneumothorax in a patient with HIV disease is usually a sign of underlying PCP.

What tests are warranted in patients with headache in the setting of HIV infection?

Workup of patients with headache and low CD4 count (<200) consists of an imaging procedure (MRI or contrast CT scan) followed by a lumbar puncture. Characteristic CT findings are listed in Table 29-6. Send CSF for cell count, protein, glucose, Gram stain, cryptococcal antigen, and bacterial culture, and strongly consider mycobacterial culture. Serum cryptococcal antigen is 99% sensitive for cryptococcal meningitis. Review if the patient has had toxoplasma titers checked—if negative, this makes toxoplasmosis an unlikely diagnosis because greater than 90% of patients with CNS toxoplasmosis have a positive IgG. You cannot diagnose CNS lymphoma noninvasively.

How should I evaluate my HIV-infected patient who has a fever?

Look for a focal process and let history and examination guide your workup. The CD4 count is the single most important factor in determining risk of opportunistic infection. Obtain CBC with differential, chest x-ray, blood cultures, urinalysis, and SGOT or serum glutamic-pyruvic transaminase (SGPT) (hepatitis C is common with IV drug use; hepatitis B is common in patients with IV drug use or male-male sex). If no focal signs exist, consider additional tests, including blood cultures for mycobacteria and serum cryptococcal antigen. Other tests, such as head CT with contrast, lumbar puncture, stool cultures, and sinus CT, should all be based on symptoms suggesting focal abnormalities. If the patient has diar-

TABLE 29-6

Patterns Seen on Head CT Scan in HIV-Related CNS Disease

DISEASE	PATTERN	ENHANCEMENT	LOCATION
Toxoplasmosis	Ring mass	++	Basal ganglia
Lymphoma	Solid mass	+++	Periventricular
Progressive multifocal leukoencephalopathy	No mass	None	Subcortical white matter

rhea, obtain stool *C. difficile* toxin, *Giardia* antigen, and stool culture for enteric pathogens and atypical mycobacteria. With pulmonary symptoms, obtain chest film, sputum Gram stain, and sputum cultures for TB. Pulmonary disease is usually one of three—bacterial pneumonia, TB, or PCP. PCP prophylaxis makes PCP unlikely, and fluconazole use makes cryptococcus unlikely.

My patient has persistent dysphagia after 2 weeks of fluconazole. What should I do next?

Obtain endoscopic biopsy with viral cultures to identify infection other than *Candida*. CMV appears on endoscopy as large, shallow, superficial ulcerations often involving most of the esophagus. Stop ddC.

TREATMENT

How do I treat PCP infection?

Treatment is with high-dose *trimethoprim/sulfamethoxazole* (first choice), *pentamidine, trimethoprim/dapsone* (for mild disease), *atovaquone,* or *clindamycin/primaquine.* All of these regimens appear to have equivalent efficacy. Side effects are common, occurring in 50% of cases treated with trimethoprim/sulfamethoxazole or pentamidine. The major side effects with pentamidine are renal insufficiency; pancreatic islet cell destruction, which can cause transient hypoglycemia or permanent hyperglycemia; and hypotension. Early use of corticosteroids in patients with moderate to severe PCP can im-

prove survival and decrease the occurrence of respiratory failure. Give steroids to patient with Po_2 less than 70 or an alveolar-arterial oxygen gradient greater than 35.

What treatments are used for the various causes of diarrhea?

Ganciclovir decreases CMV-induced nausea and diarrhea. Treat *Giardia* and *C. difficile* with oral metronidazole. Common enteric bacteria respond to appropriate antibiotics

---

Key Points ....

- Pneumothorax in an AIDS patient should make you think of *Pneumocystis pneumonia.*
- When the CD4 count is greater than 300, TB presents typically with cough, fever, sputum, and upper lobe infiltrates; when CD4 count drops, the presentation is more atypical with hilar adenopathy, lower lobe disease, or extrapulmonary TB.
- Bacterial pneumonias are common, usually caused by *Pneumococcus* and *H. influenzae;* when the CD4 count is less than 100, *Pseudomonas aeruginosa* becomes a common pathogen.
- Patients with oral candidiasis and dysphagia have a greater than 90% likelihood of candidal esophagitis and should receive empiric fluconazole or ketoconazole.
- Consider *C. difficile* as an important cause of diarrhea with HIV infection.

CASE 29-4

A 30-year-old man with C3 HIV disease (CD4 count 60) presents with severe headaches and confusion that have progressed over the past 2 weeks. He has had intermittent fevers for the past 3 weeks. His friends state that he has been more forgetful and on the day of admission he became belligerent and did not recognize his partner. Medications include AZT 200 tid, 3TC 150 bid, indinavir 800 q8h, and dapsone 100 qd. Examination shows severe seborrheic dermatitis, molluscum contagiosum, oral hairy leukoplakia, and left lower extremity weakness with a left

upgoing toe. Laboratory test results are: HCT 31, WBC 2.0, Na 134, K 3.9, Cl 98, HCO_3 26, Cr 1.0, and BUN 18.

A. What does the seborrheic dermatitis tell you?
B. What is the importance of molluscum contagiosum and oral hairy leukoplakia in patients with HIV disease?
C. What is the differential diagnosis for this patient?
D. What workup would you pursue?

with gram-negative coverage. *Cryptosporidium* is very hard to eradicate; these patients may benefit from loperamide (Imodium).

How do I treat esophagitis?

Patients with oral candidiasis and dysphagia can be given empiric ketoconazole 200 mg qd or fluconazole 100 to 200 mg qd. Treat endoscopically diagnosed CMV with ganciclovir, herpes with high-dose acyclovir, and *Candida* as above with fluconazole or ketoconazole.

How do I treat cryptococcal meningitis?

Treat initially with intravenous amphotericin B, usually for 2 weeks. Follow with chronic lifelong suppressive therapy using oral fluconazole.

MENINGITIS

ETIOLOGY

What is the definition of meningitis?

Meningitis is inflammation of the meninges from *infectious* (bacterial, viral, or fungal) or *noninfectious* causes (sarcoid, malignancy, or hemorrhage from vasculitis).

What are the most common causes of infectious meningitis?

Viral meningitis is much more common than bacterial meningitis, with enteroviruses making up 70% of all patients with viral meningitis. Herpes simplex meningitis is usually associated with primary HSV-2 infection. Acute HIV infection can cause meningitis and is under-diagnosed. In adults with bacterial meningitis, the most common etiologic agent is *Streptococcus pneumoniae*, occurring in 30% to 50% of patients. *Neisseria meningitidis* (meningococcus) is the second most common cause, occurring in 10% to 35% of adult patients. *Haemophilus influenzae*, a very common cause of bacterial meningitis in children, is quite rare in adults, causing only 1% to 2% of adult meningitis cases (Box 29-1).

What are the risk factors for the different organisms causing bacterial meningitis?

Pneumococcal meningitis may occur in the presence of pneumococcal pneumonia (15% to 25% of cases), otitis media, or CSF leaks after trauma. Risk factors for pneumococcal meningitis include alcoholism, cirrhosis, sickle cell anemia, asplenia, multiple myeloma, and chronic lymphocytic leukemia. *Neisserial meningitis* usu-

---

BOX 29-1   Causes of Bacterial Meningitis in Adults
COMMON   *S. pneumococcus*   *N. meningitidis*   **UNCOMMON**   *H. influenzae*   **SPECIAL CIRCUMSTANCES**   ***Neurosurgical Patients***   *S. aureus*   Gram-negative rods   ***Alcoholics or Immunosuppressed Patients***   *Listeria*

---

ally occurs in young adults, is rare after age 45, and is the most common cause for epidemic bacterial meningitis. Also, complement deficiency increases the risk, particularly with deficient terminal components (C5 through C8). *Listeria monocytogenes* is a gram-positive rod that is more prevalent in the setting of alcoholism, pregnancy, or hematologic malignancy. However, 20% to 30% of adults with *Listeria* infections have no risk factors.

EVALUATION

What are the typical symptoms of bacterial meningitis?

Classic symptoms seen in more than 85% of adults include fever, headache, meningismus, and mental status change. More nonspecific symptoms include nausea, vomiting, rigors, profuse sweats, weakness, myalgias, and photophobia. The presenting symptoms can be variable, depending on the infecting organism and the underlying immune status of the patient. Presence of mental status change, occurring in 95% of patients, is the single strongest indicator of bacterial meningitis.

What signs should I look for if I suspect meningitis?

Kernig's and Brudzinski's signs are present in 50% of bacterial meningitis cases. Perform these tests as follows: For Kernig's sign, attempt to extend the knee with the hip flexed. This is positive when pain in the hamstring causes resistance to further extension. For Brudzinski's sign, flex the patient's neck. In a positive test, this maneuver will produce flexion in the hip. Perform a careful skin examination because two thirds of patients with meningococcus have a violaceous rash.

TABLE 29-7
CSF Findings With Meningitis of Various Causes

ETIOLOGY	WBC	WBC DIFFERENTIAL	PROTEIN (MG/DL)	GLUCOSE* (MG/DL)	STAIN
Viral	5-500	>50% monos	30-150	Normal or lower	No organisms
Bacterial	100-2000	>90% PMNs	80-500	<35	80% gram positive
Cryptococcus	40-400†	>80% monos	40-150	Normal or lower	>90% cryptococcal Ag 50% India ink positive
Tuberculosis	100-1000	>80% monos	40-150	Normal or lower	AFB smear positive
Subdural or epidural abscess	50-300	Variable	75-300	Normal	No organisms

*Normal glucose is greater than 40 mg/dl or greater than 50% of simultaneous blood glucose.
†Lower in immunocompromised patients with HIV.

Does meningitis present differently in elderly and immunosuppressed patients?

The usual signs of meningeal inflammation (nuchal rigidity, headache, Kernig's and Brudzinski's signs, fever) may not be present in the elderly or patients with immune dysfunction, such as neutropenia or HIV disease. In the elderly, confusion and mental status changes are the single most reliable findings (in 80% to 90%).

What are the typical clinical features of viral meningitis?

The clinical features of viral meningitis include a prodrome of headache, malaise, and fever with normal mental status. Viral meningitis is particularly common in individuals older than age 40. Examination is usually unrevealing; look for genital ulcers/blisters, suggesting HSV-2; generalized adenopathy, suggesting HIV; or parotitis, suggesting mumps.

Should I obtain a CNS imaging test before lumbar puncture?

The question frequently arises whether CNS imaging is required preceding LP. Obtain a CT scan or MRI before LP in any patient with a focal neurologic examination, papilledema on funduscopic examination, or in HIV-positive patients with CD4 count less than 200. HIV-infected patients may have mass lesions resulting from toxoplasmosis, tuberculosis, or lymphoma. Look for evidence of midline shift, indicating CNS mass lesion and increased intracranial pressure; if present, risk for herniation and subsequent death with LP is approximately 6%.

What tests should I order on CSF?

Send CSF for glucose, protein, cell count with differential, bacterial culture, and Gram stain. In patients at high risk for tuberculosis or fungal meningitis, test for tuberculosis with an acid-fast bacillus (AFB) smear and culture and for cryptococcal disease with cryptococcal antigen testing and India ink preparation. It is important to remember that not all patients need AFB and fungal testing of the CSF.

What does the CSF look like in patients with bacterial meningitis?

CSF in bacterial meningitis shows greater than 500/mm³ PMNs, protein greater than 100 mm/dl, and glucose less than 40% of serum glucose (Table 29-7). About 80% of patients have a positive Gram stain.

What tests are useful if I suspect bacterial meningitis and the Gram stain is negative?

Counterimmunoelectrophoresis (CIE) can detect the presence of capsular polysaccharide from *H. influenzae*, *S. pneumoniae*, and *N. meningitidis*. This is particularly useful for evaluating patients who have received antibiotics because the polysaccharide persists after bacterial lysis.

What does the CSF test look like in a patient with viral meningitis?

In contrast to the high PMN count of bacterial meningitis, the typical pattern of viral meningitis is a total cell count less than 500/mm³ with a mononuclear predominance, protein less than 80 to 100 mm/dl, and a normal glucose level. Early in the course of viral meningitis, PMNs may predominate. A repeat LP within 6 to 8 hours will often show a shift to mononuclear predominance.

TREATMENT

What therapy should be used for suspected bacterial meningitis?

With the increase in pneumococcal resistance to penicillin, empiric therapy for meningitis must cover penicillin-resistant organisms. Vancomycin plus a third-generation cephalosporin (ceftriaxone or cefotaxime) is recommended. If the patient has risk factors for *Listeria* or if this organism is seen on Gram stain, add ampicillin, as well. A third-generation cephalosporin alone is adequate when meningococcus is seen on Gram stain, in elderly patients with probable gram-negative meningitis, or postneurosurgical patients in whom gram-negative meningitis or *S. aureus* meningitis is possible. Do not use cefoperazone or ceftazidime because they have very poor CNS penetration. Narrow the spectrum of coverage once an organism is identified.

Key Points

- Obtain CSF to look for meningitis in patients with mental status changes, headache, and fever.
- Mental status changes or seizure may be the only symptoms of meningitis in the elderly.
- Obtain contrast CT before LP for focal neurologic examination and in HIV patients with CD4 less than 200.
- Viral meningitis may elevate PMNs in the CSF early in the course of the disease; treat patients with antibiotics until CSF cultures are negative (24 hours is sufficient).
- Treat suspected pneumococcal meningitis with vancomycin plus a third-generation cephalosporin until cultures/sensitivity return.

CASE 29-5

A 73-year-old man presents to the ER with mental status changes over the past 24 hours. He has no complaints. His daughter has brought him in because of confusion. Past medical history is significant for CAD, CHF, and BPH. Examination reveals BP 100/60, P 110, T 39° C, no rash, chest is clear, heart is without murmur, and abdomen is nontender. Laboratory test values are as follows: HCT 38, WBC 23,000 with 90% polys, Na 136, K 4.9, Cl 100, HCO₃ 18, BUN 30, and Cr 2.0.

A. What tests would you order?
B. What is the most likely diagnosis for this patient?

CASE 29-6

A 37-year-old alcoholic patient presents with obtundation and fever. He was found seizing on a downtown sidewalk. His old chart shows multiple ER visits for alcohol intoxication, lacerations, and one episode of pancreatitis. On examination, BP is 90/60, P is 120, and T is 40.8° C. Skin is without rash, and neck is stiff with a positive Brudzinski's sign. Breath sounds are decreased at the right base, and heart is without murmur. He is sleepy with symmetric neurologic examination and toes upgoing bilaterally. Laboratory test values are as follows: Na 128, K 3.8, Cl 96, HCO₃ 12, HCT 39, WBC 2.9, and chest x-ray shows RLL infiltrate.

A. What tests would you order?
B. What is your differential diagnosis?
C. What treatment would you start?

PNEUMONIA

ETIOLOGY

How do people get pneumonia?

Pneumonia is inflammation of lung parenchyma from infection. Organisms reach the lung by oropharyngeal aspiration, inhalation, or hematogenous spread. Defects in host defenses often contribute, for example, impaired glottic reflex, insufficient cough, impaired ciliary function usually from smoking, or deficient immunity. Important risk factors for pneumonia are listed in Table 29-8.

What organisms cause community-acquired pneumonia?

Pneumococcus pneumoniae and then *H. influenzae* are most common; both occur in patients with predisposing conditions (see Table 29-8). *Mycoplasma pneumoniae* is probably the most common cause in young, healthy adults. Anaerobic pneumonias occur with periodontal disease because anaerobes flourish amid rotting teeth and gums; edentulous patients rarely get anaerobic infections. Anaerobic infections are also more common with aspiration of mouth flora during periods of unconsciousness or with swallowing disorders.

How is hospital-acquired pneumonia different from community-acquired pneumonia?

Hospital-acquired pneumonia occurs in up to 10% of hospitalized patients. Common culprits are gram-negative rods (often resistant to multiple antibiotics) and *S. aureus*, followed by anaerobes and *S. pneumoniae*. Gram-negative pneumonias carry high mortality (40%) because the or-

TABLE 29-8

Organisms and Mechanisms Causing Pneumonia in Patients With Specific Risk Factors for Pneumonia

RISK GROUP	SPECIFIC LIKELY ORGANISMS	MECHANISMS OF ACQUIRING PNEUMONIA
Alcoholism	*Streptococcus pneumoniae* Anaerobes *Haemophilus influenzae* *Klebsiella pneumoniae* *Mycobacterium tuberculosis*	Aspiration of oral and gastric flora due to decreased glottic reflex, seizures, or stupor Poor WBC function and humoral immunity
IV drug use	*Streptococcus pneumoniae* Anaerobes *Staphylococcus aureus* *Mycobacterium tuberculosis*	Aspiration as above Septic pulmonary emboli (tricuspid endocarditis) HIV infection
Smoking-induced lung disease	*Streptococcus pneumoniae* *Haemophilus influenzae* *Moraxella catarrhalis* *Legionella*	Impaired mucociliary transport Colonized lower respiratory tract Resistance due to prior frequent antibiotics
HIV infection	*Streptococcus pneumoniae* *Haemophilus influenzae* *Pneumocystis carinii* *Pseudomonas aeruginosa*	Impaired cellular immunity Prophylactic antibiotics and CD4 <100 make pseudomonal infection more likely
Nursing home residence	*Klebsiella pneumoniae* *Staphylococcus aureus* *Mycobacterium tuberculosis* (reactivation or primary)	Lowered immunity Predisposing illness Institutional exposures Neurologic disease or medications cause altered cognition and aspiration Colonization with gram-negative rods
Postviral superinfection	*Streptococcus pneumoniae* *Staphylococcus aureus* *Haemophilus influenzae*	Viral infections disrupt mucociliary function and interfere with cell-mediated host defense mechanisms (e.g., influenza, cytomegalovirus) Develops 7-19 days after viral infection

ganisms are aggressive and concurrent underlying medical conditions complicate recovery.

What are some uncommon causes of pneumonia?

Legionella occurs sporadically or as an epidemic; those with underlying lung disease are at greatest risk. Consider psittacosis *(Chlamydia psittaci)* with exposure to birds, especially in pet shop workers or bird keepers. *Chlamydia pneumoniae* (TWAR) occurs in young adults. Q fever from inhalation of aerosolized *Coxiella burnetii* is seen in livestock handlers.

What causes pleural effusions in patients with pneumonia?

Exudative pleural effusion accompanies about 40% of pneumonias and is caused by pleural inflammation. Most of these parapneumonic effusions are small and sterile and resolve with treatment of the pneumonia. Some become infected, creating a purulent empyema, which can cause persistent infection, sepsis, and permanent scarring if left undrained.

EVALUATION

What questions should I ask when I suspect pneumonia?

Classic symptoms of bacterial pneumonia include cough producing bloody or purulent sputum, high fever, dyspnea, or pleuritic chest pain. For example, pneumococcal pneumonia classically presents with a single shaking chill at onset followed by high fever, pleuritic chest pain, and cough productive of bloody or "rusty" sputum. *Legionella* may cause myalgias, headache, confusion, and diarrhea, as well. "Atypical" presentations are more subdued and suggest less inflammatory organisms, such as viruses, *Mycoplasma, Pneumocystis, Chlamydia,* or, uncommonly, Q fever or psittacosis. Cough, when present, is usually nonproductive, fevers are lower grade, and myalgias or severe headache may be present. Extrapulmonary manifestations may be prominent with *Mycoplasma* (meningitis, cerebellar ataxia, erythema multiforme). Hoarseness or sore throat suggests *Chlamydia pneumoniae*. Ask about occupational or animal exposures, especially when symptoms are atypical, an organism cannot be found, or patients do not respond to empiric therapy for common organisms. Foul-smelling sputum suggests anaerobes. Weight loss, anorexia, and night sweats are clues to TB infection or lung abscess.

In what situations might typical pneumonias present atypically?

Elderly patients may have few symptoms referable to the chest, and the main finding is confusion, disorientation, or anorexia. Neutropenic patients rarely have productive cough because there are no WBCs to produce sputum; their earliest and most pronounced symptom of pneumonia is isolated fever. Some lower lobe pneumonias may present with abdominal pain as a result of irritation of the diaphragm.

What examination findings support a diagnosis of typical lobar pneumonia?

Tachypnea, tachycardia, and fever are common. With early lobar pneumonia, breath sounds are decreased. Always compare breath sounds from side to side to detect subtle asymmetry. Dullness to percussion can represent consolidation or pleural effusion. Rales may be heard over the affected lobe and are most prominent with resolving pneumonia as air passages begin to open up again. Other signs of lobar consolidation include bronchial breath sounds, whispered pectoriloquy, and tactile fremitus. Bronchial breath sounds are coarse sounds of air moving in the large bronchi that transmit better through areas of consolidation to the chest wall than through normal aerated lung. Whispered pectoriloquy is elicited by having the patient whisper something (try their phone number or social security number). Transmission of sound is very good through consolidated lung, and you can easily hear the whispered words when your stethoscope is placed over the area. Elicit tactile fremitus by having the patient say "toy boat" while you place your hands symmetrically on the patient's chest; vibrations are increased over areas of consolidation and decreased when fluid or air is present in the pleural space. Use this technique when dullness to percussion is present to differentiate effusion from infiltrate.

What laboratory tests are warranted if I suspect pneumonia?

Check O_2 saturation, CBC, sputum Gram stain and culture, electrolytes, and kidney function. In typical presentations, the WBC rises, often with a left shift (excess immature forms or bands). In contrast, WBC count is often normal in viruses of *Mycoplasma or Chlamydia*. Low WBC in the presence of pneumonia is a poor prognostic sign. In particularly ill-appearing patients, consider blood cultures and ABG. Positive blood cultures occur in up to 25% of pneumococcal pneumonias and are associated with poorer prognosis (20% to 40% mortality). ABG may reveal hypoxia and respiratory alkalosis. *Mycoplasma* is suggested by hemolytic anemia or cold agglutinins (seen in 50%). You can confirm diagnosis by a rise in convalescent antibody titers. *Mycoplasma* and *Chlamydia* are often treated empirically without confirming a diagnosis. *Legionella* causes hyponatremia and a sputum Gram stain with leukocytes but no organisms. Diagnose *Legionella* by urinary antigen (type 1 only), DNA probe, direct fluorescent antibody, culture, or increase in convalescent antibody titer.

How do I interpret sputum Gram stain and cultures?

Unfortunately, sputum specimens are often contaminated with saliva and oral flora, as indicated by epithelial cells and multiple organisms on Gram stain: greater than 25 epithelial cells per low power field correlates with an inadequate specimen. An adequate specimen from deep in the chest, demonstrating one dominant organism (more the exception than the rule) can guide initial empiric therapy. Gram stain is most reliable for *S. pneumoniae* and least reliable for the difficult-to-see pleomorphic gram-negative rods of *H. influenzae*. If you see WBCs with no organisms, consider *Legionella, Mycoplasma, Chlamydia*, TB, or psittacosis. Sputum culture is less useful than stains because it is negative in up to 50% of those with blood culture–positive pneumonia. Culture is more useful in the diagnosis of TB because stains may miss this disease.

How can chest films help with the diagnosis of pneumonia?

The causative organism cannot be accurately predicted by x-ray, but certain appearances are more typical of some organisms than others (Table 29-9).

TREATMENT

How do I choose empiric treatment for a patient with pneumonia?

Identify and target the most likely organism (Table 29-10). Switch to narrow-spectrum antibiotics when sensitivities are available. For nosocomial pneumonia with gram-negative rods on sputum Gram stain, cover dually with an aminoglycoside and an extended-spectrum antipseudomonal penicillin (e.g., ticarcillin, mezlocillin, piperacillin), an antipseudomonal third-generation

TABLE 29-9

Likely Organisms as Suggested by Specific Chest Film Findings in Pneumonia

CHEST FILM FINDINGS	LIKELY ORGANISMS
Alveolar/air space lobar infiltrate with air-bronchograms*, silhouette sign†	*Pneumococcus, Haemophilus,* other typical organisms
Upper lobe infiltrates	TB, *Klebsiella*
Apical scarring	Prior TB
Bilateral lower lobe infiltrates	Anaerobes (aspiration)
Upper lobe posterior segment or lower lobe superior segment R > L	Anaerobes (aspiration) Right lung > left (right main stem bronchus more straight)
Patchy bilateral infiltrates	*Mycoplasma pneumoniae*
Patchy unilateral segmental infiltrates	*Chlamydia pneumoniae*
Diffuse interstitial infiltrates	*Pneumocystis,* viral pneumonia
Cavitation‡	*Mycobacterium tuberculosis, Staphylococcus aureus,* or gram-negative rods

*Bronchus remains aerated and dark while surrounding alveoli are fluid-filled and bright.
†Silhouette sign is the loss of a heart border or diaphragm shadow caused by focal adjacent lung consolidation.
‡Appearance of a hollow, round cavity resulting from necrosis and liquefaction of lung parenchyma.

TABLE 29-10

Empiric Antibiotic Treatment Options for Pneumonia by Risk Factor and Suspected Pathogens

	EMPIRIC THERAPY OPTIONS
RISK FACTOR	
COPD	Cefuroxime (oral) Ceftriaxone (IV) Ampicillin/clavulanate Quinolone (trovafloxacin, grepafloxacin, levofloxacin)
Aspiration	Clindamycin Amoxicillin/clavulanate or ampicillin/sulbactam
Elderly	Amoxicillin/clavulanate or ampicillin/sulbactam
Nosocomial infection	Aminoglycoside + antipseudomonal penicillin, or third-generation cephalosporin, levofloxacin or alatrovofloxacin
SUSPECTED PATHOGEN	
Pneumococcus or *Haemophilus*	Second- or third-generation cephalosporin Amoxicillin/clavulanate or ampicillin/sulbactam
Mycoplasma	Erythromycin (also, clarithromycin or azithromycin)
Legionella	Erythromycin in high dose (1 g IV q6h) Quinolones
Staphylococcus	Nafcillin + aminoglycoside Substitute vancomycin if penicillin-allergic
Anaerobes	Clindamycin Metronidazole Amoxicillin/clavulanate or ampicillin/sulbactam
Psittacosis	Tetracycline Erythromycin
Chlamydia pneumonia	Tetracycline
Q fever	Tetracycline Chloramphenicol

cephalosporin (e.g., ceftazidime, cefoperazone), or a quinolone (e.g., levofloxacin, alatrofloxacin). With clusters of gram-positive cocci on Gram stain in a nosocomial pneumonia, cover empirically for both *S. aureus* and gram-negative rods until culture results are back.

What should I know about resistance to antibiotics?

β-Lactamase production is becoming more common, leading to greater resistance to β-lactam antibiotics. Most strains of pneumococcus are penicillin-sensitive, and low-dose penicillin (600,000 to 1,200,000 U/day) is effective once the diagnosis is made. Pneumococcal resistance to penicillin and cephalosporins is up to 30% in some areas. Third-generation cephalosporins have reasonable activity against strains with intermediate resistance.

How do I manage a parapneumonic effusion?

Pleural tap is indicated to differentiate a sterile parapneumonic effusion from an infected empyema. Empyema must be drained expeditiously by chest tube or surgery to cure the infection, prevent sepsis, and avoid loculation, fibrosis, and permanent impairment of lung function. Treat for empyema if pleural fluid WBC and LDH are high, pH is less than 7.1, glucose is less than 40, or if cultures of pleural fluid grow organisms. If parameters are borderline, retap fluid in 12 hours.

Is there any way to prevent pneumonia?

Pneumococcal vaccine prevents pneumococcal pneumonia in high-risk patients, those over age 65, institutionalized elderly, HIV-positive patients, and in those with other severe underlying illnesses.

How long does it take patients to respond to treatment?

Patients generally improve after 72 hours. X-ray findings can worsen despite clinical improvement, and resolution of x-ray abnormalities lags behind clinical improvement, taking 6 weeks or more. If a patient is not responding to appropriate therapy, look for a resistant or unexpected organism, an alternate cause of fever, or a complication, such as empyema.

Who should be admitted for treatment?

Admit patients with multiple lobe involvement, low initial WBC count, multiple sites of infection, severe underlying disease, alcoholism, or advanced age. Additionally, admit for signs of early sepsis, such as hypotension, orthostasis, tachycardia, tachypnea, or hypoxia.

Key Points

- Assess patients with pneumonia for predisposing risk factors, such as HIV, alcohol use, and smoking.
- Risk factors for poor outcome include low WBC count, multiple lobe involvement, extrapulmonary infection, severe underlying disease (e.g., CHF, cancer), and advanced age.
- A good sputum Gram stain is more predictive of a true pathogen than sputum culture.
- IV drug users are at high risk of *S. aureus* pulmonary infection.
- Two common causes of pneumonia in healthy young adults are *Mycoplasma* and *Chlamydia*.

CASE 29-7

A 66-year-old woman with a long history of cigarette use and recent onset of diabetes complains of 2 days of worsening cough that started as she was gardening and became productive of purulent, rusty sputum yesterday. She had a severe shaking chill last night. T 101.9° F, HR is 80, BP is 120/60, and RR is 32.
  A. What are the most likely organisms causing her symptoms?
  B. What other information would you like?
  C. What empiric treatment is appropriate?
  D. After 36 hours, fevers continue to a temperature of 102° and WBC remains high. What should you do?
  E. Five days into her stay, her temperature reaches 103°. How do you interpret this, and what will you do?

CASE 29-8

An 80-year-old woman is brought to your office from her nursing home because she is more confused than usual today. She had been complaining of abdominal pain. T 98.5° F, and WBC 4.
  A. What could this be (list at least seven things)?
  B. Name at least seven tests to help you figure out her diagnosis.
  C. If this is pneumonia, what organisms do you need to consider?
  D. If this is pneumonia, explain her abdominal pain and lack of fever or leukocytosis.

TUBERCULOSIS

ETIOLOGY

What causes tuberculosis?

TB is an infection caused by a slow-growing aerobic bacillus, *Mycobacterium tuberculosis*, which is not decolorized by acid alcohol and is thus an acid-fast bacillus (AFB).

BOX 29-2   Risk Factors for TB Infection

MAJOR RISK FACTORS
HIV infection
Homelessness
Institutionalization (prison)
Close contact with smear-positive patient
IV drug use
Prior residence in endemic area (i.e., Africa, Southeast
Asia, Central America)

MINOR RISK FACTORS
Diabetes mellitus
Silicosis
Gastrectomy

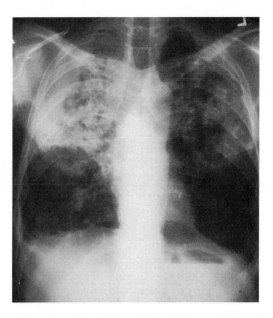

Figure 29-2 Chest film of tuberculosis. Findings of bilateral upper lobe pleural thickening, cavities, and infiltrates (more extensive in the right upper lobe).

What are the risk factors for tuberculosis?

The major risk factors for TB are listed in Box 29-2.

Who is at risk for multidrug-resistant TB?

Most multidrug-resistant TB in the United States has occurred in HIV-infected individuals and institutions.

EVALUATION

What are the typical symptoms of TB?

Classic symptoms are fever, night sweats, weight loss, and cough productive of thick sputum. Hemoptysis and dyspnea are symptoms of advanced disease. In elderly and HIV-infected patients, symptoms may be more subtle (anorexia, fatigue, confusion, weakness).

When should I include TB in the differential diagnosis?

Patients who present with typical symptoms and major risk factors should be worked up on suspicion of TB. Anyone with an upper lobe infiltrate on x-ray should also be considered for workup. Think of TB in elderly patients (especially reactivation TB) who have infiltrates on x-ray that do not respond to standard antibiotic therapy. Alcoholics are at higher risk for TB because of a higher likelihood of homelessness or incarceration.

What is the workup for TB?

Order a chest x-ray first. If infiltrates are present, especially upper lobe, obtain three sputum samples for AFB smear and culture (best collected on three separate mornings). Patients admitted to the hospital and un-

dergoing TB workup should be kept in respiratory isolation until three smears are negative. TB skin testing (purified protein derivative [PPD]) is most helpful when the presentation is atypical. In patients with typical presentations and suggestive x-ray, obtain sputum samples first to avoid a painful large positive PPD skin test. Also obtain routine annual PPD tests in HIV-infected patients, prison inmates, IV drug users, nursing home residents, homeless patients, health care workers, and prior residents of TB-endemic countries. Immunocompromised patients require concurrent use of controls (trichophyton, candida) to assess for anergy.

What are the typical x-ray findings of TB?

Most TB is reactivation TB with upper lobe infiltrates, cavitation, and pleural thickening (Figure 29-2). Patients with primary infection can develop hilar adenopathy, pleural effusions, or miliary pattern (diffuse small nodules in the lungs, named after millet seeds). HIV-infected patients can have varying x-ray presentation (see HIV Infection Complications section).

TREATMENT

What therapy should a patient with active TB receive?

Multiple drug therapy is the rule because of the risk of drug resistance. Start with 4 drugs, usually isoniazid (INH), rifampin, pyrazinamide, and ethambutol. If the organism turns out to be sensitive to INH and ri-

---

BOX 29-3 Indications for INH Prophylaxis
With Positive PPD

Close contact with smear-positive patient
HIV-infected
Chest x-ray consistent with old TB
IV drug user
Prolonged steroid use or other immunocompromise
(e.g., diabetes, silicosis, end-stage renal disease)
Recent converter within 2 years

---

fampin, then ethambutol and pyrazinamide can be discontinued after 2 months and the 6-month course finished off with INH and rifampin. Give vitamin B_6 to avoid neuropathy from INH.

Who should receive INH prophylaxis?

In general, patients with a newly positive PPD or close contacts of smear-positive patients should receive prophylaxis (Box 29-3).

Key Points ··

- Major risk factors for TB include IV drug use, HIV infection, homelessness, history of residence in a prison, and emigration from a country where TB is endemic.
- If TB is a possibility in a hospitalized patient, place the patient in an isolation room while you wait for results of three consecutive morning sputum AFB smears.
- Strongly consider TB when a patient has an upper lobe infiltrate on chest x-ray.

URINARY TRACT INFECTIONS

ETIOLOGY

My patient has dysuria. What is the likely cause?

Dysuria, urgency, frequency, and, occasionally, incontinence are symptoms of urethral irritation from urinary tract infection (UTI). These can include cystitis, prostatitis, and pyelonephritis. Similar symptoms can occur with vaginitis or urethritis (e.g., *Candida* or herpes simplex infection, respectively).

What causes UTIs?

Up to 20% of women will have a UTI during their lifetime. In young women with *acute cystitis*, the most com-

mon bacterial pathogens are *Escherichia coli* and *Staphylococcus saprophyticus*. Sexual intercourse and diaphragm use increase risk. Uncomplicated pyelonephritis is by definition community-acquired and has no urologic abnormalities and is most commonly due to *E. coli*. Complicated pyelonephritis is upper tract infection occurring in the setting of urinary catheters, stones, obstruction (e.g., BPH), or recent urinary procedures. Resistant gram-negative rods and *Enterococcus* are important organisms in this condition. Consider *Pseudomonas* with indwelling catheters and recent urologic procedures (TURP, cystoscopy) and *Enterococcus* when broad-spectrum antibiotics, such as cephalosporins, have been used recently.

EVALUATION

How is urinalysis interpreted?

In patients with dysuria, obtain clinic dipstick and laboratory microscopic analysis of a spun urine sediment. Many dipstick results include leukocyte esterase (LE), which correlates with the presence of pyuria with 95% sensitivity. LE and white blood cells are present in UTIs but are nonspecific, occurring also in cervicitis, vaginitis, and urethritis. Microscopic hematuria is present in 40% to 60% of patients with acute cystitis and is uncommonly found in other causes of acute dysuria, making it a modestly specific indicator of cystitis.

When is urine culture useful?

There is no role for culture in acute cystitis. Send urine for culture and sensitivity in suspected pyelonephritis, recurrent urinary tract infection, or if the urinalysis is equivocal. A positive culture is defined as greater than 100,000 colonies. Lower counts, 10^2 to 10^4, can still be associated with infection; this is termed acute dysuric syndrome.

How is pyelonephritis different from cystitis?

Pyelonephritis commonly presents with fever, back or abdominal pain, and costovertebral angle or flank tenderness. Other symptoms seen with pyelonephritis are nausea, vomiting, headache, and malaise. Fever is not a symptom of isolated cystitis.

TREATMENT

What is the best antibiotic for acute cystitis?

For cystitis in young women, short-course therapy with 3 days of trimethoprim/sulfamethoxazole DS bid or ciprofloxacin 250 mg bid has an excellent cure rate and few side effects. Short-course therapy is not recommended for elderly women, patients with diabetes, or men; treat these patients for 7 days.

What treatment is appropriate for community-acquired pyelonephritis?

The major treatment decision is whether to hospitalize. Admit when vomiting makes it impossible to take oral medications, likelihood of noncompliance, and need for IV fluids. For uncomplicated pyelonephritis, choose antibiotics with good gram-negative activity, such as trimethoprim/sulfamethoxazole, aminoglycosides, third-generation cephalosporins, or quinolones. Amoxicillin is a poor choice because 25% to 35% of community-acquired *E. coli* are resistant. Duration of therapy is controversial; most physicians treat acute uncomplicated pyelonephritis for 2 weeks. Bacteremia and persistent fevers several days into therapy are common and should not change treatment.

How does treatment for complicated UTI differ?

Treat complicated infections with drugs effective against resistant gram-negative rods, including *Pseudomonas*. If urine Gram stain shows gram-positive cocci, cover for *Enterococcus*, as well. For empiric therapy, use an aminoglycoside and an antipseudomonal third-generation cephalosporin. For patients at risk for *Enterococcus*, use an extended-spectrum penicillin. Remove urinary catheters if possible. Once cultures are available, narrow antibiotics. For *Pseudomonas*, use two drugs to limit emergence of resistance. Septic shock often accompanies complicated UTIs. Support blood pressure with IV fluids and refractory hypotension with vasoactive medications. Relieving any urinary obstruction is a critical part of therapy.

How are recurrent cystitis managed?

Recurrence is caused by either relapse of the same organism or reinfection with a new organism. Relapse immediately after short-course therapy warrants 2-week treatment for presumed upper tract disease. For reinfection, self-treatment by patients is reasonable because studies show excellent correlation between patients' symptoms and bacteriologic evidence of UTI. For patients with two to three recurrences per month, prophylactic therapy with daily trimethoprim/sulfamethoxazole has been shown to decrease infections by 95%.

Key Points

- Cystitis does not cause fever.
- In young women with cystitis, 3-day trimethoprim/sulfamethoxazole is the preferred treatment.
- Patients with Foley catheters or recent instrumentation of the urinary tract are at high risk for resistant gram-negative rods or enterococcal infection.
- Obtain urine culture for recurrent cystitis, UTIs in men, and pyelonephritis.

CASE 29-9

A 25-year-old woman presents with 24 hours of fever, nausea, vomiting, and abdominal pain. She denies urinary frequency, dysuria, or hematuria. She is sexually active with one male partner. T is 39.9° C, P is 120, and BP is 90/60. Skin is without rash, chest is clear, heart sounds are without murmur, abdomen is soft and nontender, and right flank pain is present. Laboratory test results are: HCT 36, WBC 20,000, Na 138, K 3.9, Cl 96, and HCO_3 16. Urinalysis shows many WBCs/HPF and RBCs 0-5/HPF.
  A. What other tests would you order?
  B. Would you admit this patient? Why?
  C. What organism do you suspect?
  D. What therapy would you offer?

CASE 29-10

A 73-year-old man is hospitalized for hip fracture. He is treated with narcotics for pain and develops acute urinary retention requiring placement of a Foley catheter. He also develops an aspiration pneumonia and is successfully treated with ceftriaxone. The day before planned discharge, he develops fever, diaphoresis, and chills. His examination shows clear lungs, no heart murmur, and no rash. Laboratory test results are: HCT 33, WBC 26,000, Na 133, K 4.0, Cl 98, and HCO_3 20. WBC 20-30/HPF, and RBC 5-10/HPF. Urine Gram stain shows gram-positive cocci and gram-negative rods.
  A. What are the most likely causes of the patient's symptoms?
  B. What empiric therapy would you start?

30

Nephrology

ACID-BASE DISTURBANCES

ETIOLOGY

What causes acid–base disturbances?

The body normally keeps arterial blood pH at 7.4. Respiratory or metabolic derangements can alter pH. Hyperventilation removes carbon dioxide (CO_2) and hydrogen ions, creating a respiratory alkalosis. Hypoventilation or airway obstruction raises the partial pressure of carbon dioxide (P_{CO_2}) and creates a respiratory acidosis. Metabolic derangements altering pH include ingestion of particular substances; changes in renal bicarbonate processing; or production of endogenous acids, such as ketones or lactate (Table 30-1).

What do the terms *acidemia* and *alkalemia* mean?

These terms refer to arterial blood pH. Patients with pH lower than 7.4 are acidemic; those with pH greater than 7.4 are alkalemic. In contrast, the terms *acidosis* and *alkalosis* refer to processes that cause excess accumulation of acid or alkali. Multiple processes can coexist, each affecting pH (Table 30-2).

What are the causes of metabolic acidosis?

Metabolic acidosis is divided into anion gap and non–anion gap acidosis. *Anion gap acidosis* occurs when an unmeasured anion lowers pH. The mnemonic MULE PAK may help you remember the causes of anion gap acidoses: *M*ethanol, *U*remia, *L*actic acidosis, *E*thylene glycol, *P*araldehyde, *A*spirin, *K*etoacidosis. Most common on this list are lactic acidosis (e.g., sepsis) and ketoacidosis, which can be from uncontrolled type 1 diabetes, starvation, or alcohol ingestion. *Non–anion gap acidosis* is caused by loss of bicarbonate through the gut or kidney (see Table 30-1).

What is renal tubular acidosis?

Renal tubular acidosis (RTA) occurs when kidneys waste bicarbonate because of malfunctioning tubules. RTA is proximal (type 2) or distal (types 1 and 4), depending on which tubules are affected. Type 4 is most common and is seen with diabetes; type 1 is often associated with nephrolithiasis.

What causes metabolic alkalosis?

Metabolic alkalosis is either sodium chloride responsive or sodium chloride resistant, depending on whether it corrects with sodium chloride volume infusion. Sodium chloride–responsive alkalosis is common and occurs with vomiting, nasogastric suction, or diuretic-induced volume contraction. In these conditions, urine chloride is low. Sodium chloride–resistant metabolic alkalosis is quite rare and causes elevated urine chloride. Examples of this hormonally driven chloride wasting include hyperaldosteronism, Cushing's syndrome, and Bartter's syndrome.

What are primary and compensatory acid–base processes?

The primary process is the main alteration in pH. The term *acidemia* implies a primary acidosis; *alkalemia* implies a primary alkalosis. Compensatory processes occur when the kidney or respiratory system reacts to correct an altered pH. Respiratory compensation is immediate, whereas renal compensation takes 12 to 24 hours to start.

EVALUATION

Is there a systematic way to approach acid–base problems?

Absolutely (Box 30-1). Routinely calculate anion gap in all hospitalized patients. Suspect an acid-base derangement when you see an abnormal respiratory rate, altered bicarbonate, elevated anion gap, poor oxygenation, suspected CO_2 retention, or unexplained altered mental status. If any of these are present, draw an ABG for pH and P_{CO_2}. This combined with chemistry panel (sodium, chloride, and bicarbonate [HCO_3^-]) allows you to calculate anion gap and identify primary, compensatory, and other concurrent acid-base processes.

TABLE 30-1
Causes of Acid-Base Derangements

RESPIRATORY		METABOLIC	
ACIDOSIS PCO$_2$ > 40	**ALKALOSIS PCO$_2$ < 40**	**ACIDOSIS HCO$_3^-$ > 24**	**ALKALOSIS HCO$_3^-$ > 24**
Hypoventilation	Pulmonary embolus	Anion gap acidosis	Chloride sensitive
Asthma	Pneumonia	Lactic acid (sepsis)	Vomiting
COPD	Pulmonary edema	Uremia	Volume contraction
	Aspirin	Aspirin	Diuretics
	Hepatic insufficiency	Ketoacidosis	Chloride resistant
	Fever	With osmolar gap:	Cushing's
	Anxiety	Methanol	Hyperaldosteronism
	Pregnancy	Ethylene glycol	Bartter's syndrome
		Paraldehyde	
		Non–anion gap acidosis	
		Diarrhea	
		Acetazolamide	
		Renal tubular acidosis	

TABLE 30-2
Interpretation of Key Laboratory Tests in Patients With Acid-Base Disorders

VALUE	NORMAL	INTERPRETATION IF HIGH	INTERPRETATION IF LOW
pH	7.4	Alkalemia	Acidemia
HCO$_3^-$	24 mEq/L	Metabolic alkalosis	Metabolic acidosis
PCO$_2$	40 mmHg	Respiratory acidosis	Respiratory alkalosis

My patient's pH is 7.3, PCO$_2$ is 60, and HCO$_3^-$ is 30. How do I identify the primary process?

Here are a few key principles:

1. Patients never overcompensate for the primary acid-base derangement.
2. Respiratory processes alter PCO$_2$ (PCO$_2$ > 40 is acidosis, < 40 is alkalosis).
3. Metabolic processes alter HCO$_3^-$ (HCO$_3^-$ > 24 is alkalosis, < 24 is acidosis).
4. Change in pH is inversely related to change in CO$_2$ and directly related to change in HCO$_3^-$.

The pH of 7.3 reveals an acidemia, so the primary process is an acidosis. Now you are ready to decide whether the source of the low pH is respiratory (true if PCO$_2$ is high) or metabolic (true if HCO$_3^-$ is low). In this case the high PCO$_2$ of 60 reveals the primary respiratory acidosis.

So I found the primary process. How do I identify a compensatory process?

Using the same example, look next at the HCO$_3^-$. The high bicarbonate reveals a metabolic alkalosis, which is compensating for the respiratory acidosis. Here is another example: pH = 7.2, PCO$_2$ = 20, HCO$_3^-$ = 15. The pH reveals acidemia, and low HCO$_3^-$ reveals a primary

BOX 30-1   Systematic Steps to Interpreting Acid-Base Problems (see text for details)

1. Identify the primary process.
2. Identify the compensatory process.
3. Calculate anion gap correcting for low albumin (even if pH is normal or high).
4. If anion gap is elevated, calculate osmolar gap.
5. If anion gap is elevated, use delta-delta to find simultaneous metabolic derangements.
6. Use clues in history and physical to determine specific conditions causing alterations.

metabolic acidosis. The low PCO$_2$ reveals the compensatory respiratory alkalosis.

How can I tell if a patient has compensated or uncompensated respiratory acidosis?

With sudden-onset respiratory acidosis, pH falls before the kidney has time to compensate. In uncompensated respiratory acidosis, pH falls 0.08 for each PCO$_2$ rise of 10. In compensated respiratory acidosis, the drop in pH will be less due to renal bicarbonate production.

How do I calculate the anion gap?

To calculate the anion gap, subtract anions from cations: anion gap = sodium − (chloride + bicarbonate). The normal anion gap is 8 to 12. This number represents unmeasured negative charges, mostly on albumin. When unmeasured anions appear, the anion gap increases. It is significant when anion gap rises by more than 8 points.

What does a low anion gap mean, and why is this important?

Multiple myeloma, hypoalbuminemia, and cations such as lithium lower the anion gap. This can mask a significant anion gap acidosis. If albumin is low, estimate baseline anion gap as 3 times the albumin level. For example, a calculated anion gap of 14 when albumin is 2 represents a significant anion gap acidosis (i.e., a change from a baseline anion gap of $2 \times 3 = 6$, to 14).

When and how do I calculate the osmolal gap?

When your patient has an anion gap acidosis, calculate the osmolal gap (Osm gap):

Osm gap = (measured serum Osms) − (calculated Osms)

where calculated Osms = 2(sodium) + BUN/2.8 + glucose/18. If the osmolar gap is greater than 10, suspect methanol or ethylene glycol ingestion. Look for oxalate crystals in the urine, seen with ethylene glycol ingestion. Blood levels of these agents can be measured but will not be available soon enough to be useful.

What is a "triple ripple," and how do I use the delta–delta?

A triple ripple occurs when multiple acid-base disorders coexist. Use the "delta-delta" when an anion gap acidosis is present to find a concurrent metabolic alkalosis or non–anion gap acidosis. In an isolated anion gap acidosis, the anion gap should rise from baseline (delta-AG) by the same amount that the HCO_3^- falls (delta HCO_3^-). If delta-AG is not the same as delta-HCO_3^-, another metabolic process is present. People put this concept to use in various ways. One way is to add the change in anion gap (measured gap minus normal gap) to the measured HCO_3^- to see if you get a number estimating a normal HCO_3^-. If the result is greater than 24, there is a concurrent metabolic alkalosis. If the result is less than 24, there is a concurrent non–anion gap acidosis (Table 30-3). Practice this on Case 30-2.

What are pertinent history and examination clues in my patient with a low pH?

You must use clues from history and examination to decide what specific conditions are causing the acid-base disturbances. Alcoholism increases the likelihood of al-

TABLE 30-3
Finding Concurrent Metabolic Processes Using the Delta-Delta Concept

WHEN:	THEN THE PATIENT HAS:
Change in anion gap* + HCO_3^- = 24	Isolated anion gap acidosis
Change in anion gap + HCO_3^- > 24	Anion gap acidosis plus metabolic alkalosis
Change in anion gap + HCO_3^- < 24	Anion gap acidosis plus non–anion gap acidosis

*Change in anion gap = measured anion gap − normal anion gap.

coholic ketoacidosis, methanol or ethylene glycol ingestion. Elderly patients are at increased risk for lactic acidosis (sepsis, bowel necrosis) or inadvertent aspirin overdosage. Patients with a history of suicide attempts are at risk for aspirin, methanol, or ethylene glycol ingestion.

TREATMENT

Treat the underlying disorder.

Key Points

- When pH is less than 7.4, there is a primary acidosis; when pH is greater than 7.4, there is a primary alkalosis.
- A low baseline anion gap from low albumin or myeloma may mask significant gap acidosis.
- If you find a patient breathing deeply and rapidly with no immediately apparent cause, suspect respiratory compensation for sepsis or other metabolic acidosis.
- If a significant anion gap is present, check for an osmolal gap.

CASE 30-1

A 45-year-old man with a long history of chronic low back pain presents with several days of melena and the following laboratory test results: Na 140, Cl 103, HCO_3^- 15, glucose 108, BUN 28, measured Osm 295, pH 7.5, Pco_2 20, and Po_2 90. He asks for morphine for his pain.

A. What is his primary acid-base derangement?
B. Is there a compensatory acid-base adjustment, and if so, what is it?
C. Are there any other acid-base derangements present?
D. What do you think is going on clinically to cause his acid-base derangements?

<table>
<tr><td>

CASE 30-2

A 21-year-old woman is found unresponsive. Her friends report that she was going to the bathroom all the time and was vomiting profusely earlier in the day. Laboratory test results are: Na 130, Cl 88, HCO_3^- 10, pH 7.1, Pco_2 32, Po_2 88, BUN 28, glucose 720, and Osm 315.

   A. What is her primary acid-base derangement?

   B. Is there a compensatory acid-base adjustment, and if so, what is it?

   C. Are there any other acid-base derangements present?

   D. What do you think is going on clinically to cause her acid-base derangements?

</td></tr>
</table>

ACUTE RENAL FAILURE

ETIOLOGY

What causes acute renal failure?

Acute renal failure (ARF) is rapid deterioration of renal function resulting in azotemia (elevated BUN and creatinine) and possibly oliguria with less than 400 ml urine output in 24 hours. Causes are divided into prerenal (40% to 80%), intrinsic renal, and postrenal, based on the site of injury (Table 30-4).

What causes prerenal ARF?

Prerenal azotemia occurs with inadequate blood supply to glomeruli. This can be caused by decreased cardiac output (CHF), hypovolemia (bleeding, diarrhea, burns), or changes in renal perfusion from stenosis or medications. ACEIs dilate efferent arterioles, and NSAIDs block prostaglandins, resulting in afferent arteriolar narrowing. Prolonged prerenal states can cause renal ischemia, leading to acute tubular necrosis (ATN).

What causes intrinsic renal disease?

Intrinsic renal failure can occur in the glomeruli (glomerulonephritis), the interstitium (interstitial nephritis), or the tubules (acute tubular necrosis). Glomerulonephritis, injury to the glomeruli from any cause, is most commonly immune-mediated. Examples include systemic lupus erythematosus, post-streptococcal glomerulonephritis, Goodpasture's syndrome, and hepatitis C. Interstitial nephritis is inflammation in the interstitial space and is caused by allergic reactions to NSAIDs, antibiotics (e.g., penicillins and cephalosporins), or infectious diseases. Patients are asymptomatic or may present with fever, rash, and joint pain. Toxins such as NSAIDs are important mediators of renal injury and can cause damage by multiple mechanisms.

TABLE 30-4
Common Causes of Acute Renal Failure

LOCATION OF INJURY	COMMON CAUSES
Prerenal (40%-80%)*	Hypovolemia: bleeding, diarrhea, sepsis, diuretics Poor perfusion: renal artery stenosis, ACEI, NSAID Poor cardiac output: CHF
Postrenal (10%)	Bladder outlet obstruction: BPH, cancer Medications: anticholinergics, narcotics
Intrinsic renal (30%-50%) Glomeruli	Immune: IgA nephropathy, lupus, Wegener's, Goodpasture's Infectious: Hepatitis B/C, post-strep, HIV, endocarditis Toxic: Heroin
Interstitial nephritis	Drugs: NSAIDs, penicillins, sulfa Infection: pyelonephritis
Acute tubular necrosis	Toxins: radiocontrast, aminoglycosides, myoglobin Tubular obstruction: myoglobin Tubular ischemia: sepsis, hypotension

*% of total ARF cases.

What is acute tubular necrosis (ATN)?

This common cause of ARF occurs with tubular ischemia from any severe prerenal state, such as septic shock. Nephrotoxins, such as radiocontrast dye and aminoglycosides, are the second major cause. Prehydration and nonionic dye minimize dye toxicity. Once-daily dosing decreases aminoglycoside toxicity. Another cause of ATN is tubular deposition of myoglobin from rhabdomyolysis. Renal function frequently recovers after ATN.

What postrenal cause of acute renal failure is most common?

Postrenal azotemia is caused by obstruction. Bladder outlet obstruction is most common, resulting from benign prostatic hypertrophy or prostate cancer. Once a Foley catheter is placed, postobstructive diuresis can produce severe volume and electrolyte depletion. Other causes include neurogenic bladder dysfunction and obstruction caused by papillary sloughing, stones, or abdominal tumor.

What toxins damage the kidneys?

Toxins can injure the kidney at various sites. NSAIDs cause acute interstitial nephritis and nephrotic syndrome. NSAIDs also decrease renal blood flow by blocking the dilating effect of prostaglandins on the afferent arterioles, a particular problem in patients with low intravascular volumes, such as CHF, cirrhosis, or nephrotic syndrome.

What is nephrotic syndrome?

Nephrotic syndrome is a common final pathway of many intrinsic renal diseases, including diabetes and hepatitis B. Massive protein loss (>3.5 g in 24 hours) leads to hypoalbuminemia, edema, hyperlipidemia, and hypercoagulability resulting from loss of antithrombin III in the urine.

Why are patients with diabetes at particular risk for acute renal failure?

Diabetic nephropathy is common in patients with diabetes (50% of type 1, somewhat less in type 2) and increases risk for ARF from other cause, especially toxins. High rates of atherosclerosis in patients with diabetes also increase the likelihood of renal artery stenosis. Further, diabetic neuropathy may result in atonic bladder, urinary retention, and postrenal azotemia.

EVALUATION

What are the signs and symptoms of ARF?

What are the nonspecific and are due to accumulation of nitrogenous wastes or volume overload. Patients may have nausea, vomiting, anorexia, or cardiopulmonary symptoms, such as chest pain from pericarditis or dyspnea from pulmonary edema. Patients may also report fatigue, confusion, or pruritus. Look for signs of volume overload, such as elevated jugular venous pressure, cardiac murmur, or gallop. Bladder obstruction can sometimes be detected by abdominal mass or suprapubic dullness from a distended bladder. Chronic renal failure may cause pallor from anemia and skin excoriations resulting from pruritus.

What are the first steps in diagnosing the cause of acute renal failure?

For acute oliguric renal failure, first rule out obstruction by placing a Foley catheter, or by ultrasound looking for hydronephrosis (dilation of ureters or calyces). Then, use fluid challenge (or diuretics if volume overloaded) to establish urine output. Review medications and remove nephrotoxins. Collect a fresh urine sample for urine sediment evaluation. Send BUN and creatinine; a ratio greater than 20:1 suggests a prerenal state.

What is an "active" urine sediment?

An active urine sediment refers to the presence of cells or casts in a fresh, centrifuged urine and indicates presence of intrinsic renal disease. In contrast, urine sediment in prerenal and postrenal injury is usually without cells or casts. Exceptions to this rule occur when bladder obstruction leads to infection with white cells or when persistent prerenal ischemia causes ATN with muddy brown casts. When intrinsic disease is present,

---

TABLE 30-5
Characteristic Urine Findings and Special Laboratory Tests for Major Types of ARF

LOCATION OF INJURY	URINE DIPSTICK	URINALYSIS	OTHER LABORATORY TESTS
Prerenal	Negative*	Hyaline casts	FeNa < 1 BUN:Cr ratio > 20:1
Postrenal	Negative	Negative	FeNa > 2
Intrinsic renal			
Glomerulonephritis	3+ blood 3+ protein	Red cell casts Dysmorphic red cells	Consider: antistrep Ab, ANA, ANCA, SPEP, ESR, HIV, uric acid, glucose, hepatitis serology, renal biopsy
Interstitial nephritis	1+ blood 1+ protein†	Eosinophils White blood cell casts	Serum eosinophils
Tubular injury	Negative‡	Muddy brown casts Tubular cells	Myoglobin

SPEP, Serum protein electrophoresis; *ANCA,* antineutrophil cytoplasmic antibody; *ANA,* antinuclear antibody; *ESR,* erythrocyte sedimentation rate.
*Persistent prerenal azotemia can cause ATN, so the urinalysis findings will be those of ATN.
†Proteinuria <1.5 g/day = interstitial nephritis, >3.5 g/day = nephrotic syndrome.
‡If ATN is due to rhabdomyolysis, the urine dipstick will be positive for blood because of cross-reacting myoglobin, but microscopic urinalysis will be negative for red blood cells.

specific laboratory tests may be useful (Table 30-5), but renal biopsy may be required to make final diagnosis.

What is a "FeNa," and how does it help diagnose prerenal states?

FeNa is the fractional excretion of sodium from serum into the urine, as determined in the following equation:

$$FeNa = \frac{Cr^S \times Na^U}{Cr^U \times Na^S} \times 100$$

If the FeNa is less than 1, the nephron is working hard to retain salt and water, so the cause of acute renal failure is likely prerenal. On the other hand, if the FeNa is greater than 2, the nephron is not able to retain sodium, indicating an intrinsic renal process. Diuretics may falsely increase the FeNa.

What laboratory tests can help me distinguish chronic from acute renal failure?

Patients with chronic renal failure usually have anemia due to decreased erythropoietin, low calcium, and small kidneys on ultrasound. With ARF, anemia is less likely and kidneys are not small.

TREATMENT

How is ARF managed?

Most patients require hospitalization for diagnosis and volume management. Decide whether volume depletion or overload exists. Then use daily weights, "ins and outs," including free water losses (~10 ml/kg per day), and examination to guide volume repletion or diuresis. Watch for infection, an increased risk in patients with renal failure. Nutrition is a priority because anorexia is common. Do a renal dose for all medications based on calculated creatinine clearance, as determined by the following equation:

$$Creatinine\ clearance = \frac{(140 - age) \times ideal\ weight\ (kg)}{72 \times serum\ creatinine}$$

Multiply by 0.85 for women to correct for lean body mass.

What laboratory tests should I follow?

In oliguric ARF, expect daily increases in creatinine of 0.5 to 1.0 mg/dl and BUN of 10 to 20 mg/dl. Acidemia and hyperkalemia are common, so follow electrolytes at least daily. Obtain CBC, uric acid, calcium, magnesium, and phosphate at admission. If renal failure persists, consider rechecking these levels. Check ABG as needed to monitor pH and acidosis.

When is dialysis required?

When symptomatic renal failure is present, dialysis may be needed, especially in oliguric patients. The indications for emergent dialysis are listed in Box 30-2.

BOX 30-2 Indications for Dialysis

Severe volume overload with CHF
Life-threatening acidosis
Severe electrolyte abnormalities, especially hyperkalemia
Pericarditis
Toxins that can be removed by dialysis

Key Points

- With the workup for ARF, consider prerenal, intrarenal, and postrenal causes.
- Acidemia, hyperkalemia, and CHF are common in ARF and may necessitate dialysis.
- Treatment involves careful volume and electrolyte management; all medications must be dosed based on creatinine clearance.

CASE 30-3

A 60-year-old woman presents with bloody emesis and black, tarry stools for 24 hours. Her blood pressure is 75/palpable, and her pulse is 120. Vigorous hydration with normal saline is begun. HCT 20, BUN 40, Cr 1.2, Na 144. Despite a catheter, urine output is low at 350 m over 24 hours. Also, urine Na 4 mEq/L, urine Cr 97 mEq/L. The following Cr rises to 2.0.

A. What is the most likely diagnosis, and what workup would confirm your diagnosis?
B. Calculate a FeNa.
C. What problems might she develop over the next few days, and how will you monitor for them?
D. Does she need dialysis?

CASE 30-4

A 75-year-old man recently started diphenhydramine (Benadryl) for sleep. He reports increasing grogginess, fatigue, and mild nausea. On examination, you palpate a suprapubic mass, and his prostate is enlarged. BUN 65, Cr 3.6, and CBC normal.

A. What is your first diagnostic step?
B. What subsequent complications might he develop?

CASE 30-5

A 26-year-old man presents with fatigue, fever, and sore throat for 10 days. He reports a history of IV drug use. He was seen at an outside clinic and started on cephalexin 7 days ago for presumed strep throat. Now, he continues to have fever and fatigue, but his throat is improved. BP is 164/94, there is a scaling rash in his nasolabial folds, and oropharynx without exudate. BUN 36, Cr 2.8, and urinalysis reveals moderate proteinuria, rare red blood cells, and moderate eosinophils.
A. What is the differential diagnosis?
B. What is appropriate management?

CASE 30-6

A 54-year-old man seeks a second opinion from you about his chronic sinusitis. He has had multiple sinus infections, two sinus drainage procedures, and two episodes of "pneumonia." He is currently on trimethoprim/sulfamethoxazole, pseudoephedrine, and nasal beclomethasone spray. His BP is 150/94. Examination is unremarkable except for poor maxillary sinus transillumination and crackles at his left lung base. His WBC is normal, his hematocrit is 35, and his creatinine is 1.9.
A. What is the differential diagnosis for his elevated creatinine?
B. What additional history, examination, and tests would you like?
C. Predict what his urinalysis will show.

CASE 30-7

A 30-year-old man complains of increasing edema. He used heroin until 3 months ago. His PMH is otherwise negative, and he takes occasional ibuprofen for headaches. BP is 160/100; pulse is 80. His examination shows old needle track marks, bibasilar crackles, and 3+ pitting edema to the knees. He has 4+ protein on UA, a creatinine of 2.4 and a BUN of 20. His cholesterol is 346. A 24-hour urine shows 6 g of protein.
A. What is his diagnosis, and what are the possible causes?
B. What workup should he have?
C. List two findings you expect to see on his sediment examination.

ELECTROLYTE DISTURBANCES: CALCIUM

ETIOLOGY

What causes hypercalcemia and hypocalcemia?

The causes of hypercalcemia and hypocalcemia are listed in Boxes 30-3 and 30-4. Apparent hypocalcemia may result from hypoalbuminemia because most serum calcium is bound to albumin. Total calcium drops by 0.8 mg/dl for every 1 mg/dl fall in albumin.

BOX 30-3   Causes of Hypercalcemia (From Most to Least Common)

Primary hyperparathyroidism
Drug-induced (thiazide diuretics)
Malignancy:
  Osteolytic metastasis (breast cancer)
  PTH-like hormone production (lung cancer)
  Direct bone invasion (lymphoma)
Granulomatous disease (TB, sarcoid)
Immobilization

BOX 30-4   Causes of Hypocalcemia

Hypoalbuminemia (apparent hypocalcemia)
Renal failure
Hypoparathyroidism
Low magnesium
Pancreatitis
Multiple blood transfusions (citrate binds calcium)

EVALUATION

When should I suspect hypercalcemia or hypocalcemia?

Hypercalcemia causes nonspecific symptoms or may be discovered inadvertently. Check calcium in any older patient with confusion, recalcitrant constipation, or polyuria. Other nonspecific signs include lethargy, nausea, vomiting, anorexia. and abdominal pain (from renal stones or pancreatitis). Severe hypercalcemia causes dehydration by diuresis and/or vomiting. Severe or rapidly acquired *hypocalcemia* causes painful tetany (muscle spasms). Classic findings are Trousseau's sign (carpal spasm with a blood pressure cuff inflated just above systolic pressure) and Chvostek's sign (facial twitching elicited by tapping just anterior to the ear). Lethargy, confusion, or seizures may also occur.

What evaluation is warranted in patients with calcium abnormalities?

With hypercalcemia, obtain history and examination for signs of malignancy; pursue focal findings with further evaluation. When no signs of cancer are present, check complete blood count, renal function, and intact parathyroid hormone (PTH). For hypocalcemia, ask about neck surgery (inadvertent parathyroid removal) and other autoimmune disorders that may be associated with hypoparathyroidism. Obtain albumin, magnesium, phosphorous, PTH, vitamin D, and creatinine. PTH is low with primary hypoparathyroidism and hypomagnesemia but elevated with other causes of hypocalcemia.

What ECG findings suggest calcium abnormalities?

The QT interval is shortened with hypercalcemia and prolonged with hypocalcemia. Hypocalcemia also worsens ECG findings of digoxin toxicity.

TREATMENT

How do I treat hypercalcemia?

Treat the underlying cause. For severe hypercalcemia (>13 mg/dl) or symptoms, start with hydration. After volume replete, add furosemide, then a bisphosphonate or calcitonin if needed.

How do I replace calcium in patients with hypocalcemia?

Give IV calcium gluconate to acutely symptomatic patients. Replace low magnesium. Find and treat underlying causes. Give oral vitamin D and calcium carbonate for hypoparathyroidism.

Key Points
- Hypercalcemia presents nonspecifically; check for it in any confused older patient.
- Hypocalcemia potentiates digoxin toxicity.

ELECTROLYTE DISTURBANCES: POTASSIUM

ETIOLOGY

What causes elevated potassium?

Pseudohyperkalemia commonly occurs when red blood cells lyse during sample collection, releasing intracellular potassium. Redraw blood with a larger-gauge needle and make sure the tourniquet is not on too long. True hyperkalemia occurs with renal failure, rhabdomyolysis (muscle cell injury releases intracellular potassium), extracellular shift of potassium with acidosis, potassium-sparing diuretics (e.g., spironolactone), ACEIs, and trimethoprim/sulfamethoxazole.

What causes hypokalemia?

Most results from diuretics; vomiting and diarrhea are also common. Magnesium depletion can cause hypokalemia, especially in alcoholic patients. Medications causing potassium depletion include diuretics, cisplatin, theophylline, aminoglycosides, and amphotericin.

EVALUATION

What evaluation is warranted in patients with hypokalemia?

Patients on diuretics may not need further tests. Check magnesium when hypokalemia resists replacement. With hypertension and hypokalemia, consider an adrenal hormone excess.

What clues on ECG suggest a potassium abnormality?

Hyperkalemia causes peaked T waves, progressing to widened QRS complexes and sine waves as potassium continues to rise. Hypokalemia causes T wave flattening and U waves.

TREATMENT

How should I treat a patient with hyperkalemia?

ECG changes mandate emergent treatment. First, give IV calcium gluconate to stabilize cardiac membranes, then IV glucose, insulin, and bicarbonate to drive potassium into the cells. If the patient can make urine, give IV furosemide. Kayexalate, a sodium/potassium exchange resin, is given orally or as an enema but acts slowly. In extremely urgent situations, use dialysis.

How do I replace potassium?

Replace orally with KCl or KPO_4. If IV replacement is required, give no faster than 10 mEq/hr.

Key Points
- Hyperkalemia is due to excess intake, shift from the intracellular compartment (acidosis, cell injury), or inability to excrete potassium (renal failure, drugs).
- Refractory hypokalemia may be due to coexistent hypomagnesemia.

ELECTROLYTE DISTURBANCES: SODIUM

ETIOLOGY

What leads to hypernatremia?

Hypernatremia is commonly caused by lack of water. Patients unable to get to water become hypernatremic (e.g., from acute CVA when home alone or in coma). Occasionally, fluid requirements are too great to keep up enough intake (e.g., diabetes insipidus).

What causes hyponatremia?

Causes are categorized by volume status as hypovolemic, euvolemic, or hypervolemic. In hypovolemic hyponatremia, both water and sodium are missing and sodium losses exceed volume losses. With hypervolemic hyponatremia, patients actually have total body excess sodium with even greater excess water in edematous states such as CHF, cirrhosis, or severe hypoalbuminemia from nephrotic syndrome. Euvolemic hyponatremia is most often from the syndrome of inappropriate ADH secretion (SIADH) release (Table 30-6). Patients with hyponatremia resulting from SIADH usually have low BUN and uric acid levels. Thiazide diuretics are a common cause of euvolemic hyponatremia, with the exact pathogenesis unclear. Pseudohyponatremia occurs with severe hyperlipidemia, hypergammaglobulinemia, or hyperglycemia. For each increase of glucose by 100 mg/dl over a normal glucose level of 100, the serum sodium decreases by 1.6 mEq/l.

EVALUATION

When should I suspect sodium disturbances?

Patients with hypernatremia are often volume depleted and may have altered consciousness, preventing them from drinking. Symptoms of hyponatremia include confusion, disorientation, and anorexia. Seizures or coma may occur with severe or rapidly developing hyponatremia. For patients with any sodium derangement, first establish volume status (see below).

TREATMENT

How do I treat hypernatremia?

First, replace volume deficit with normal saline, then replace free water deficit with D5W over 36 hours, reducing sodium by 0.5 to 1 mEq/hr. Calculate the free water deficit, which is equal to $[(\text{serum sodium}/140) - 1] \times$

TABLE 30-6 Causes of SIADH	
CAUSE	EXAMPLES
Severe pulmonary disease	Lung abscess, severe pneumonia, mechanical ventilation with PEEP
Tumor	Small-cell lung carcinoma
CNS disorders	Meningitis, encephalitis, tumor
Drugs	Morphine, tricyclic antidepressants, sulfonylureas, carbamazepine
Endocrine disorders	Hypothyroidism, primary adrenal failure

PEEP, Positive end-expiratory pressure; *SIADH,* syndrome of inappropriate ADH secretion.

$0.6 \times$ weight in kg. For central diabetes insipidus, replace antidiuretic hormone (ADH).

How do I treat hyponatremia?

Use water restriction for mild euvolemic hyponatremia. For seizures or coma, correct more rapidly with normal (0.9%) or hypertonic (3%) saline and furosemide. Treat hypovolemic hyponatremia with IV normal saline. Treat hypervolemic hyponatremia with both salt and water restriction along with diuretics as needed. Bring the serum sodium level up by at most 1 mEq/hr to avoid central pontine myelinolysis.

> **Key Points**
> - Categorize hyponatremia by volume status.
> - Treat most euvolemic hyponatremia with free water restriction.
> - Correct sodium imbalances slowly by no more than 1 mEq/hr.

FLUID MANAGEMENT

ETIOLOGY

In which situations do patients need fluid administration?

Hospitalized patients unable to drink because of illness or procedures need maintenance fluid, electrolytes, and glucose replacement. Volume-depleted patients need volume resuscitation.

TABLE 30-7

Electrolyte Concentrations in Various Intravenous Solutions (in mEq/L)

FLUID	SODIUM	POTASSIUM	CHLORIDE	BICARBONATE	LACTATE
½ normal saline (0.45%)	77		77		
Normal saline (0.9%)	154		154		
Ringer's lactate*	130	4	110		28
Sodium bicarbonate (per amp)	44.5			44.5	
5% dextrose in water (D5W)†					

*Also contains 3 mEq calcium/L.
†Has 50 g of dextrose per liter of water and no other electrolytes.

EVALUATION

How do I evaluate volume status?

Look for volume depletion by weight loss, postural hypotension, poor skin turgor, dry mucous membranes, oliguria, and tachycardia. An increased BUN/creatinine ratio greater than 20 is also a clue. Look for fluid overload (often a preventable iatrogenic occurrence) by weight gain, jugular venous distension, edema, and rales. Evaluate volume status daily in hospitalized patients.

TREATMENT

How do I design maintenance fluid and electrolyte therapy?

Patients unable to eat need approximately 2 L/day of fluid as ¼ or ½ normal saline with glucose for calories. Standard basal requirements for electrolytes are about 1 mEq/kg/day of Na, K, and Cl with adjustments as needed for excess losses.

How do I choose appropriate resuscitation fluid for a dehydrated patient?

Fluid therapy is an exercise in balancing input and output of electrolytes and water. Know the electrolyte content of various solutions (Table 30-7). For volume resuscitation in patients with dehydration or low blood pressure, choose a fluid with high saline content that will stay in the intravascular space (normal saline or lactated Ringer's). Remember, lactated Ringer's has potassium, so do not give large volumes to anuric patients. Giving fluid in boluses is preferable to running fluids at a high rate (and forgetting about them). This lowers the risk of iatrogenic volume overload. Frequent examinations of fluid status are mandatory in patients receiving volume resuscitation to evaluate their response and plan further fluid therapy.

Key Points ··
- Assess fluid status at least once daily in all hospitalized patients.
- Use ½ normal saline with glucose and potassium for maintenance fluids.
- Fluid resuscitate with normal saline boluses, and reassess fluid status between boluses.

CASE 30-8

A 50-year-old man with a history of poorly controlled hypertension and renal failure requiring dialysis 3 times a week comes to the ER because he feels weak and short of breath. He has missed his last three dialysis appointments. Examination shows HR 90, BP 180/100, RR 22, T 98.4° F, oxygen saturation 93%, JVP elevated to 10 cm, bibasilar rales, an S₃, and 1+ leg edema. Na 130, K 8.0, HCO₃ 18, Cl 100, BUN 60, and creatinine 8.5. Chest film shows prominent vessels in the upper lung fields.
   A. What is this patient's most life-threatening problem, and why?
   B. What would this man's ECG show?
   C. Name the interventions you could use to manage his hyperkalemia, and state how each works.

CASE 30-9

A 67-year-old woman with a long history of heavy smoking, hypertension, and alcohol use is brought to clinic. She lives in a nursing home and has become more disoriented over the last week. She always has a rattly cough, but her sputum has increased. Today, she is breathing hard and not making sense. Her only medication is hydrochlorothiazide. Laboratory tests show: WBC 15, Hct 37, Na 118, K 3.5, Cl 85, and HCO₃ 23.
   A. List possible causes of hyponatremia in this patient.
   B. What aspects of the examination will help you categorize this patient's hyponatremia?
   C. On examination, she is euvolemic with bronchial breath sounds and dullness to percussion over the left lower lung field. What is the likely cause of her hyponatremia, and how should you treat it?

HYPERTENSION

ETIOLOGY

Why is hypertension important?

Untreated severe hypertension can reduce life expectancy by 10 to 20 years. Persistent hypertension produces end-organ damage with cardiomegaly, retinopathy, renal failure, and strokes appearing in over 50% of patients after just 7 to 10 years of untreated disease.

What causes hypertension?

Approximately 90% of hypertension is "essential" and cannot be attributed to any specific cause. Onset of essential hypertension is usually between ages 35 and 55; most patients have a family history of high blood pressure. Excessive alcohol use is probably the most common secondary cause of hypertension. Sleep apnea and thyroid disease can also contribute, as can renal insufficiency (3% of all cases), renal artery stenosis (2%), oral contraceptives (2%), and hyperaldosteronism (1%). Pheochromocytoma causes less than 1%.

EVALUATION

My patient has a blood pressure today of 154/94. Is this hypertension?

The upper limit of normal BP is 140/90. However, a single measurement does not qualify as hypertension. The diagnosis can only be made after two measurements at two different visits. One exception: a single very high BP of greater than 200/110. So-called "high-normal" blood pressure of 130-140/85-90 confers a risk of developing true hypertension, so these patients should be followed with annual BP checks. Because hypertension has important implications for life expectancy, patients' life insurance rates will be affected by this diagnosis. Write "elevated blood pressure" instead of "hypertension" in the chart until you have confirmed the diagnosis. Once you have made the diagnosis, encourage your patients to buy their own blood pressure cuffs to help engage them in their care.

How reliable is in-clinic measurement of blood pressure?

"White coat" hypertension is blood pressure increased simply because of being in the clinic. This can increase blood pressure by an average of 10 mmHg systolic and 8 mm Hg diastolic. Data suggest that white coat hypertension is essentially benign. Have your patient measure blood pressures at neighborhood fire stations and drug stores. A recent innovation is ambulatory blood pressure cuffs, which take intermittent measurements throughout the day away from clinic and allow you to investigate for white coat hypertension.

Are there any tricks to measuring blood pressure?

Measuring BP should be a therapeutic, "I-am-your-doctor" maneuver; practice until you are facile. To be accurate, make sure the cuff is the right size. The inflatable portion should go around at least 80% of the arm. The patient should be seated for 5 minutes before BP is checked.

What questions are important in the initial evaluation of hypertension?

Establish whether the patient has end-organ damage, if reversible causes of hypertension are likely, and if comorbid conditions exist that make complications of hypertension more likely, such as diabetes or high cholesterol (Box 30-5).

What should I look for on examination?

BP: Always recheck the measurement in both arms
Skin: Abdominal striae, hirsutism or purpuric bruises of Cushing's disease
HEENT: Funduscopic examination for hypertensive changes of AV nicking, arterial narrowing, hemorrhages, exudate, or papilledema
Neck: Carotid bruit of atherosclerosis, goiter of hyperthyroidism
Lungs: Rales of congestive heart failure from prolonged hypertension
Heart: S_3/S_4, heave, indicating left ventricular hypertrophy or enlargement
Abdomen: Bruit of renal artery stenosis, mass of polycystic kidney disease
Extremities: Edema from congestive heart failure or medication side effect, proximal muscle weakness from Cushing's disease

---

BOX 30-5 Questions to Ask of Patients With Newly Diagnosed Hypertension

Family/personal history: Hypertension, stroke, diabetes, high cholesterol, or heart disease?
Diet history: Salt and fat content
Substance history: Alcohol, cigarettes, illicit drugs (especially cocaine)
Medications: Including naturopathic medications
Review of symptoms: Chest pain, headache, visual changes, neurologic symptoms, sleep apnea, thyroid symptoms

---

What tests are useful in the initial evaluation of hypertension?

The initial evaluation, aside from history and examination, is limited to ECG, urinalysis, basic chemistry panel, and lipid panel. LV hypertrophy on ECG is associated with increased mortality and indicates longer-standing disease. This should prompt you to start medications. The ECG also serves as baseline for future ischemia. An active urine sediment with casts, red blood cells, or protein suggests kidney disease, which may be either the cause or result of hypertension. A creatinine greater than 1.5 also indicates renal disease. Glucose screens for diabetes. Low potassium suggests hyperaldosteronism or Cushing's disease and may itself worsen BP control. Lipid panel stratifies further risk for atherosclerosis.

When and how should I screen for the uncommon, reversible causes of hypertension?

Look further with judicious use of tests (Table 30-8) in these three circumstances:

- New hypertension in age less than 35 or greater than 55
- Compliant patient with severe continuing hypertension, particularly on more than three drugs
- Examination or laboratory test suggesting reversible causes (e.g., Cushing's habitus, hypokalemia, alkalosis)

TREATMENT

When should a patient be started on blood pressure medications?

Once antihypertensive medications are started, patients will likely be on them for the rest of their lives. Therefore, try nonpharmacologic measures first. A 3- to 12-month trial is adequate, with the shorter duration if more risk factors are present, such as diabetes. (Recent data on diabetes supports early aggressive blood pres-

sure management, with goal of <135/85). Weight loss of only 10 pounds can reduce BP by 10 points. Although a low-sodium diet (<2 g/day) can lower BP by 10 mmHg, this occurs only in salt-sensitive patients, less than 50% of all hypertensives. Elderly and African-American patients are the most likely to be salt-sensitive. Although these changes will not normalize a BP of 160/105, the amount of medication required may be lower.

Why should I start with a β-blocker or diuretic?

The Joint National Committee (JNC), a national panel that reviewed evidence on hypertension treatment, recommends nonpharmacologic measures first, followed by either a diuretic or a β-blocker. These are the only medications shown in long-term trials to reduce not only blood pressure but also the more important measures of morbidity and mortality. Also, as older drugs, they are as much as 30 times cheaper than newer medications. There are a few important exceptions: use ACEIs as first-line treatment in patients with CHF or diabetes (reduces risk of nephropathy).

How do I change or increase antihypertensive medications?

Keep things simple. Pick one medication and go to the highest tolerated dose before adding another agent. The key here is the notion of tolerance. Even a mild side effect will have a significant impact on compliance. New JNC guidelines also endorse the option of dual drug therapy at low doses to avoid side effects. Become familiar with one or two drugs in each class and their dosage, cost, and side effects (Table 30-9). Many patients have more than one disease, so if you need to change or add a medication, choose one with multiple benefits. For example, in an elderly gentleman with benign prostatic hypertrophy, an α-adrenergic blocker will relieve symptoms of outlet obstruction. Second key point: do not make anything worse. Diuretics may aggravate urinary incontinence, so consider β-blockers.

What improvement should I expect with each type of intervention?

Blood pressure improvement is roughly the same for lifestyle modifications and starting medication doses: 5 to 10 mmHg. With higher doses of medications, you should be able to normalize most patients' blood pressure, up to 40 to 50 mmHg decrease.

How often should my patient follow up?

While you are initiating or changing therapy, every 4 to 6 weeks is a good interval. Once stable, 3 or 6 months is an adequate interval. Ideally, patients should check and record their blood pressure 2 to 3 times per week when changes are being made.

TABLE 30-8
Tests to Use Selectively to Look for Reversible Causes of HTN

CONDITION	TEST
Alcohol use	CAGE questions,* serum GGT
Hypo/hyperthyroidism	TSH
Sleep apnea	Nocturnal pulse oximetry or sleep study
Cushing's disease	24-hour urine cortisol
Hyperaldosteronism	Serum aldosterone/renin ratio
Renovascular disease	Renal artery duplex
Pheochromocytoma	24-hour urine catecholamines

*See Box 35-1, p. 220.

TABLE 30-9

Once-Daily Dosed Antihypertensive Medications, Relative Cost, and Side Effects

DRUG	COST	IMPORTANT SIDE EFFECTS	ALSO TREATS
Diuretics Hydrochlorothiazide Chlorthalidone	$	Frequent urination Decreased potassium Increased lipids at high doses Increased uric acid	Volume overload Leg edema
β-Blockers Atenolol Nadolol Propanolol SR	$	Fatigue Decreased exercise tolerance Impotence Asthma Bradycardia	Prevents MI recurrence Migraine prophylaxis Angina
ACE Inhibitors Benazepril Lisinopril	$$$	Renal insufficiency Hyperkalemia Cough (10%-20%) Life-threatening angioedema	CHF Diabetic nephropathy
α-Blockers Doxazosin Terazosin Tamsulosin	$$	Postural hypotension Headache Weakness	Benign prostatic hypertrophy
Calcium-channel blockers Felodipine Amlodipine Nifedipine SR Diltiazem CD	$$$$	Bradycardia and negative inotropy (only with diltiazem) Constipation Leg edema Reflux	Angina

---

What should I do at follow-up appointments?

Review goals and intervening BP records. Reinforce compliance and lifestyle modification. Screen for side effects of medications. Change, add, or increase medication for continued poor control or side effects. For patients on ACEI, check electrolyte and renal function panel 1 week after starting or changing dose. Review whether end-organ damage has occurred (ECG, UA, eye examination, electrolyte and renal function panel) at an interval of several years.

Why is blood pressure hard to control?

Compliance is a big issue. Most people feel fine despite their high blood pressure; medications often make them feel worse. Other factors that can worsen control include alcohol use; too much salt; weight gain; pregnancy; and other medications, including NSAIDs, tricyclic antidepressants, oral contraceptives, appetite suppressants, nasal decongestants, and naturopathic medications.

When should I admit someone for BP?

Admit the patient with elevated BP and acute symptoms or signs of end-organ strain, such as confusion, chest pain, papilledema, hematuria/proteinuria, or pulmonary edema. A reading greater than 240/130 is associated with significant mortality, so even asymptomatic patients should be admitted.

A nurse calls to tell me an inpatient has high blood pressure. What should I do?

The reflex response has been to give sublingual nifedipine. This treats you and the nurse but not the patient; it may even be harmful because it abruptly drops blood pressure. Look for other causes, such as pain. If hypertension persists, treat with a regular, daily medication.

Key Points

- Hypertension should only be diagnosed after several readings.
- Treatment will be lifelong, so start with education and lifestyle changes.
- Compliance is hard for patients, so keep medications simple and ask about side effects.
- Look for and aggressively treat comorbid conditions, such as diabetes and high cholesterol.
- Obtain baseline ECG, chemistry panel, and urinalysis in patients with new hypertension.
- Reversible causes of hypertension are uncommon, so be selective in whom you screen.

CASE 30-10

A 27-year-old woman with a recent ankle sprain has no personal or family history of hypertension. She takes ibuprofen and oral contraceptives. She drinks 4 beers a night. On examination, BP is 146/92.

A. What could be elevating her blood pressure?

B. How soon would you like to see her again?

C. What changes would you like to ask her to make before her next visit?

CASE 30-11

A 72-year-old woman comes to see you for the first time. Aside from chronic constipation and occasional gout, she is remarkably healthy. Her only real medical problem is high blood pressure that has been present "for years and years." Her medications are Metamucil, milk of magnesia, and nifedipine 20 mg tid. From time to time she takes a "water pill" for her swollen legs. Her blood pressure is 150/84, and her pulse is 59.

A. Would you recommend a change in her BP medication, and why or why not?

B. What evaluation will you do?

C. What medication would you choose for her?

CASE 30-12

A 57-year-old woman with obesity, diabetes, and depression sits in your office crying because you have just told her she has hypertension. When she is depressed, she eats potato chips and has gained 30 pounds over the past year. She is extremely tired all the time; in fact, she fell asleep while driving over to see you. In her family, all her siblings have hypertension and diabetes. On examination, her blood pressure is 166/117. She has stretch marks on her stomach and lower extremity swelling. Her ECG and UA are normal. Her laboratory tests show low potassium.

A. Name at least five possible causes of, or contributors to, hypertension in this patient.

B. Would you order any further tests, and if so, why?

C. How would you start to treat her?

31

Neurology

THE NEUROLOGIC EXAMINATION

What should I cover with the neurologic examination?

Perform a screening neurologic examination on all new inpatients and on clinic patients who request a "full physical." This includes assessment of mental status, cranial nerves, strength, sensation, coordination, and reflexes. A sample normal screening examination is provided in Box 31-1. This should take no more than 5 minutes to perform on an alert, cooperative patient. To facilitate the examination, tell your patient why you are doing each step. For example, you can say, "I'm going to test your strength now. Push against me with your . . . pull against me with your . . .," or, "I'm going to test your coordination now. Touch my finger, now touch your nose, now go back and forth." The motor strength examination is graded on a scale from zero to five (Box 31-2).

When do I need to perform a more detailed neurologic examination?

If screening neurologic examination is abnormal, or if the patient presents with a neurologic problem, a more detailed examination is warranted and can be tailored to fit the circumstances (Table 31-1).

Key Points
- Master a 5-minute screening neurologic examination for inpatient admits and outpatient physicals.
- Focus the neurologic examination depending on the clinical situation.

ALTERED MENTAL STATUS

ETIOLOGY

What causes altered mental status?

Coma requires an abnormality affecting both cerebral cortexes or in the reticular activating system (midline brainstem). Lesser degrees of altered mental status can arise from metabolic or toxic derangements or structural problems (Box 31-3).

EVALUATION

What terms are used to accurately describe level of consciousness?

Avoid imprecise terms, such as lethargic, stuporous, or obtunded. Instead, describe the level of stimulus required to arouse the patient (e.g., wakens to voice, unarousable to noxious stimuli) and the degree of drowsiness (e.g., falls asleep after several minutes of conversation).

How do I evaluate comatose patients?

Prioritize your approach as outlined (Box 31-4). Focus neurologic examination on level of consciousness, pupillary responses, motor response to noxious stimuli (tickling the nose hairs is noxious enough), deep tendon reflexes, and on oculovestibular testing, performed by watching eye movements when the head is rotated laterally. Eyes that appear painted on ("doll's eyes") imply loss of brainstem function. Eyes that rotate to stay focused on an object during head turning reveal intact oculocephalic processing. Obtain standard initial labo-

BOX 31-1 Sample Normal Screening Neurologic Examination

Mental status: Alert and oriented to person, place, and time
Cranial nerves: Intact smell and visual acuity; pupils 3 mm bilaterally and reactive to light to 2 mm, intact ocular movements, facial sensation, motor strength, palate elevation, shoulder shrug, and midline tongue
Sensation: Intact to light touch and sharp sensation in all four extremities
Motor: 5 out of 5 strength in all extremity muscle groups
Coordination: Intact to finger-nose-finger, gait normal
Deep tendon reflexes: 2+ at the biceps, triceps, knee and ankles; Babinski's reflex absent

BOX 31-2 Grading Motor Strength

0 = No movement
1 = Trace movement
2 = Movement when the force of gravity removed
3 = Able to move against gravity but not resistance
4 = Able to move against resistance but weaker than expected for age and size
5 = Full strength against resistance

BOX 31-3 Causes of Altered Mental Status

METABOLIC OR TOXIC
Common causes
Drugs (prescription, nonprescription, illicit)
Infection (e.g., meningitis, pneumonia)
Electrolytes (Ca^{++}, Na^+, glucose)
Anoxia (hypoperfusion, hypoxia)
Myocardial infarction

Less common causes
Hypertensive encephalopathy
Adrenal insufficiency
Hypothyroidism
Vitamin B_{12} deficiency

STRUCTURAL
Common causes
Ischemic stroke
Hemorrhage
CNS trauma

Less common causes
CNS tumor
CNS abscess

TABLE 31-1
Tailoring the Neurologic Examination for Specific Conditions
(add the following tests to usual screening examination)

CONDITION	NEUROLOGIC EXAMINATION	OBSERVE AND RECORD
Coma	Responsiveness	Level of stimulus required to rouse patient: voice, shaking, noxious stimuli (tickle nose hairs)
	Motor response	Avoidance or posturing with noxious stimulus
	Pupil size, response	Size in mm, ipsilateral and contralateral response to light
	Oculocephalic reflex	Abnormal if eyes fixed with head, normal if eyes roll to stay focused on a fixed point; clear C-spine first!
	Corneal reflexes	Blink elicited when cornea touched with cotton swab
Stroke	Simultaneous double stimuli	Touch both arms at once, ask which arm is being touched; patient has neglect if cannot feel both
	Stereognosis	Ability to identify coin in hand with eyes closed
	Graphesthesia	Recognize number drawn on hand with eyes closed
	Romberg's sign	Stand up straight with eyes closed
	Pronator drift	Keep arms extended out at shoulder height with palms up; abnormal if one palm or arm turns downwards and inwards
	Gait	Symmetry, stride, arm swing, stance (wide or narrow)
Memory loss	MMSE	30-point mini-mental status examination
Neuropathy	Pain/temperature	Sharp toothpick, cold metal
	Proprioception	Toe up or down
	Light touch	Identify pattern: dermatomal, stocking-glove

ratory tests: ABG, CBC, electrolytes, renal and liver function, glucose, and urinalysis.

What historical clues are helpful in determining the cause of confusion?

Ask family, friends, and emergency medical staff for clues. Abrupt *onset* suggests a discrete event, such as stroke, more gradual onset a diffuse metabolic process. Onset with a worst-ever headache, suggests subarachnoid hemorrhage (SAH). *Progression* from an initial focal deficit is a clue to the location of a structural problem. Ask about potential *precipitating factors,* such as trauma, alcohol withdrawal, or drug overdose. Obtain pill bottles from the patient's home, if possible. *Past medical problems,* such as recent trauma, diabetes, seizures, drug overdose, or heroin or alcohol use, are also clues to possible causes of altered mental status.

What studies should I order in a confused patient?

Use initial laboratory tests (listed above) to detect a metabolic cause for altered mental status. If no abnormality is found initially, further testing can include alcohol level, toxicology screening, carboxyhemoglobin levels, drug levels, or head CT, as indicated by the specific case. Most mass lesions or bleeds in the cerebral hemispheres are easy to detect, although 5% of SAHs can be missed when imaged early by CT scan. Negative CT in a patient thought to have SAH requires LP to look for bloody CSF. Perform LP in any patient with fever and altered mental status unless a good explanation for both is quickly found.

How do I recognize the difference between delirium and dementia?

Delirium is transient, fluctuating confusion, usually accompanied by agitation and adrenergic signs, such as tachycardia and diaphoresis. It usually resolves with treatment of the causal metabolic derangement. Psychosis may look like delirium but has no underlying metabolic derangement. In contrast, *dementia* is a confusional state in which patients remain attentive. It is chronic, persistent, and slowly progressive, with loss of memory as a prominent feature (Table 31-2).

What information helps determine likely outcome in a comatose patient?

Use prognostic information to counsel families. Good prognosis is associated with drug intoxication (90% survival), intact pupillary and oculovestibular reflexes, and in patients showing rapid initial clinical improvement. Poor prognosis is associated with loss of pupillary, corneal, and oculovestibular reflexes for longer than

---

BOX 31-4 Evaluation and Management of the Comatose Patient

IMMEDIATE ISSUES FOR STABILIZATION
ABCs*
C-spine films
Glucose 25 g IV
Thiamine 100 mg IV
Naloxone 0.4-1.2 mg IV
Rapid examination
ABG, CBC, renal and liver function, electrolytes, urinalysis

URGENT ISSUES AFTER STABILIZATION
History
Thorough neurologic examination
Head CT with/without contrast
LP if indicated
ECG
Antibiotics if meningitis suspected

LATER ISSUES
Correct electrolytes
Correct acid-base disorder
Toxicology screen
Chest x-ray
EEG
Other laboratory tests if indicated

*See Chapter 6, How to Approach the Acutely Ill Patient section.

TABLE 31-2
Features Distinguishing Delirium From Dementia

FEATURE	DELIRIUM	DEMENTIA
Level of consciousness	Impaired	Normal*
Clinical course	Acute, fluctuates over hours	Slowly progresses over years
Autonomic hyperactivity	Present	Absent
Prognosis	Usually reversible	Usually irreversible

*Patients usually retain normal level of consciousness until very late in the course of dementia.

6 hours after onset of insult (95% mortality); unwitnessed cardiac arrest; prolonged resuscitation; nontraumatic coma with failure to improve after 4 days; and traumatic coma in the elderly. Mortality is 75% in comatose patients with SAH; 50% with head injury; and 40% to 50% from cardiac arrest, tumor, infection, or metabolic insult. Permanent, severe impairment occurs in 15% to 25% of coma survivors.

TREATMENT

How do I treat a comatose or confused patient?

With coma, start empiric treatment with thiamine, glucose, and naloxone. Consider intubation when confusion is severe enough to impair airway protection. For comatose and confused patients, treat the underlying cause. If meningitis is suspected, give immediate IV antibiotics even before LP is completed, if necessary, to optimize outcome.

> **Key Points** ·······························
> - Patients with coma need rapid, prioritized evaluation and management.
> - Altered mental status with fever is meningitis until proven otherwise and requires early antibiotics and LP.
> - Tickling the nose hairs is a painless way of administering a noxious stimulus.
> - Delirium is an acute alteration in mental status that may fluctuate and is usually caused by a reversible metabolic or toxic abnormality.

STROKE

ETIOLOGY

What causes stroke?

Strokes are either ischemic or hemorrhagic disruption of blood flow to the brain. *Ischemic strokes* occur from occlusion or hypoperfusion of a blood vessel. Occlusion can arise from a local process, such as atherosclerotic plaque with or without thrombosis, vessel wall changes resulting from hypertension called lipohyalinosis, vessel injury from vasculitis, or hyperviscosity syndromes (e.g., polycythemia vera, sickle cell anemia, thrombocytosis). Occlusion can also occur with an embolus originating at a remote site, such as the carotid artery, heart, or even peripheral circulation via a patent foramen ovale. Hypoperfusion can occur during too rapid a fall in blood pressure, as with the use of sublingual nifedi-

pine, or with a cardiac arrest. *Hemorrhagic strokes* are classified as either subarachnoid or intracranial, depending on the location of bleeding. Although most subarachnoid bleeds are the result of trauma rather than stroke, spontaneous rupture of a congenital aneurysm is considered a form of stroke. These aneurysms are usually located in the vessels of the circle of Willis and may go undetected for years. Intracranial hemorrhage usually occurs as the result of long-standing hypertension. Other causes include trauma, amyloid angiopathy (recently recognized and common), and bleeding disorder. Ischemic stroke may transform into hemorrhagic stroke if necrosis or reperfusion causes bleeding.

What are the risk factors for stroke?

The most important risk factor for stroke is hypertension. Diabetes, smoking, sedentary lifestyle, elevated cholesterol, atrial fibrillation, valvular disease, and cocaine use are also risk factors.

EVALUATION

What historical information is useful in evaluating patients with stroke?

History should focus on the type and distribution of deficits; timing of onset; and associated symptoms, such as headache, vomiting, neck stiffness, or visual disturbances. Existence of risk factors should be sought, including hypertension, hypercholesterolemia, diabetes, other vascular disease, valvular disease, atrial fibrillation, prior transient ischemic attack symptoms, or cocaine use.

How are timing of onset and associated symptoms helpful?

Timing of onset lends important clues. Brief episodes of ischemic neurologic deficits, called transient ischemic attacks (TIAs), often last minutes to hours and are completely resolved within 24 hours of onset. Symptoms of a TIA may include transient monocular blindness, loss of speech, or loss of motor or sensory function of a hand or leg. TIAs often herald a more severe ischemic event. Maximal deficits at onset suggest embolic stroke. Evolution over minutes to a maximal deficit with associated headache and altered alertness suggests hemorrhage. "Stroke in evolution" with deficits worsening or fluctuating over hours to days suggests a propagating thrombus, recurrent emboli, development of edema, or an enlarging hematoma. Associated symptoms are also helpful. Subarachnoid bleed from a ruptured berry aneurysm often presents with "the worst headache of my life" and may be accompanied by vomiting or rapid loss of consciousness. Severe warning headaches may occur days to weeks before a catastrophic SAH. In comparison, headache is rarely a feature with stroke. Vomiting may accompany posterior circulation strokes, although it is unlikely to accompany strokes in other distributions. An altered level of consciousness frequently accompanies hemorrhagic stroke resulting from the immediate mass effect of the bleeding, whereas ischemic strokes rarely cause initial changes in consciousness, although they may cause progressive changes as edema develops over hours to days.

What are some patterns of neurologic deficits seen with types of strokes?

Lacunar strokes are associated with hypertensive changes in small vessels, which cause vascular occlusion deep in the brain in areas such as the thalamus or internal capsule. Lacunes typically cause isolated hemisensory or hemimotor loss. Hypertensive hemorrhages and embolic strokes can also occur in similar distributions as lacunar infarcts. *Proximal middle cerebral artery* (MCA) occlusion causes contralateral weakness and sensory loss, often involving the arm and face more than the leg, and homonymous hemianopsia (loss of the contralateral field of vision in both eyes). When MCA occlusion occurs in the dominant hemisphere, there is an associated aphasia (speech deficit). If the nondominant hemisphere is involved, a contralateral hemineglect or even denial of deficit may occur. *Basilar artery* occlusion can lead to a combination of vertigo, ataxia, visual disturbances, and cranial nerve palsies. *Subarachnoid bleeding* causes meningeal irritation with neck stiffness and meningeal signs, although these may be lost with coma. Focal neurologic deficits are rarely seen with SAH.

How is physical examination helpful?

In addition to performing a thorough neurologic examination, evaluate for increased intracranial pressure by funduscopic examination, evaluate for meningeal signs, auscultate for carotid bruits or valvular disease, look at extremities to detect venous thrombosis, and palpate pulse to detect atrial fibrillation.

What laboratory studies should I order?

Obtain CBC, platelet count, chemistries, glucose, cholesterol, sedimentation rate, VDRL, PT, and PTT. If the diagnosis of TIA or ischemic stroke is confirmed by history and imaging, order carotid Doppler, echocardiogram, and ECG for arrhythmias. This workup may be performed as an outpatient in those with a single TIA but should be performed in the hospital if symptoms are escalating, or if stroke is suspected. If SAH is suspected but CT scan is negative, perform LP to look for xanthochromia or blood.

What imaging is helpful in patients with stroke?

Head CT without contrast differentiates between an ischemic and a hemorrhagic process. A normal CT scan does not rule out ischemic stroke; a repeat CT in 48 hours may reveal focal edema as a darkened area with loss of normal fissures and gray-white borders. Hemorrhagic stroke looks bright white on noncontrast CT scan. If contrast is given with the initial CT, hemorrhage cannot be distinguished from a contrast-enhanced intracranial mass. MRI or MR angiography may be useful in specific situations in which atypical forms of vascular pathology are suspected and should be obtained only after specialty consultation.

TREATMENT

What general things can be done to treat stroke patients?

Several general principles apply to the treatment of stroke. Do not lower arterial pressure too aggressively. The reasoning behind this is that higher blood pressures are likely required to perfuse brain tissues near areas of injury in the days after a stroke. Systolic pressures above 210 can be treated with gentle diuresis. Use maintenance fluids with isotonic solutions if patients are not eating, but avoid overhydration so as not to worsen cerebral edema. For all stroke patients, perform frequent vital signs and neurologic examinations in the first hours to days to monitor for extension or complications of the initial stroke.

What medications help patients with stroke?

Patients presenting less than 3 hours after onset of a completed (nonprogressing) ischemic stroke may be candidates for thrombolysis with tissue plasminogen activator (tPA). Outcomes at 3 months with this strategy show a decrease in disability but not mortality. The major drawback of using tPA is the tenfold-greater risk of intracerebral hemorrhage (6.4% with tPA, compared with 0.6% in those treated more traditionally). Additionally, over 20 exclusion criteria exist for the use of tPA (see Table 23-6). Patients with ischemic "stroke in evolution," especially in the basilar artery distribution, may benefit from IV heparin, although the data are only suggestive at best. Intraarterial thrombolysis by interventional radiology is available and used in basilar artery circulation occlusion but remains to be fully tested for benefits and risks. Patients with a documented cardiac or peripheral source of clot require anticoagulation (see Chapter 28, Clotting Disorders section, for details). Give patients with TIA symptoms antiplatelet therapy with aspirin (325 mg/day). If aspirin is unsuccessful at this dose and TIAs continue, increase the dose or start ticlopidine. Ticlopidine is more effective and expensive than aspirin and carries a risk of leukopenia, rash, and diarrhea. Patients with subarachnoid bleeds benefit from bed rest, sedation, blood pressure control, and calcium channel blockade, specifically with nimodipine before definitive surgical ablation. Amyloid angiopathy has no known prevention or therapy.

When is surgery indicated?

Refer patients with TIAs and greater than 70% carotid artery stenosis to an experienced surgeon for carotid endarterectomy; complication rates significantly alter risk/benefit profile. Surgical evacuation of bleeding is reserved for severe hemorrhage. Intracranial bleeding at any site of more than 80 ml associated with deep coma will likely lead to death, and heroic measures to evacuate the blood are unlikely to change the outcome.

Key Points ·······························
- Hypertension is the leading risk factor for stroke.
- Prevent stroke with aspirin.
- Strokes are categorized as hemorrhagic or ischemic by noncontrast head CT scan.
- Do not aggressively lower blood pressure in patients presenting with stroke.

SEIZURE

ETIOLOGY

What causes seizures?

Seizures are paroxysmal, transient discharges of groups of neurons within the brain. More than 10% of the population will experience one or a few seizures, often related to a structural or metabolic derangement, such as CNS infection, childhood fever, stroke, hypoglycemia, electrolyte disturbance, hypoperfusion, alcohol or benzodiazepine withdrawal, CNS tumor, or drug overdose (cocaine, tricyclic antidepressant, theophylline). Only about 0.2% to 2% of the population has true idiopathic epilepsy usually presenting before age 18 and defined as recurrent seizures with characteristic EEG findings and no identifiable structural or metabolic cause. Seizures are further broadly classified as generalized or partial, as determined by EEG.

What types of seizures are there?

Generalized seizures include tonic-clonic, absence, and atonic seizures. The classic tonic-clonic seizure begins with a stiff phase of tonic muscle contraction lasting several seconds, followed by generalized rhythmic jerking movements (clonus) during which consciousness is lost. Incontinence of stool or bladder or tongue trauma may occur, although these are nonspecific features of loss of consciousness from any cause. With absence seizures, patients stare blankly without loss of consciousness. With atonic seizures, also known as *drop attacks,* patients abruptly lose postural tone. With tonic-clonic seizures, there may be a prolonged postictal period of extreme sleepiness and confusion. In contrast, there is no postictal state after absence or atonic seizures and patients are able to return to normal function immediately. *Partial seizures* occur in a focal distribution and may or may not cause loss of consciousness.

EVALUATION

What workup is warranted in patients presenting with their first seizure?

For first-time seizure, rule out treatable causes. Determine the exact sequence of events to help classify the episode as generalized or partial, with or without loss of consciousness or postictal confusion. Ask about possible precipitants, such as alcohol or benzodiazepine withdrawal, drug overdose, or cocaine use. Look for signs of trauma, tongue laceration, or incontinence. Note vital signs. Look for papilledema by dilated retinal examination and for focal neurologic deficit as a clue to an underlying structural lesion, such as stroke or tumor. Obtain CBC, chemistry panel, toxicology screen, alcohol level, and head CT scan without contrast to detect acute CNS bleeding, and then with contrast to detect mass lesions. LP is recommended for patients with first seizure and may show postictal pleocytosis caused by the seizure alone, with up to 80 WBC/ml persisting for 1 to 5 days after the event (neutrophils or mononuclear cells).

When a patient has known epilepsy and seizes, what workup is warranted?

Obtain antiseizure drug level. If drug level is subtherapeutic and no new focal deficits are apparent on examination, no further workup is required.

TREATMENT

A single tonic-clonic seizure from an identifiable structural or metabolic cause should be managed with correction of the underlying problem and does not warrant anticonvulsant medication. Use anticonvulsants if seizures are recurrent resulting from slow resolution of the underlying derangement. Phenytoin is the drug of choice in this setting, administered by a loading dose of 1000 mg IV over several hours. Side effects include hypotension with rapid loading, rash, and rare but potentially life-threatening leukopenia or hepatitis. Treat continuous seizing, or status epilepticus, with a more rapid-acting drug, such as diazepam in 5 mg IV boluses. True epilepsy can be treated with a number of different anticonvulsant medications, most of which require titration to therapeutic drug levels. Phenytoin is commonly the first drug tried for tonic-clonic seizures. Carbamazepine, phenobarbital, and valproic acid are other common choices used as second-line agents or for other types of seizures.

MOTOR WEAKNESS

See Table 31-3 for the presentation and diagnosis of some diseases causing motor weakness.

Key Points

- Obtain careful history to classify a seizure as partial or generalized with or without loss of consciousness or postictal state.
- First-time seizures require evaluation to rule out a structural or metabolic cause.
- Monitor patients starting phenytoin for hypotension, hepatitis, and leukopenia.

TABLE 31-3
Motor Deficit Syndromes

SYNDROME	PRESENTATION	DIAGNOSIS
Amyotrophic lateral sclerosis (ALS)	Mixed upper and lower motor neuron deficits cause easy fatigability, twitching, wasting and muscle cramps; may involve tongue, palate, gag reflex; spares extraocular muscle involvement; steadily progressive disability to death after 3-5 years	Clinical picture, normal CSF, abnormal EMG
Botulism	Fulminating weakness 12-72 hours after ingestion of contaminated food (usually home-canned food); begins with diplopia, ptosis, facial weakness, dysphagia, progresses to respiratory difficulty; no sensory or DTR deficits	Test food for *Clostridium botulinum;* EMG repetitive stimulation increases motor response
Guillain-Barré syndrome	Symmetric ascending weakness beginning in legs and progressing upwards at varying rates; may be accompanied by sensory complaints, autonomic disturbances, respiratory muscle involvement	CSF shows increased protein, normal cell count; EMG shows slowing of sensory and motor conduction
Multiple sclerosis	Focal, usually transient episodes of weakness, numbness, unsteadiness, or visual change; episodes remit and relapse, may be progressive with persistent deficits, hyperreflexia	MRI shows focal scattered plaques from demyelination of periventricular white matter in brain, cord, and optic nerves
Paralytic shellfish poisoning	Rapidly progressive paralysis with accompanying sensory symptoms beginning 30 minutes after eating poisonous shellfish	Saxitoxin blocks sodium channels; diagnosis made by history
Poliomyelitis	Prodromal flulike illness followed by focal, asymmetric, rapid-onset weakness, aseptic meningitis, myalgias	RNA virus can be isolated from nasal cultures, stool, CSF

CASE 31-1

A 75-year-old woman is sent to the ER by her nursing home for worsening confusion over the last week. She is unable to give history. On examination, she is only oriented to her name and falls asleep several times during the interview and examination. Her mucous membranes are dry and vital signs show orthostatic changes with a sitting pulse of 110, BP of 95/60, and temperature of 36° C. Neurologic examination shows intact reactive pupils at 2 mm, and cranial nerves appear to all work, although she cannot comply with testing. She is moving all four extremities symmetrically, although she appears weak. She has difficulty standing for measurement of orthostatic vital signs.

A. Is this delirium or dementia, and why do you think so?
B. What could be causing her altered mental status?
C. What evaluation do you wish to pursue (see answer for results)?
D. From results of tests, what is causing altered mental status?
E. What further tests and treatment does she need?

CASE 31-2

A 27-year-old man is brought to the ER after seizing. His girlfriend reports he cried out, went stiff, and then began shaking all over for about a minute or two. As far as she knows, he has never done this before. On examination, he is dazed, drooling, and breathing heavily. HR 120, BP 150/100, RR 24, fundi show no papilledema, and reflexes are brisk but symmetric. No focal deficits are apparent, although he is not awake enough to actively participate in the neurologic examination.

A. What is the differential diagnosis for his presentation?
B. What more do you want to ask his girlfriend?
C. What other tests are warranted?
D. What treatment do you want to give him?

32

Psychiatry

DEPRESSION AND ANXIETY

ETIOLOGY

How common is depression?

When all of the causes of death and disability in the entire world are ranked, depression comes in fourth, behind lower respiratory infections, diarrhea, and perinatal conditions. This statistic is reflected in primary care clinic populations, where prevalence of depression ranges from 20% to 40%. That means, at a minimum, you should diagnose depression in 1 out of 5 patients. In fact, primary care physicians only recognize about half of the cases of depression that they see.

Can medical conditions cause depression?

Although the reason for the association is unknown, hypothyroidism and Cushing's syndrome are both associated with depression. If there are signs of these conditions by history or examination, screen for them (TSH and 24-hour urine cortisol).

Do medications cause depression?

Many medications can cause depression, but only very rarely. More frequent associations are seen with a subset (Box 32-1). Although antihypertensives are on this list, β-blockers are not included because the evidence for causality of depression is weak at best. If your patient is depressed, review the medication list.

When should I be concerned about bipolar disorder?

Manic-depressive illness, or bipolar disorder, usually presents at a younger age than unipolar major depression. Symptoms of concern are hyperactivity, irritability, flight of ideas, and grandiosity. Antidepressants may trigger an acute manic episode, so refer patients with a suggestive history to a psychiatrist.

What is "atypical depression"?

An "atypical" depression is characterized by carbohydrate craving, weight gain, and excessive sleep. An example is seasonal affective disorder, more common in northern regions where winter days are shorter. Women account for 60% to 80% of cases. The diagnosis is confirmed when the depression spontaneously improves with the onset of spring. Therapy can include full-spectrum light boxes.

EVALUATION

What are the criteria for diagnosis?

Because depression is common but frequently missed, be certain to include at least one question on this topic in your review of symptoms. For diagnosis, the patient should have five of the listed criteria for 2 weeks or more (Box 32-2). In the elderly, irritability, agitation, diminished cognitive function, and sleep disruption are more likely than frank depressed mood. This is also true in adolescents, where irritability may be the predominant mood state. Be certain to ask about thoughts of suicide, as well as symptoms suggesting a history of mania or psychosis.

How can I ask my patients about depression without making them defensive?

It is helpful to question patients about the more objective measures of depression, such as sleep, food intake, and concentration. For example, "How are you sleeping?" investigates the classic pattern of early morning awakening. You can then define depression as a physiologic state that causes the symptoms the patient is experiencing before entering into discussion of mood. This avoids the pitfall of patients thinking that you are telling them it is "all in their head."

BOX 32-1 Medications Commonly Causing Depression

Central-acting antihypertensives: Reserpine, methyldopa, and clonidine
Hormones: Oral contraceptives, progesterone, and corticosteroids
CNS depressants: Alcohol, sedatives, opiates, and psychedelics

---

BOX 32-2 Criteria for Major Depression*

Depressed mood
Anhedonia (loss of interest in most, if not all, activities)
Weight loss or gain (5% of body weight in 1 month) or appetite loss or gain
Insomnia or hypersomnia
Psychomotor agitation or retardation
Fatigue or loss of energy nearly every day
Feelings of worthlessness or inappropriate guilt
Trouble concentrating, indecision
Recurrent thoughts of death or suicide

*Five out of nine for over 2 weeks required for a diagnosis of major depression.

BOX 32-3 Risk of Depression With Selected Medical Conditions

Stroke: 50%
Diabetes with end-organ damage: 70%
Cancer varies with type and severity:
    Pancreatic: 50%
    Acute leukemia awaiting transplant: <2%

What medical conditions require careful screening for depression?

Some conditions have particularly increased rates of depression (Box 32-3).

If I ask about suicidal thoughts, will this make my patient more likely to try suicide?

There is no evidence that asking patients about thoughts of suicide makes them more likely to commit suicide. These thoughts are not uncommon in depression; ask about specific plans and access to means (e.g., guns). If a patient is actively suicidal, contact a social worker or psychiatrist right away so that they can assist in admitting the patient for acute inpatient care.

TREATMENT

Why is depression important to treat?

In addition to the death and disability from depression itself, evidence is mounting that depression has a significant effect on other medical conditions. In one study of patients with myocardial infarction, depression was an independent risk factor for mortality equivalent to left ventricular dysfunction. Whether this is due to decreased compliance with medications or other factors is not known.

Can I treat depression without a psychiatrist's help?

Internists can and should treat uncomplicated cases of depression. For suicidal thoughts, poor response to medicine, and complicating psychiatric conditions, such as personality disorder or mania, refer the patient to a psychiatrist.

Is psychotherapy helpful?

Evidence exists that psychotherapy and medications achieve equivalent response rates. Also, there appears to be a synergistic effect with psychotherapy and medications. Some data suggest that relapse rates are decreased when a patient receives cognitive therapy. Medications are generally cheaper, however.

What medication should I use?

The selective serotonin reuptake inhibitors (SSRIs) are extremely effective and well-tolerated antidepressants and so are first-line therapy. Although these medications are more expensive than the older tricyclic antidepressants, patients stay on them longer and have fewer physician visits, so the costs are equivalent in the end. Also, SSRIs are relatively safe in overdose, in contrast to the tricyclic antidepressants. Start SSRIs at full dose except in the elderly and in anxious patients, for whom half the usual starting dose is better.

How should I counsel my patient about starting medications?

On the whole, the SSRIs have minimal side effects, but sexual dysfunction, especially delayed orgasm, is most common. Other side effects are gastrointestinal distress. Time required for improvement of symptoms varies. Prepare your patient for the fact that SSRIs take from 2 days to 4 weeks to have effect. The side effects begin immediately but often subside after 1 to 2 weeks. Have your patient contract to take at least a full month of the prescription. Compliance is improved if you have the patient come for a return visit in 1 to 2 weeks. Other antidepressants are effective and have different side effect profiles (Table 32-1).

When should I combine medications?

For marked sleep disturbance, add a low dose of a sedating antidepressant at bedtime, such as 10 to 25 mg of doxepin or 50 mg of nefazodone. Depression refractory to higher doses of SSRIs warrants referral to a psychiatrist.

When I should start an antidepressant other than an SSRI?

In patients with chronic pain, start with a tricyclic antidepressant; this class of medication is effective for neuropathic pain in particular. SSRIs will treat the depression that often accompanies chronic pain but are less effective than tricyclic antidepressants for the pain itself. If there is a history of significant sexual dysfunction, consider selecting another class of drug, such as bupropion or nefazodone. Recent data also supports bupropion as an aid to smoking cessation.

I seem to have a lot of anxious patients. Should I be prescribing benzodiazepines?

Generalized anxiety disorder is a relatively uncommon condition. By contrast, depression masquerading as anxiety is quite common. A patient who seems anxious or overly concerned about his or her medical condition needs an evaluation for depression. Benzodiazepines can be used to treat a patient's insomnia and agitation in the short term until the antidepressant begins to take effect. Because of addiction, this should be done cautiously.

What is my depressed patient's prognosis?

Most depression resolves at 1 year without any intervention. Antidepressants or psychotherapy shorten this interval to 1 to 2 months. The recurrence rate is 50%. Of those patients who recur, another 50% will never have another episode. About 10% of patients with depression will suffer from chronic symptoms.

Key Points ··

- Depression is common and responds well to SSRIs.
- Most patients can be managed in the primary care setting.
- Suicidal thoughts, symptoms of mania, and poor response to therapy require referral to psychiatry.

CASE 32-1

A 75-year-old man is brought in by his daughter. For several months, he has been eating poorly and losing weight and is more ornery than usual. When you ask how he is sleeping, he says that, as usual, he has to get up at night to urinate. Regarding concentration, he says that he cannot read a book because of his poor eyesight. He no longer enjoys his golf game because of his bad back.

A. What further questions do you want to ask regarding depression?
B. Does he require any further testing?
C. If you decide that he is depressed, what medication and dose would you choose?
D. If his insomnia is particularly bothersome, what additional medication would you give?

CASE 32-2

A 52-year-old woman comes to your office in tears on the anniversary of her husband's death. She is having trouble concentrating at work and has put on 10 pounds. She believes that she is not a good mother to her children. She does not have the energy to get out of bed in the morning and always feels tired. She drinks at least glass of wine a night and recently has been started on hormone replacement therapy for postmenopausal state. She was suicidal a week ago and in fact took out her husband's gun and held it on her lap.

A. What may be contributing to her depression?
B. What treatment do you recommend?

TABLE 32-1
Common Antidepressants

DRUG	SIDE EFFECTS
SSRIs	Class effects: GI distress, sexual dysfunction
Sertraline	Very mild sedation
Fluoxetine	Agitation
Paroxetine	Mild sedation, mild A/C
Tricyclic antidepressants	Class effects: cardiac arrhythmias, sedation
Doxepin	A/C, strong sedation
Nortriptyline	A/C, mild sedation
Other	
Nefazodone	Mild sedation
Bupropion	Lowers seizure threshold

A/C, Anticholinergic: dry mouth, constipation.

33

Pulmonary

ASTHMA

ETIOLOGY

What is asthma?

Asthma causes chronic inflammation of the airways and affects people of all ages. Patients with asthma have higher levels of inflammatory mediators in their airways, even when asymptomatic. This leads to reversible bronchoconstriction, the hallmark of asthma. In the early stages, reversible bronchoconstriction is the rule. If left untreated, however, chronic remodeling occurs and leads to irreversible airway narrowing. Most asthmatic patients fluctuate between good days with minimal symptoms and bad days with aggravation of symptoms. Hospitalization is often necessary for acute exacerbations because patients can unpredictably and rapidly progress to respiratory failure and death.

What are the common forms of asthma?

Proper characterization of asthma allows you to maximize treatment (Table 33-1). Any patient may have more than one form. Most asthmatic patients have exacerbations of their symptoms with viral upper respiratory infections (URIs). Viral URIs can also prompt 6 to 8 weeks of wheezing or cough in patients without asthma. Aspirin-intolerant asthma often presents as a triad of nasal polyps, chronic rhinitis, and wheezing. Occupational asthma can be due to low-level intermittent exposure at work, such as welder's flux, or high-level exposure that precipitates more generalized airway hyperresponsiveness in reaction to a variety of precipitants.

What other disease can cause reversible bronchoconstriction?

Chronic bronchitis and emphysema often respond to the same treatment as classic asthma. Congestive heart failure can cause cardiogenic wheezing ("cardiac asthma"), which reverses with treatment of the pulmonary edema. Lymphangitic spread of some tumors, such as breast cancer, can present as wheezing and cough. Less common causes include endobronchial neoplasms, cystic fibrosis, and allergic bronchopulmonary aspergillosis (ABPA).

What is cough–variant asthma?

In this form, cough predominates over wheezing or chest tightness, even with severe exacerbations. Precipitants, classification of severity, and treatment are the same.

Why is asthma classified by severity?

The National Asthma Education and Prevention Program (NAEPP) suggests categorizing asthma severity to guide therapy as mild-intermittent, mild-persistent, moderate-persistent, or severe-persistent (Table 33-2). Although these categories describe the chronic condition, even patients with mild-intermittent disease can have exacerbations severe enough to warrant hospitalization.

EVALUATION

What are the common symptoms of asthma?

The clinical presentation of asthma varies, but common symptoms include chest tightness, wheezing, cough, and exercise intolerance. Sputum production is common with acute exacerbations, even in the absence of infection. Symptoms can wax and wane and may be difficult to distinguish from respiratory infections, congestive heart failure, and COPD. Some patients have other symptoms of allergic disease (allergic rhinitis, atopic dermatitis, urticaria).

How do I document reversible airway constriction?

Document reversible airway constriction with office spirometry. Asthmatic patients commonly have an ob-

---

TABLE 33-1

Precipitants and Special Interventions for Different Types of Asthma

TYPES OF ASTHMA	PRECIPITANT	SPECIAL INTERVENTION BEYOND USUAL ASTHMA THERAPIES
Allergen-induced*	Animal dander, dust mites, cockroaches, pollen, molds	Allergen avoidance
Exercise-induced	Exertion	Preexercise bronchodilator
Stress-induced	Stressful situations	Preexposure bronchodilator
Cold-air–intolerant	Cold air	Preexposure bronchodilator
URI-related wheezing	Viral respiratory infection	Bronchodilator for URI
Aspirin-intolerant	NSAIDs, aspirin	Avoid NSAIDs and aspirin
Occupational	Occupational irritant	Respirator, avoid irritant
GERD-induced	Gastroesophageal reflux	GERD treatment and prevention measures (see Chapter 13)

*Formerly termed "extrinsic" asthma and associated with elevations in serum IgE; is now characterized by a wide range of allergens that can induce asthma without elevations in serum IgE or serum eosinophils.

TABLE 33-2

NAEPP Classification of Asthma

CLASSIFICATION	SYMPTOM FREQUENCY	EXACERBATIONS	NIGHTTIME SYMPTOMS	USUAL SYMPTOMS	FEV$_1$ AND PEFR	PEFR VARIABILITY
Mild intermittent	≤2×/wk	Brief	≤2×/mo	Asymptomatic with normal lung function	≥80% predicted	<20%
Mild persistent	>2×/wk, <1×/day	Limit activity	>2×/mo	Asymptomatic with normal lung function	≥80% predicted	20%-30%
Moderate persistent	Daily	>2×/wk	>1×/wk	>1×/wk	Need daily short-acting β-agonist	>30%
Severe persistent	Continuous	Frequent	Frequent	Limits activity	≤60%	>30%

---

structive pattern such that the ratio of forced expiratory volume in 1 second over forced vital capacity (FEV_1/FVC) is less than 75%. After two puffs of a β_2-agonist, such as albuterol, both FEV_1 and FEV_1/FVC increase toward normal. Commonly, even asthmatic patients with an FEV_1 considered normal demonstrate significant increases in FEV_1 with albuterol.

What if a patient has a history suggestive of asthma but normal spirometry?

This is not uncommon. For cases like this, reversible bronchoconstriction can be documented in other ways. One approach is to have patients come to see you at "their worst." Often morning bronchoconstriction is missed at afternoon office appointments. Another option is to have patients keep a diary of peak expiratory flow rate (PEFR) and symptoms. Variability of morning and evening PEFRs can often be diagnostic. Methacholine challenge, in which patients are given increasing concentrations of a histamine-like substance, can show increased sensitivity to low concentrations in asthmatic patients, but this test is not usually necessary to make a diagnosis.

What key questions should I ask a patient with asthma?

- *Description of symptoms:* Symptoms, when they occur (day or night, season of the year, during final exams, etc.), how long they last, what brings them on, what makes them better, and where they occur (at work, at home, on the softball field, etc.); symptoms at nighttime, exercise intolerance, cough, or symptoms suggestive of GERD

- *Past asthma history:* Prior ER visits, hospitalizations, intubations, childhood symptoms
- *Other allergy history:* Allergic rhinitis, atopic dermatitis, urticaria, previous skin testing
- *Family medical history:* Asthma or other allergy-like syndromes in parents and siblings
- *Home environment:* Carpets, dust collectors (books, stuffed animals, etc.), plants, pets
- *Work environment:* Chemical exposures, animal exposures
- *Medication use:* Current and past prescriptions, over-the-counter, and alternative therapies
- *Use of tobacco or inhaled street drugs:* These often make asthma more difficult to treat

What are the key features of outpatient evaluation for asthma?

Perform history as above to gauge severity of symptoms. Physical examination usually shows normal vital signs and breath sounds that range from normal to diffuse end-expiratory wheezing. The expiratory phase time may be prolonged. There may be signs of other allergic disease. Also use the examination to rule out cardiac disease or other significant lung disease. Office spirometry is essential; many patients with seemingly mild symptoms can have alarmingly compromised lung function. A sputum examination may help rule out bacterial bronchitis and often shows significant eosinophilia (>2% total cell counts), although not all laboratories are able to identify this. A WBC differential may show elevated eosinophils, although this is neither sensitive nor specific. Ask the patient to keep an asthma diary, including PEFR monitoring, to assist with diagnosis and guide treatment. Allergy skin testing may help identify specific allergens to avoid.

TREATMENT

What are the goals of asthma therapy?

The goals of asthma therapy are to give patients more symptom-free days, better quality of life, and fewer days of missed productivity, and to prevent the chronic remodeling of the airways that occurs with age. There is no cure for asthma. Even an asthmatic patient with excellent control of symptoms will have occasional exacerbations.

What is the best therapy for chronic asthma?

The best therapy for asthma uses a three-pronged approach: (1) avoid precipitants, (2) relieve acute bronchoconstriction, and (3) control inflammation (Tables 33-3 through 33-5). Do not use one approach without the others. Add medications one at a time and monitor for response to minimize the number required. β_2-

Agonists (e.g., albuterol, long-acting salmeterol) relax airway smooth muscles and relieve acute bronchoconstriction. Salmeterol is particularly useful in preventing nocturnal wheezing. Theophylline is an oral smooth muscle relaxant that has a narrow therapeutic window and is much less potent. Corticosteroids target inflammation, are the only agents proven to decrease chronic airway modeling, and are therefore the mainstays of therapy for all but mild-intermittent disease. Inhaled steroids have fewer systemic side effects and are available in a range of potencies (see Table 33-5). Mast cell stabilizers reduce allergen-induced asthma for 20% of adults. Antileukotriene agents benefit about 60% of adults with asthma of all types; a 4- to 6-week trial of either of these last two agents is warranted for patients whose symptoms are inadequately controlled with standard therapy.

How do you treat an acute asthma exacerbation?

The cornerstone of treatment for acute asthma exacerbations is systemic corticosteroids. When a patient presents to an emergency room, give oral prednisone 60 mg PO (or 1mg/kg) or IV methylprednisolone 120 mg immediately. This usually takes 4 to 8 hours to take effect. In the meantime, give repeated nebulized albuterol treatments. Epinephrine can be given for patients in status asthmaticus. The use of IV aminophylline and magnesium has fallen out of favor. Teach patients to use steroid inhalers as directed and to seek medical assistance with any exacerbation. Observe the patient for signs of improvement before discharging them. Oral steroids should be continued and rapidly tapered over the ensuing week or so beginning at 40 to 60 mg daily to prevent recurrent exacerbation.

What medications should I avoid in patients with asthma?

Aspirin, NSAIDS, and β-blockers can worsen bronchospasm to varying degrees in patients with asthma. Inquire about use of these agents, and do not forget eye-drops as a source of β-blockers.

What can be done for a patient whose asthma does not respond to usual therapy?

Review the patient's known asthma precipitants and try to identify others. GERD is thought to aggravate asthma symptoms, so H_2-blockers or proton-pump inhibitors can be tried. Observe the patient's use of the metered-dose inhaler (MDI). Is the patient not receiving the medication because of noncompliance or improper technique? Reconsider the diagnosis. Undiagnosed endobronchial lesions or other undiagnosed disease may be the culprit. Bronchoscopy is often useful in this setting. There are rare asthmatic patients who are insensitive to corticosteroids. These patients can be treated with other immunosup-

---

TABLE 33-3
The Three Fundamental Components of Asthma Therapy

COMPONENT	EXAMPLES	WHEN TO USE
Avoid precipitants	Polyurethane mattress covers for dust mites GERD therapy	Use as an adjunct to medications
Symptom relief	Albuterol inhaler (short-acting for daytime) Salmeterol inhaler (long-acting for night) Theophylline tablets (not as potent)	Use as needed for bronchospasm
Inflammation controllers	Corticosteroids, inhaled, oral, or IV Mast cell stabilizers Antileukotrienes	Use daily for all but mild-intermittent asthma

---

TABLE 33-4
Symptom Relievers Used for Treating Bronchoconstriction

DRUG	DOSAGE
SHORT-ACTING β_2-AGONISTS	
Albuterol (Proventil, Ventolin)	2-4 puffs q4-6h prn sx or before exercise
Terbutaline (Brethine, Brethaire)	2-4 puffs q4-6h prn sx; 5 mg PO tid (in adults)
Pirbuterol (Maxair)	1-2 puffs q4-6h prn asthma sx
Metaproterenol (Alupent)	2-3 puffs q3-4h prn asthma sx
LONG-ACTING β_2-AGONISTS	
Salmeterol (Serevent)	2 puffs qd bid (NEVER exceed 4 puffs/24 hr)
METHYLXANTHINES	
Theophylline (Theo-Dur and others)	100-400 mg PO bid; follow serum levels

---

TABLE 33-5
Inflammation Controllers Used for Treating Asthma

DRUG	DOSAGE
INHALED CORTICOSTEROIDS*	
Beclomethasone (Vanceril, Beclovent)	2-4 puffs bid-qid
Triamcinolone (Azmacort)	4-8 puffs bid
Flunisolide (AeroBid)	2 puffs bid
Budesonide (Pulmicort)	2 puffs bid
Fluticasone (Flovent)	2 puffs bid (44, 110, 220 µg)
MAST CELL STABILIZERS	
Cromolyn (Intal)	2-4 puffs qid
Nedocromil (Tilade)	2 puffs qid
ANTILEUKOTRIENE AGENTS	
Zileuton (Zyflo)	600 mg PO qid (check LFTs for the first 3 mo)
Zafirlukast (Accolate)	20 mg PO bid 1 hour before or 2 hours after meals
Montelukast (Singulair)	10 mg PO qd

*Listed from minimum to maximum potency.

---

pressives, but this should be used only as a last resort when other diagnoses have been ruled out.

What are the side effects of steroids?

Short-term oral steroids can cause psychosis, hypertension, hypokalemia, and glucose intolerance. Long-term use causes osteoporosis, osteonecrosis, immunosuppression, and cataract formation.

When should an asthmatic patient with an acute exacerbation be hospitalized?

There are no clear guidelines, but concerning signs include prior hospitalizations or intubations, inability to speak in full sentences, use of accessory muscles, loss of wheezes resulting from absent air movement, hypercarbia or hypoxemia on ABG, or sluggish response to initial treatment. When deciding whether to hospitalize, always err on the side of patient safety.

Key Points

- Asthma is a disease of chronic airway inflammation triggered by a wide array of precipitants.
- Treatment for asthma should always include modification of the precipitants, an inhaled corticosteroid or other antiinflammatory, and symptom relief with bronchodilators.
- Treat asthma exacerbations with systemic steroids and increased bronchodilators.

CASE 33-1

A 20-year-old college basketball player comes to you because she is unable to complete a game. Usually, after 20 minutes of exertion, she begins to cough and experience chest tightness. She states that she often feels poorly the next day as well.
  A How would you begin to evaluate her?
  B. What studies would you order?
  C. What treatment would you suggest?

CASE 33-2

A 52-year-old grandmother with asthma calls you stating that for the last 3 days she has been feeling wheezy and short of breath. About 1 week ago she had URI symptoms after visiting her grandchild. You try to ask her some questions on the phone, but she is only able to answer you in short two- to three-word answers.
  A. What do you do?
  B. How should she be evaluated?
  C. Should this patient be hospitalized?

CHRONIC OBSTRUCTIVE PULMONARY DISEASE

ETIOLOGY

What is COPD?

Chronic obstructive pulmonary disease, or COPD, is a group of disorders characterized by airflow obstruction, chronic cough, and expectoration. Under the general term of COPD are the specific disorders of chronic bronchitis and emphysema. Chronic bronchitis is defined clinically by a chronic or recurrent productive cough on most days for at least 3 months per year for at least 2 successive years. Emphysema is a pathologic diagnosis based on lung biopsy or chest CT. These two disorders often coexist in the same patient. Both result in airflow obstruction, exertional dyspnea, and bronchospasm. Whereas the bronchospasm of asthma is usually reversible and responsive to steroids, the airway obstruction of COPD is fixed and progressive. Along with the fixed defect of COPD, some patients have a reversible component to the airway obstruction.

What is cor pulmonale?

In severe COPD, chronic hypoxia and destruction of pulmonary vascular beds result in pulmonary hypertension, with increased work for the right ventricle. With time and increasing severity, patients develop signs of right heart failure: lower extremity edema, elevated jugular venous pressures, and hepatic congestion. This condition is termed *cor pulmonale.*

What are the risk factors for COPD?

Tobacco use is the greatest risk factor, present in 85% to 90% of cases. Other risk factors include family history, recurrent pulmonary infections, environmental pollution, occupational exposures, and α_1-antitrypsin deficiency.

What causes COPD exacerbations?

A COPD exacerbation is any significant decrement in function or increase in symptoms. Respiratory tract infections, either viral or bacterial, often set off an exacerbation. Behavioral factors, such as underuse of medications or continued smoking, may play a role. Drugs such as β-blockers can trigger bronchospasm, as can environmental irritants, such as pollen, fumes, and weather changes. Be on the lookout for other causes of acute decompensation, such as congestive heart failure (left or right), angina, pneumonia, pulmonary embolism, anemia, renal dysfunction, or pneumothorax. Arrhythmia, aspiration, pleural effusion, and sedation can also play a role.

EVALUATION

How do patients with COPD present?

Chronic cough and sputum production suggest the diagnosis of chronic bronchitis. As the disease progresses, patients are more affected by chronic dyspnea, wheezing, and exercise limitation. Worsening obstruction causes wheezing, increased dyspnea on exertion, and increased inhaler use. On examination, look for tachypnea and tachycardia. Examine for use of accessory muscles, retraction of chest wall soft tissues, poor airflow, rales, wheezes, and rhonchi. Look for signs of right heart failure, including edema, neck vein distention, or a right-sided S_3 gallop.

What tests help evaluate patients with COPD?

Pulmonary function tests (PFTs) reveal obstruction by a reduced FEV_1 and FEV_1/FVC ratio. Unlike with asthma, obstructive changes on PFTs generally do not normalize with bronchodilator therapy, although some patients with COPD have a component of reactive/reversible obstruction. A chest x-ray screens for pneumonia and pulmonary masses and may show the classic signs of increased lung volumes, flattened diaphragms, upper lobe bullae, and increased retrosternal air space. Basilar emphysema on chest film suggests α_1-antitrypsin deficiency or prior IV Ritalin use. ABG may show low Po_2 and high Pco_2 or may be normal. CBC may show polycythemia, a sign of chronic hypoxia. WBC may be elevated because of infection or steroid use.

TREATMENT

What are nonpharmacologic therapies for COPD?

Prevention of worsening disease is key: aggressively pursue smoking cessation, and vaccinate against influenza annually and against pneumococcus. Control environmental triggers. Pulmonary rehabilitation, like cardiac rehabilitation, is a multidisciplinary approach to maximizing patient quality of life, with education, exercise training, psychologic support, and close medical follow-up. Surgical options are also under development, including lung transplant and lung reduction surgery in appropriate patients.

What is a basic medication regimen for COPD?

Begin with a β-agonist inhaler, and layer on further therapy as disease requires (Figure 33-1).

When is oxygen therapy warranted?

For *chronic* disease, provide continuous oxygen to patients with severe hypoxia ($Pao_2 \leq 55$, or oxygen saturation < 88%). If cor pulmonale or polycythemia is present, use slightly higher cutoff values for oxygen ($Pao_2 \leq 59$). Alternately, oxygen may only be required intermittently, for example, during exercise- or sleep-induced hypoxia. In any patient with a terminal illness, oxygen may be palliative and should be provided, regardless of oxygen level. In *acute* exacerbations, use oxygen to maintain a saturation of at least 90%. Although administration of excessive oxygen may result in worsened CO_2 retention in some COPD patients, this risk has been overstated in the past. In the tachypneic, cyanotic patient, aggressive oxygen use is appropriate. Begin with 1 to 1.5 L/min per nasal cannula and adjust to maintain saturation level at least 90%.

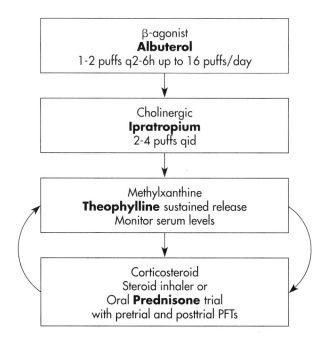

Figure 33-1 Stepped care approach to COPD.

What therapies are used for COPD exacerbations?

For patients presenting in distress to the emergency room, proceed with oxygen therapy as outlined above. Begin with nebulized *albuterol* and *ipratropium bromide* (these can be combined) every 20 minutes in the first hour, decreasing to every 4 to 6 hours as the patient's condition allows. MDIs can also be used. If obstruction will not reverse and is life-threatening, consider subcutaneous *terbutaline* if there is no underlying cardiac disease. When patients do not respond to initial nebulized treatments, add corticosteroids, even though these are not as effective as in asthma patients. Use IV *methylprednisolone*. The dose is controversial, but a reasonable choice is 2 mg/kg IV bolus, and 0.5 mg/kg every 6 hours thereafter. Finally, consider *methylxanthines*. Although this class of drug is well-supported in the chronic management of COPD, its use in the acute setting is less clear. For patients already on theophylline, be sure to check serum drug levels before adding more methylxanthine. (CAUTION: methylxanthine metabolism is affected by smoking, liver disease, and many medications, including cimetidine, oral contraceptives, erythromycin, and ciprofloxacin. Monitor serum levels carefully, and consult a pharmacist for recommended infusion rates.) For signs of infection, such as fever, chills, or pulmonary infiltrate on x-ray, treat with *antibiotics*. The role of antibiotics when infection is less clinically evident is controversial.

When is intubation indicated?

In the patient with fulminant, unresponsive respiratory failure, mechanical respiratory support may be necessary. Noninvasive positive-pressure ventilation may suffice. Whether to intubate for mechanical ventilation is a complex and multifactorial decision. Important considerations include progressive respiratory acidosis, worsened hypoxia despite maximal medical therapy, altered mental status, cardiovascular dysfunction, and patient preference.

Key Points

- COPD is a fixed obstructive pulmonary disease and is frequently not steroid responsive.
- Albuterol and ipratropium are the baseline treatment.
- Treat chronic hypoxia with oxygen therapy to avoid cor pulmonale.

CASE 33-3

A 61-year-old man comes to your clinic for the first time complaining of neck and upper back pain. He has smoked 2 packs a day for 40 years and drinks 3 to 6 beers daily. He has been told before that he has "emphysema." He gets short of breath walking up any hills and he admits to a chronic dry smoker's cough. He takes no medicines. BP 150/90, HR 90, R 20, and T 97° F. He is thin with deep creases in his face, nicotine stains on his right hand, and a barrel chest. Breath sounds are distant, his chest is resonant to percussion, and expiratory-to-inspiratory time is 3:1. You hear distant heart sounds only over his epigastric area. His fingers and toes are clubbed.

A. What tests would help you confirm his diagnosis of "emphysema"?
B. How would you determine if he has chronic bronchitis?
C. What is likely to be causing his clubbing?
D. What chest x-ray findings do you expect to see in a patient with emphysema?
E. What other workup does this man need, and how does each test help you?
F. What interventions might help a patient with COPD?

PULMONARY EMBOLISM

ETIOLOGY

What causes pulmonary embolism?

PE is an underrecognized and potentially fatal condition. Most occur when a DVT breaks off from its site of origin and lodges in a pulmonary artery. Risk factors (similar for DVT) include Virchow's triad of hypercoag-

---

BOX 33-1 Risk Factors for Pulmonary Embolus

Age > 60
Oral contraceptive use
Congestive heart disease
Hypercoagulable state
Malignancy
Nephrotic syndrome
Prolonged immobilization
Pregnancy
Recent surgery

---

ulability, immobility, and endothelial injury (Box 33-1). Greater than 10% of those with PE have no identifiable risk factors. Occasionally, embolus is not clot, amniotic fluid, or air, but fat released from a bone fracture.

EVALUATION

How do patients with PE present?

Up to 40% of patients with PE are asymptomatic. If symptoms are present, they are often nonspecific: chest pain (may be pleuritic), dyspnea, cough, hemoptysis, sweating, or syncope. Ask patients with any of these symptoms about risk factors for PE. Findings on examination may include any combination of tachypnea, tachycardia, fever, cyanosis, diaphoresis, an accentuated second heart sound, S_3 or S_4 gallop, right ventricular heave, or a pulmonary friction rub if a PE has infarcted lung tissue at the pleural surface. Massive PE may cause hemodynamic collapse with critically low blood pressure or cardiac arrest. Look for unilateral lower extremity edema as a clue to the original DVT (measure calf diameters if necessary) when you suspect PE.

What initial tests should I order when I suspect PE?

Initially obtain standard tests for dyspnea, including CBC, chemistry panel, ABG, chest x-ray, and ECG. *ABG can be normal with PE (in 13%) but usually shows a significant A-a gradient and respiratory alkalosis (hypoxia causes patients to breathe faster, drops CO_2, and raises pH). Calculate A-a gradient using the following equation:

$$\text{A-a gradient} = P_{A}O_2 - P_{a}O_2$$

where $P_{A}O_2$ = Alveolar oxygen concentration = $F_{I}O_2 (PB - 47) - P_{CO_2}/0.8$
(approximately 100 at sea level with normal P_{CO_2})

$P_{a}O_2$ = Arterial oxygen concentration = blood gas P_{O_2}

$F_{I}O_2$ = Fraction of oxygen in inspired air
(0.21 for sea level)

PB = Atmospheric pressure (760 mm Hg at sea level)

Normal A-a gradient is less than 10 if younger, less than 20 if older. Chest film may be normal, may reveal another condition, such as pneumonia or CHF, or may show a triangular infarct from occlusion of a pulmonary artery. *ECG* may show an alternate diagnosis, such as MI, PE can cause sinus tachycardia, atrial arrhythmia, right heart strain, right axis deviation, right bundle branch block, or an "S1, Q3, and T3" pattern (S wave in lead I, Q wave and flipped T wave in lead III). Consider drawing blood for a hypercoagulability workup.

When should I pursue further testing for PE, and what tests should I order?

Your level of clinical suspicion based on risk factors, history, examination, and initial tests is key in guiding further workup. *Doppler ultrasound* of the lower extremities detects 95% of proximal leg clots and obviates the need for further tests if positive. A *D-dimer* ELISA test is sensitive (>85%) for thromboembolic activity. If D-dimer and Doppler are both negative, PE is highly unlikely and you can forgo further testing in patients with low clinical suspicion for PE. If noninvasive tests cannot clearly rule out DVT, obtain *ventilation/perfusion scan* (V/Q), a nuclear medicine test that looks for perfusion defects resulting from PE that are not matched by lung ventilation defects. V/Q scans are read as normal, nondiagnostic (formerly called *low* and *intermediate probability*) or high probability for embolus. The likelihood of PE based on V/Q scan results depends on clinical suspicion for PE. Data from the Prospective Investigation of Pulmonary Embolus Diagnosis study (PIOPED study) have provided estimates of PE likelihood combining the clinical suspicion and V/Q result (Table 33-6). From this information, you can see that a low probability V/Q scan does not rule out PE when clinical suspicion of PE is intermediate or high (16% and 40%, respectively, will have PE); this situation warrants further testing. *Pulmonary angiogram* makes the diagnosis of PE definitively and is underused. Indications for pulmonary angiogram are listed in Box 33-2. High-resolution CT scan is an emerging option for further evaluation and best detects large proximal pulmonary emboli.

TREATMENT

How do I treat PE?

Stablize the ABCs (see How to Approach the Acutely Ill Patient section in Chapter 6). Give oxygen and blood pressure support. Start heparin if there are no contraindications (Box 33-3), even before definitive diagno-

---

BOX 33-2   Indications for Pulmonary Angiogram

Nondiagnostic V/Q and Doppler with high clinical suspicion for PE
Nondiagnostic V/Q and Doppler with poor cardiopulmonary reserve
High probability V/Q with contraindications for anticoagulation
Hemodynamic instability to be evaluated for use of intraarterial thrombolytics
Failed anticoagulation, considering surgery for PE

BOX 33-3   Contraindications to the Use of Heparin

ABSOLUTE CONTRAINDICATIONS
Active internal bleeding
Intracranial bleeding
Intracranial lesions likely to bleed
Severe heparin-induced thrombocytopenia
Malignant hypertension

RELATIVE CONTRAINDICATIONS
Recent stroke
Recent major surgery
Severe hypertension
Bacterial endocarditis
Thrombocytopenia
Peptic ulcer disease

TABLE 33-6
Likelihood of PE Based on Level of Clinical Suspicion and V/Q Scan Results

CLINICAL SUSPICION (PRETEST PROBABILITY)	NORMAL V/Q	INDETERMINANT V/Q FORMERLY "LOW PROBABILITY"	FORMERLY "INTERMEDIATE PROBABILITY"	HIGH PROBABILITY V/Q
Low	2%	4%	16%	56%
Intermediate	6%	16%	28%	88%
High	0%*	40%	66%	96%

*Number of patients in this category were too small to be conclusive.

sis is made when clinical suspicion is high for PE. Start warfarin once PE is confirmed and all anticipated procedures are completed. Therapy for 6 months is required, assuming a risk factor is identified and modifiable. Warfarin may be continued indefinitely if risk is not modifiable (e.g., cancer, inherited hypercoagulable state).

What other options for treatment exist?

Thrombolytic therapy is used when patients with massive PE are hypotensive. This therapy produces rapid clot lysis and improves hemodynamics more quickly than heparin, but overall mortality for these patients remains high. Inferior venacaval filters can be placed when patients have contraindications to anticoagulation (see Box 33-3) or recurrent PE on appropriate anticoagulation. The filter is a wire barrier that is placed under angiographic guidance into the inferior vena cava. It allows blood flow but stops larger clots from proceeding to the lungs. Surgical embolectomy is controversial and used only when patients have persistent severe hypotension resulting from a massive, life-threatening PE and thrombolytic therapy is contraindicated or ineffective.

Key Points

- PE is frequently missed and life threatening; you can only find it if you think to look.
- Anticoagulate with heparin as you pursue PE workup.
- Use risk factors, history, examination, and noninvasive tests to guide your clinical suspicion for PE.
- Use clinical suspicion and PIOPED data to interpret likelihood of PE from V/Q scan.

CASE 33-4

A 44-year-old woman reports dyspnea and fatigue. She recently returned from Bolivia, where she was volunteering. She also reports pleuritic right chest pain and cough with pink sputum. She denies fevers, chills, nausea, diaphoresis, orthopnea, or prior medical problems. BP is 110/70, HR is 130 and irregular, T is 99° F, and RR is 32. She looks moderately uncomfortable, she speaks full but short sentences, neck shows jugular venous pulsations elevated to 8 cm (normal is 5 cm), lungs are clear, heart sounds reveal an accentuated S_2, and her right leg is swollen.

A. What is your differential for this patient's dyspnea?
B. What studies would you like to order?
C. How will you manage her problem?
D. As you are hanging her heparin, she suddenly becomes very dizzy, diaphoretic, and extremely dyspneic. What is happening? How will you assess and treat her now?

34

Rheumatology

GOUT

ETIOLOGY

What causes gout?

Patients with gout either underexcrete uric acid (most common) or overproduce uric acid. Risk factors for gout include medications, alcohol use, obesity, and hereditary predisposition (extremely common in individuals from Samoa and the Philippines).

What medications cause increases in uric acid?

The most commonly used medications that trigger gout are diuretics. Low-dose aspirin, cyclosporine, and niacin are also important precipitants of gout.

What are common triggers for a gouty attack in patients with a history of gout?

Hospitalization triggers acute gout attacks in up to 85% of those with a prior history of gout. The stress of surgery, medical illness, addition of medications that decrease uric acid excretion, or fluid shifts are contributing factors. Acute gout attacks occasionally can be precipitated or worsened by starting allopurinol. For this reason, allopurinol is not started during an acute attack.

EVALUATION

What is the typical presentation of gout?

The most common first site of involvement is the metatarsophalangeal (MTP) joint of the great toe (>50% of initial gout attacks). The pain is great and is exacerbated by minimal pressure, even of bedsheets, on the joint. Erythema and warmth of the affected joint are typical. The onset of pain is usually sudden and often involves only one joint.

What symptoms and signs are seen with a severe attack of gout?

Fever, multiple joint involvement, tachycardia, and a high WBC mimic infection. These patients are frequently misdiagnosed.

How do I diagnose gout?

The gold standard is to tap the involved joint and look for microscopic urate crystals, which are needle-shaped and strongly birefringent under polarized light. Most patients with gout have a high uric acid level (>7 mg/dl). Occasionally uric acid levels are depressed during an acute attack; repeat the uric acid level in those patients once the attack subsides. In patients with an established diagnosis of gout and recurrent episodes, there is no need to tap the joint again.

TREATMENT

How should I treat an acute attack of gout?

The mainstay for treatment is nonsteroidal antiinflammatory medication, for example, indomethacin 50 mg 3 times a day. Be extremely careful to avoid using NSAIDs in patients with contraindications, such as congestive heart failure, renal insufficiency, history of gastric of peptic ulcer disease, or allergy to aspirin or NSAIDs. The alternatives for treatment of acute gout are prednisone (a 3- to 5-day course) or colchicine. When colchicine, NSAIDs, and systemic steroids are contraindicated, joint injection with steroids is a good option.

Who should receive chronic medication to prevent gouty attack?

Patients who have had more than two attacks of gout are reasonable candidates. After a first attack, 75% of patients will have a second attack within 2 years, so patients with more than two attacks are likely to continue to have problems.

What therapy should be used for preventing attacks?

Allopurinol and probenecid are both effective. Probenecid only works with intact renal function. Do not start either drug during an acute attack because they both can prolong or worsen the attack.

Key Points

- Common medications that trigger gout are diuretics and niacin.
- Do not start allopurinol during an acute attack.
- Treat acute gout with NSAIDs except in patients with renal insufficiency, CHF, or PUD.

CASE 34-1

A 39-year-old man with type I diabetes presents with severe pain in his left MTP joint. On examination, he has erythema over the first MTP joint of the left foot. Laboratory test results are as follows: BUN 39, Cr 3.3, glucose 350, HCT 35, and WBC 4.6. Joint fluid crystals are consistent with urate. Uric acid is 8.8, and Hgb_{alc} is 10.0.

What therapy would you use?

RHEUMATOID ARTHRITIS

ETIOLOGY

What is rheumatoid arthritis?

Rheumatoid arthritis (RA) is a chronic autoimmune disease of unclear cause that causes synovial inflammation with erosion of adjacent cartilage and bone. Worldwide prevalence is 1%, with women developing RA 3 times as frequently as men. It occurs in all age-groups, although it generally increases with age. The course of RA is highly variable, but it usually causes significant morbidity and decreased longevity.

EVALUATION

What are the most common symptoms?

RA is usually a symmetric polyarthritis involving characteristic peripheral joints, especially the metacarpophalangeal (MCP) and MTP joints (Figure 34-1). Lumbosacral and distal interphalangeal joints are hardly ever involved. Movement of inflamed joints produces a deep, gnawing discomfort. The pain is most severe in the morning or after periods of inactivity ("gelling"). Joint deformities such as flexion contractures and subluxation (incomplete dislocations) are common. Constitutional symptoms may precede overt arthritis and include weight loss, low-grade fever, and fatigue. Some 20% of patients develop extraarticular manifestations (Figure 34-2).

What questions should I ask to assess disease severity?

Ask questions to determine which joints are involved and pain severity ("Is the pain so severe it prevents you from sleeping?"). Assess how long morning stiffness takes to resolve ("After you have gotten up, how long does it take until you're feeling as good as you're going to feel?"). Identify an activity that the patient can perform only marginally well (e.g., combing hair, slicing bread, walking more than two blocks). Describe the level of function with this activity in every clinic note. This helps you compare functional level between visits (questions courtesy of Dr. Ronald Anderson, Brigham and Women's Hospital, Boston).

What should I look for on the musculoskeletal examination?

Look for effusions or swollen joints. Check pressure points and extensor tendons (elbows, Achilles tendon) for rheumatoid nodules. Watch for common deformities, including ulnar deviation of fingers, subluxation of MCP joints, swan neck, and boutonniere deformities of the fingers and cock-up deformities of the toes (Figure 34-3). Palpate each joint for effusions, and try to distinguish boggy synovium from soft tissue swelling. If the joint is inflamed (compared with periarticular structures), all aspects of the joint will be tender to palpation. Squeezing the MCPs and MTPs will elicit pain if these joints are inflamed. Also check active and passive range of motion (ROM). With joint involvement (rather than periarticular structure), passive ROM is as limited as active ROM. Detailed measurements of ROM are rarely necessary. Describe ROM as normal; slightly, moderately, or markedly limited; or fused. Asymptomatic flexion contractures (easily noticed in peripheral joints like the elbow) suggest active synovitis.

What might I see on neurologic examination of a patient with RA?

Check for paresthesias of the hands and feet because entrapment neuropathies are common as a result of active synovitis. If the cervical spine is involved, making C1-C2 instability likely, perform a careful neurologic examination at every visit.

How do I diagnose RA?

RA is a clinical diagnosis requiring presence of at least four of seven criteria (Box 34-1).

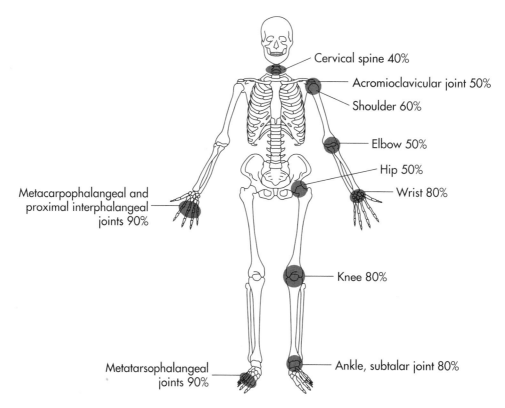

Figure 34-1 Joints commonly involved in RA (pattern of involvement is usually symmetric and involves the MCP, MTP, and PIP joints).

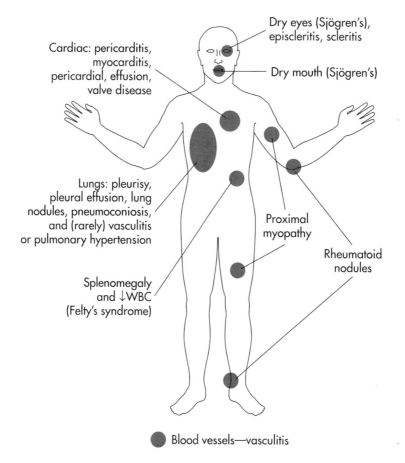

Figure 34-2 Extraarticular manifestations of RA.

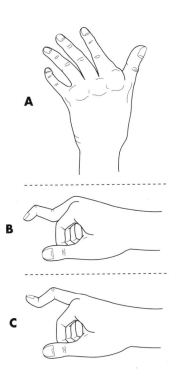

Figure 34-3 Characteristic joint deformities seen in RA. **A,** Ulnar deviation; **B,** swan neck deformities; **C,** boutonniere's deformities.

BOX 34-1   Revised Criteria (1987)
for the Diagnosis of RA

Four criteria are required for diagnosis; criteria numbers 1-4 must be present for 6 weeks or more:

1. Morning stiffness lasting at least 1 hour
2. Arthritis in at least three joints
3. Arthritis of the hand joints
4. Symmetric arthritis
5. Rheumatoid nodules
6. Positive serum rheumatoid factors
7. X-ray changes typical of rheumatoid arthritis

What laboratory tests should I order if I suspect RA?

Order rheumatoid factor (RF), an IgM antibody specific for IgG. Although RF is present in 70% of adults with RA, it is nonspecific (found in many other inflammatory conditions) and suggests RA only if other clinical criteria are present (see Box 34-1). High titers are associated with worse joint disease and extraarticular manifestations (see Figure 34-2). Once it is positive, you never need to check it again because it does not correlate with disease activity or response to treatment. Other helpful laboratory tests to monitor include hematocrit (anemia of chronic disease is common in active RA) and ESR, which is typically elevated and roughly correlates with disease activity (although a normal ESR does not rule out RA).

What will I see on a joint aspiration with RA?

Joint aspirations in RA show 5000 to 25,000 PMNs. Tap a joint if you are uncertain of the diagnosis of RA (looking for evidence of another disease process, such as gout) or if you think the joint might be infected. Have a low threshold for tapping joints that are persistently or excessively inflamed because patients with RA are at risk for joint infections.

Are x-rays helpful in diagnosis of RA?

Do not order x-rays early in the disease. Small erosions at the joint margins and joint space narrowing take months to years to develop.

TREATMENT

How is RA treated?

There is no cure for RA, but early medical therapy alleviates pain and delays joint deformities. There are two main categories of medications: NSAIDs and disease-modifying antirheumatic drugs (DMARDs). NSAIDs relieve symptoms but do not delay joint destruction. The focus is on early treatment with DMARDs to halt inflammation and delay joint destruction. No DMARD is universally effective. They frequently are discontinued because of side effects. Therefore they are tried in a stepwise manner, from least to most toxic, until inflammation is suppressed. Hydroxychloroquine is the first DMARD tried. If it is not effective, then methotrexate is the next choice and can be used in combination with hydroxychloroquine for severe disease. Gold, sulfasalazine, and azathioprine are other possibilities. It takes weeks to months for DMARD therapy to achieve full effect, and even then, pain relief is rarely complete. Therefore many patients also take NSAIDs. Steroids are used only during painful flares because they have a questionable disease-modifying effect and significant side effects with long-term use.

Is surgical therapy effective?

Advances in orthopedic surgery have had a profound effect on the quality of life of patients with RA. Early in the disease, most symptoms are caused by active synovitis, but joint destruction begins after 1 to 2 years. Eradicating active synovitis will then only partially improve symptoms (see Figure 34-3). Because the vast majority of patients develop at least some degree of structural damage, orthopedic surgery is usually required to maximize functional ability in long-standing disease. Total joint replacement (hips and knees) has revolutionized the treatment of RA.

Key Points

- RA causes symmetric arthritis of peripheral joints, especially MCP and MTP joints.
- Pain and stiffness are most severe in the morning or after periods of inactivity.
- Extraarticular manifestations occur in 20% of patients (usually with high RF).
- Early treatment with a DMARD is essential to prevent destructive changes.
- Surgical therapy (such as joint replacement) is effective in advanced disease.

CASE 34-2

A 35-year-old woman reports gradual onset over the past 2 months of fatigue, pain involving the MCP joint, proximal interphalangeal (PIP) joint, and wrist joints, and morning stiffness lasting 1 hour. On examination, MCPs, PIPs, and wrists are swollen bilaterally. The joints are tender and slightly warm.

    A. What is your differential diagnosis?
    B. What laboratory tests would you order?
    C. What do you recommend for treatment?

CASE 34-3

A 45-year-old woman is taking 7.5 mg of prednisone a day for seropositive RA with multiple joint deformities. She reports that she cannot raise her left foot. On examination, she is slightly cushingoid. There is 2+ swelling of the MCPs, PIPs, wrist, and ankles, and ulnar deviation and boutonniere and swan neck deformities. Flexion and extension of the wrist are markedly reduced. Her toes are cocked up. She cannot dorsiflex her left foot.

    A. What is the differential diagnosis of her left footdrop?
    B. What tests would you obtain?
    C. What do you recommend for treatment?

SYSTEMIC LUPUS ERYTHEMATOSUS

ETIOLOGY

What is lupus?

Lupus is a chronic immune disorder that involves many organ systems, with a wide variety of symptoms. The severity ranges from nearly asymptomatic to life-threatening. Many patients have mild disease with a variety of skin lesions, alopecia, or arthritis, but some patients have serious complications, such as renal failure, organic psychosis, or vasculitis. Survival rate in SLE is approximately 90% over the first 10 years. Involvement of the kidneys or CNS is an unfavorable prognostic sign. Major causes of death are renal failure, infection (often resulting from the use of immunosuppressive drugs), and coronary artery disease.

Who gets lupus?

Lupus is most common among women of childbearing age, with a 9:1 female-to-male ratio. Black women are affected 3 times more commonly than white women. It usually develops between ages 13 and 40 but can occur at any age. Genetic factors are important because lupus is more common in relatives of affected patients.

What causes lupus?

Lupus is an autoimmune disease. For unidentified reasons, autoantibodies (Table 34-1) cause tissue injury when they are directed at a specific cell type (such as red blood cells) or if they form antigen-antibody (immune) complexes. Circulating immune complexes are deposited in blood vessels, initiating a cascade of complement-mediated injury. Certain drugs can cause a reversible drug-induced lupus (see below).

TABLE 34-1

Frequency of Important Autoantibodies in Systemic Lupus Erythematosus

ANTIBODY	FREQUENCY	COMMENTS
Anti–double-stranded DNA	70%	If positive, it is likely patient has lupus (high specificity) Often increases with flares (doubling or increase of 30 in less than 10 weeks suggests disease flare)
Anti-Smith antibody	30%	Nearly pathognomonic for SLE when present
Anti-RNP antibody	40%	Can be present in other rheumatologic conditions
Anti-Rho antibody (SS-A)	30%	Children of mothers with anti-Ro are at risk of neonatal lupus and congenital heart block
Anti-La antibody (SS-B)	10%	Can be present in other rheumatologic conditions
Anti-histone antibody	70%	Positive in 95% of patients with drug-induced SLE, 20% of patients with idiopathic SLE

Does pregnancy exacerbate lupus?

Active disease at conception is likely to worsen during pregnancy, but patients in remission usually complete pregnancy without a clinical exacerbation. Nearly half of all lupus patients deliver prematurely, often by emergency cesarean section. Patients with a positive anti-Ro antibody are at risk of delivering a child with neonatal lupus or congenital heart block. Phospholipid antibody syndrome may occur in association with lupus and can cause fetal loss.

EVALUATION

What are the most common manifestations of lupus?

The most common presenting symptom is arthritis in a similar distribution as RA and with similar morning stiffness. Other common manifestations are fatigue, skin rashes (some photosensitive), renal insufficiency, and hematologic cytopenias. Less common but interesting manifestations of disease include pericarditis, pleuritis, oral ulcers, and psychiatric disturbances.

What questions should I ask if I think a patient may have lupus?

If the patient answers "yes" to three or more of the following questions, further testing with an ANA is warranted:

1. Have you ever had arthritis or rheumatism for more than 3 months?
2. Do your fingers become pale, numb, or uncomfortable in the cold?
3. Have you had any sores in your mouth for more than 2 weeks?
4. Have you been told that your have low blood counts (anemia, low WBCs, or low platelets)?
5. Have you ever had a prominent rash on your cheeks for more than 1 month?
6. Does your skin break out after you have been in the sun (not sunburn)?
7. Has it ever been painful to take a deep breath for more than a few days (pleurisy)?
8. Have you ever been told that you have protein in your urine?
9. Have you ever had rapid loss of a lot of hair?
10. Have you ever had a seizure, convulsion, or fit?

What are features of drug-induced lupus?

Renal and CNS manifestations are extremely rare in drug-induced lupus, but arthralgias, pleuritis, and pericarditis are common. Common offending drugs include hydralazine, procainamide, and isoniazid. The syndrome typically resolves with discontinuation of the drug. Nearly all patients with drug-induced lupus have a positive anti-histone antibody, but the anti–double-stranded DNA, found in 70% of patients with idiopathic lupus, is almost always absent.

How do I diagnosis lupus?

No one clinical abnormality or laboratory test establishes the diagnosis of lupus. In 1982, the American College of Rheumatism developed a classification system of 11 criteria (Table 34-2). Lupus is diagnosed when patients meet at least 4 of these 11 criteria, either serially or at the same time. The ANA is positive in nearly all patients with lupus and is the best screening test, although it can also be positive with many other chronic inflammatory conditions.

TABLE 34-2
Diagnosing Lupus (1982 American Rheumatism Association Criteria)*

SYMPTOM, SIGN, OR LABORATORY ABNORMALITY	FREQUENCY
Serositis—pleuritis, pericarditis	56%
Oral or nasopharyngeal ulcers—painless	27%
Arthritis—nonerosive, two or more peripheral joints	86%
Photosensitivity—erythematous skin rash, raised or flat	43%
Blood dyscrasias:	
Hemolytic anemia (with reticulocytosis)	30%
Leukopenia (WBC < 4000) on 2 or more occasions	40%
Lymphopenia (<1500) on 2 or more occasions	
Thrombocytopenia (<100,000) in the absence of offending drugs	30%
Renal—proteinuria, casts	50%
Antinuclear antibody—in absence of drugs known to cause lupus	>95%
Immunologic disorders:	
Anti–double-stranded DNA	70%
Anti-Smith: antibody to Smith nuclear antigen	30%
False-positive VDRL × 6 months, negative FTA-ABS	
Neurologic disorder—seizures, psychosis	50%
Malar rash—flat or raised erythema, spares nasolabial folds	
Discoid rash—raised erythematous, scaling, follicular plugging, atrophic scarring	

*Four of eleven criteria required in research setting to have diagnosis of SLE.

What complications can occur?

Infection can be difficult to distinguish from a lupus flare. ESR, double-stranded DNA, and complement may be less abnormal with infection than with flare. Osteonecrosis, osteoporosis, and premature coronary artery disease all occur because of long-term steroid use. Congenital heart block and neonatal lupus can occur when maternal anti-Ro antibodies are present.

TREATMENT

There is no cure for lupus. The goal of treatment is to relieve symptoms, suppress inflammation, and prevent future pathology (Table 34-3). The risk-benefit ratio of potentially toxic drugs must be tailored to each individual. General measures involve rest and avoidance of stressful emotional experiences, sunlight, and drugs that can trigger lupus flares, such as oral contraceptive pills. Patients with lupus should always wear sunscreen when they are exposed to sunlight.

CASE 34-4

A 30-year-old African-American woman reports 6 months of fatigue and painful swollen wrists, fingers, knees, and ankles, which are worst for the first 30 minutes after she gets out of bed. In the past she has had intermittent episodes of rash after sun exposure, sharp chest pain, painless sores on the roof of her mouth, and a spontaneous abortion. Examination reveals normal vitals signs, an erythematous rash over her cheeks and nose that spares the nasolabial folds. Joint examination reveals tender but mild spongy swelling of the wrists, MCP joints, and ankles bilaterally.

A. What is the most likely diagnosis, and what are some other possible diagnoses?
B. Which of the 11 criteria of lupus does this patient meet?
C. Which laboratory tests should you send next, and how will they affect your management of this patient?
D. What initial therapy would you recommend for this patient?

VASCULITIS

ETIOLOGY

What causes vasculitis?

Vasculitis is inflammation and necrosis of blood vessels, usually resulting from immune complex deposition. It can occur as a primary process or in association with various systemic diseases. Size or charge of the immune complexes may be important in determining which vessels and organ systems are involved. Additionally, antibodies may be directed against epitopes on vascular endothelium in certain forms of vasculitis. The types of cells involved (i.e., lymphocytes, neutrophils, eosinophils) also help determine the pattern of vascular in-

---

Key Points

- SLE is diagnosed clinically by satisfying at least 4 of 11 diagnostic criteria.
- The ANA is nearly always positive with lupus (>95% sensitivity), but some patients with a positive ANA do not have lupus (not very specific); only 70% of SLE patients have anti–double-stranded DNA, but when it is present, the patient usually has lupus (high specificity).
- Double-stranded DNA levels predict flares when they are elevated, but ANAs do not.

TABLE 34-3

Drugs Commonly Used to Treat Systemic Lupus Erythematosus

DRUG	USE
NSAIDs	Mild arthritis or serositis
Steroids	
High dose	Potentially life-threatening severe neuropsychiatric conditions, pulmonary hemorrhage, rapidly progressing renal failure
Low dose	Hemolytic anemia, thrombocytopenia, NSAID-resistant arthritis, mild glomerulonephritis
Hydroxychloroquine	Mild disease, dermatitis, arthritis; steroid-sparing
Cyclophosphamide*	Severe organ involvement, glomerulonephritis, CNS disease
Azathioprine†	Potentially life-threatening disease, severe vasculitis, nephritis

*Cyclophosphamide can cause GI and bone marrow toxicity. Intravenous treatment can cause nausea and vomiting. Reversible alopecia occurs in 50% of patients. Infertility can also result.

†Azathioprine is less effective but safer than cyclophosphamide and takes up to 3 months for the full effect. It can cause GI or bone marrow toxicity. Long-term use may result in a slightly higher rate of certain malignancies.

flammation. Some systemic diseases are associated with vasculitis (Box 34-2).

How are the various forms of vasculitis classified?

Classification is currently based on size of the vessels involved (i.e., large, medium, and small) with 3 major syndromes in each category (see Box 34-2).

What illnesses can mimic vasculitis?

Atrial myxoma can present with fever, weight loss, stroke-like symptoms, purpuric rash, Raynaud's phenomenon, and a high ESR. Cholesterol emboli may cause livedo reticularis (a diffuse, lacy, violaceous skin discoloration) and nonpalpable purpura, along with an elevated ESR, renal insufficiency, active urinary sediment, and eosinophilia. Bacteremia with *Neisseria gonorrhoeae, N. meningitidis,* or rickettsia can cause a cutaneous vasculitis.

EVALUATION

When should I consider vasculitis in the differential diagnosis?

Involvement of several organ systems at the same time, such as the kidneys, skin, and nerves, is a classic feature of many forms of vasculitis. Systemic symptoms, such as fever, anorexia, and weight loss, are common. Diagnosis usually hinges on a biopsy showing vessel inflammation.

How does large-vessel vasculitis present?

Giant cell arteritis (temporal arteritis) is seen in people over age 55, especially in those of Northern Euro-

---

| **BOX 34-2** | Examples of Vasculitis Categorized by Size of Vessel Typically Affected |

LARGE VESSEL
Giant cell/temporal arteritis
Takayasu's arteritis
Systemic disease: RA, ankylosing spondylitis, Reiter's syndrome, syphilis

MEDIUM VESSEL
Polyarteritis nodosa
Churg-Strauss vasculitis
Connective tissue disease–associated: RA, lupus

SMALL VESSEL
Hypersensitivity: drugs, hepatitis C, HSP, SBE
Wegener's granulomatosis
Microscopic polyarteritis nodosa

RA, Rheumatoid arthritis; *HSP,* Henoch-Schönlein purpura; *SBE,* subacute bacterial endocarditis.

---

pean extraction. Symptoms include headache, jaw claudication (pain in the jaw muscles with chewing), transient or permanent loss of vision, tenderness over the temporal scalp, fever, and weight loss. Polymyalgia rheumatica occurs in 50% of patients with temporal arteritis and is characterized by proximal muscle weakness and pain. ESR is usually greater than 100. Diagnosis is suggested by clinical picture and confirmed by temporal artery biopsy. Takayasu's arteritis is most often reported in young women (especially Asian) and is one of the major causes of renovascular hypertension in Asian young adults. Inflammation and stenosis occurs in the aorta and vessels arising from the aortic arch. Renal and CNS arteries can also be affected. ESR is high. Diagnosis is by arteriogram. Large artery involvement, especially of the proximal aorta, can be seen in miscellaneous systemic diseases, such as ankylosing spondylitis; Reiter's disease; syphilis; relapsing polychondritis (a rare but fascinating disease); and, rarely, rheumatoid arthritis.

How does medium-vessel vasculitis present?

Polyarteritis nodosa (PAN) affects small and medium-sized muscular arteries. Target organs include the CNS, peripheral nerves, bowel, and kidneys. Joint and skin manifestations may also occur, and an isolated cutaneous form exists. PAN may be associated with chronic hepatitis B, hairy cell leukemia, HIV infection, or amphetamine abuse. ESR is often high, and an active urinary sediment is frequently present. Diagnosis is based on arteriographic demonstration of vasculitis, with or without aneurysms, especially in renal arteries. Biopsy of nerve, muscle, or testicular tissue is often useful. Churg-Strauss vasculitis affects similar vessels as PAN with less renal and much more pulmonary involvement. Distinctive features include a history of asthma in almost all patients, formation of granulomas, and eosinophilic infiltrates in the lungs and vessels. Diagnosis is similar to PAN. Connective tissue diseases, such as rheumatoid arthritis or lupus, may have an associated PAN-like vasculitis.

How does small-vessel vasculitis present?

Wegener's granulomatosis classically involves a triad of upper respiratory tract, lung, and kidneys but may present in a more limited fashion. Skin, eyes, and joints may also be involved. Antineutrophil cytoplasmic antibody is usually positive, with a cytoplasmic pattern of staining, called c-ANCA. This serology has not replaced the need for open lung biopsy to confirm diagnosis. Wegener's can be a culprit causing chronic sinusitis or a saddle-nose deformity. Microscopic polyarteritis nodosa (MPAN) is a small-vessel version of PAN with similar organ involvement. Both c-ANCA and p-ANCA (perinuclear antineutrophil cytoplasmic antibody) patterns are seen in these patients. Hypersensitivity vasculitis is a group of different diseases that typically cause a leuko-cytoclastic vasculitis of the skin, characterized by neu-trophilic infiltrate with neutrophil fragmentation in and around the small capillaries and venules. Skin is most often involved, showing petechiae or purpura, especially on the lower extremities. Kidneys and bowel can also be involved, depending on the cause. Causes include drugs (penicillin, sulfa) and other causes of serum sickness, subacute bacterial endocarditis (SBE), Henoch-Schönlein purpura (HSP), mixed essential cryoglobu-linemia (now known to be caused primarily by hepatitis C), and other connective tissue diseases.

What other vasculitis syndromes should I be aware of?

Primary CNS vasculitis is a small- and medium-vessel vasculitis limited to the CNS that can cause stroke in young adults. It is seen in patients who abuse amphet-amines, after recent herpes infection involving the eye, or in patients with Hodgkin's lymphoma. *Thromboangiitis obliterans* (Buerger's disease) occurs most often in men who smoke and may represent a hypersensitivity to nicotine. It is characterized by panarteritis or pan-phlebitis with thrombosis and typically involves medium and small vessels of the lower extremities. Symptoms may include claudication (painful leg muscles with walking), Raynaud's-like phenomena, and su-perficial thrombophlebitis.

TREATMENT

Treat giant cell arteritis with high-dose steroids to prevent blindness that can occur suddenly. Steroids are also used for Takayasu's arteritis, with surgery if necessary to bypass stenotic vessels. Treat PAN, MPAN, and primary CNS vasculitis with steroids or, if resistant, cyclophosphamide. Cyclophosphamide is the drug of choice for Wegener's; methotrexate may be useful also. Some patients with mild, limited disease may also respond to trimethoprim/sulfamethoxazole. For Buerger's disease, counsel patients to stop smoking; surgery and immunosuppressive therapy may be of benefit to some of these patients.

Key Points

- Headache or fever of unknown origin in the elderly could be from giant cell arteritis.
- Polymyalgia rheumatica is an important cause of shoulder or neck pain and stiffness in elderly patients; about 10% to 20% of these patients develop giant cell arteritis.
- Acute onset of footdrop or wrist-drop could be polyarteritis nodosum.
- Petechiae or purpura associated with vasculitis are raised and palpable; in contrast, noninflammatory disorders, such as platelet abnormalities, cause non-palpable purpura.
- Think about primary CNS vasculitis in a young person with a stroke.
- Hepatitis B and C can be associated with vasculitis.

CASE 34-5

A 63-year-old Caucasian woman with a history of hypothyroidism and hypertension reports feeling unwell for 1 month. She has lost 5 pounds and has had frequent low-grade fevers, as well as stiffness in the shoulders and low back when she awakes in the morning. She has a past history of migraine headaches, but over the last month she has had a more persistent right-sided headache. She attributes her weight loss to the fact that her jaw gets tired as she eats. She takes estrogen, proges-terone, thyroxine, and acetaminophen with codeine. Exam reveals BP 140/85 in both arms, weight 154 pounds, temperature 38° C, mild ten-derness of the right temporal scalp, and mildly reduced range of motion in both shoulders.

  A. *What is the most likely diagnosis?*
  B. *What are the appropriate diagnostic tests?*
  C. *What would you recommend for treatment?*

chapter

35

Substance Abuse

ALCOHOL

ETIOLOGY

How common are alcohol-related problems?

Up to half of all men have temporary alcohol-related problems. Between 10% and 20% of men and 5% to 10% of women have persistent alcohol-related problems, defined as alcohol use causing legal, marital, physical, or interpersonal problems.

Why do patients with alcoholism develop alcoholic ketoacidosis?

Alcoholic ketoacidosis occurs in the patient who habitually drinks heavily but has stopped drinking 1 to 2 days before presenting for medical care. The patient usually has not had anything to eat or drink over the preceding 12 to 24 hours because of nausea and abdominal pain. Blood gas shows a moderate acidosis, chemistry shows a low HCO_3, and serum ketones are elevated with predominance of β-hydroxybutyrate. During the starvation state, counterregulatory hormones produce a marked increase in serum free fatty acids. Alcohol suppresses ketogenesis initially, but as the alcohol level falls, rapid conversion of fatty acids to ketones occurs.

Why do patients who use alcohol have electrolyte problems?

Chronic use of alcohol causes renal magnesium wasting from tubular cells. Magnesium is important in maintaining a normal potassium level; low magnesium levels lead to potassium loss and hypokalemia. Adequate magnesium levels are also important in normal parathyroid hormone production and release. With hy-

pomagnesemia, inadequate parathyroid hormone levels lead to low 1,25-dihydroxyvitamin D, calcium, and phosphate levels. Poor nutrition decreases phosphate intake, and phosphate loss in the urine occurs in the setting of hypomagnesemia.

EVALUATION

How can I recognize and diagnose alcohol-related problems?

Suspect alcohol abuse when you see patients with trauma, motor vehicle accidents, or unexplained abdominal pain. Also, consider alcohol use in patients with hypertension. Ask all patients if they consume alcohol. If the answer is no, ask if they have had problems with alcohol in the past. Patients who are currently using alcohol can be screened with CAGE questions (Box 35-1). CAGE questions have a sensitivity of 80% and a specificity of 85% if a cutoff of two or more positive responses is used; they are less sensitive in women and ethnic minorities.

What cardiovascular abnormalities are seen with alcohol abuse?

There is a firm link between chronic alcohol consumption and hypertension. This is seen in people who drink three or more drinks a day and is a common cause of secondary hypertension. "Holiday heart" is a syndrome of paroxysmal arrhythmias, the most common of which is atrial fibrillation, described in alcohol binge drinkers. Other arrhythmias include atrial flutter, paroxysmal atrial tachycardia, and ventricular tachycardia. Alcohol is an important cause in up to 50% of congestive cardiomyopathies. There is some reversibility with cessation of alcohol use.

What are the acute and chronic effects of alcohol on the liver?

Alcoholic hepatitis from an acute alcohol binge presents variably from asymptomatic LFT abnormalities to a florid, acute, life-threatening liver failure. Usually, it is insidious with anorexia, nausea, vomiting, abdominal pain, and low-grade fever. Physical examination usually reveals an enlarged, tender liver. Evidence of portal hypertension (severe hemorrhoids, ascites, GI bleeding from esophageal varices) and hepatic encephalopathy may be present in severe cases. Liver enzymes are mildly or moderately elevated, AST more so than ALT (Table 35-1). Cirrhosis develops in 10% to 20% of chronic alcoholic patients. It develops at a lower daily alcohol intake in women because women have 50% less alcohol dehydrogenase in their stomachs, resulting in decreased immediate metabolism of alcohol. In many patients, cirrhosis is unrecognized until a life-threatening complication occurs, such as esophageal variceal bleeding. Check liver synthetic function with pro-time and albumin.

What are the different CNS complications seen with alcohol use?

Acute intoxication can cause ataxia, incoordination, and drowsiness. Large amounts of alcohol, especially in individuals without chronic use, can cause coma. Wernicke-Korsakoff syndrome is a nutritional neurologic disorder caused by thiamine deficiency. It commonly goes unrecognized. The clinical manifestations of Wernicke's encephalopathy are acute onset of oculomotor abnormalities (bilateral abducens palsy, nystagmus, total ophthalmoplegia), ataxia, and global confusional state. Other symptoms that can occur include hypothermia, hypotension, and coma. All of these symptoms may reverse with administration of thiamine. Approximately 80% of patients with Wernicke's encephalopathy who survive will develop Korsakoff's psychosis, which is char-

---

BOX 35-1   CAGE Questions Used to Screen for Alcohol Abuse

Have you ever felt you should Cut down on your drinking?

Have people Annoyed you by criticizing your drinking?

Have you ever felt Guilty about your drinking?"

Have you ever started the day by having a drink as an Eye opener to get going or calm your nerves?

TABLE 35-1
Laboratory Abnormalities Seen With Heavy Regular Alcohol Use

LABORATORY ABNORMALITY	CAUSE
HEMATOLOGY	
Anemia:	
Microcytic	Iron deficiency resulting from GI blood loss
Macrocytic with mildly increased MCV	Liver disease/direct effect on stem cells
Macrocytic with markedly increased MCV	Folate deficiency
Thrombocytopenia	Decreased platelet survival and/or hypersplenism resulting from cirrhosis
Leukopenia	Decreased marrow production of WBC
ABDOMINAL	
Increased SGOT (AST) > increased SGPT (ALT) (SGOT rarely ever > 300)	Alcoholic hepatitis
Increased GGT	"Alcohol use test," very sensitive to alcohol use
Decreased albumin	Alcoholic hepatitis or cirrhosis
Increased PT	Decreased clotting factor production
Increased amylase	Pancreatitis
MINERALS/ELECTROLYTES	
Decreased magnesium	Renal tubular magnesium wasting
Decreased potassium	Renal potassium loss worsened by magnesium deficiency
Decreased calcium	Hypomagnesemia decreases parathyroid hormone release, causing poor GI calcium absorption
Decreased phosphate	Poor nutrition, increased urinary loss

acterized by retrograde and anterograde amnesia. Confabulation, the fabrication of stories, may be present. A significant proportion of patients with Korsakoff's psychosis do not recover and require long-term institutionalization. Chronic alcohol use can cause peripheral neuropathy, which involves the feet first and then the hands in a "stocking and glove" distribution.

What are the symptoms of alcohol withdrawal?

Most patients with chronic alcohol use have mild withdrawal symptoms of tremor, sleep disturbance, and increased anxiety. In addition, tachycardia and increased temperature can occur. A small number (<5%) can have severe withdrawal with marked confusion and hallucinations (delirium tremens). Alcohol withdrawal seizures occur in a small percentage of patients, usually in the first 2 days after cessation of alcohol. A prior history of withdrawal seizures increases the risk of recurrence with subsequent episodes of withdrawal.

TREATMENT

How is alcohol withdrawal treated?

For mild withdrawal symptoms of tachycardia and jitteriness, a β-blocker can be helpful. Benzodiazepines are the mainstay of treatment of alcohol withdrawal. Longer-acting benzodiazepines, such as diazepam, are effective but are more likely to cause prolonged sedation because of drug accumulation. Lorazepam has an intermediate half-life and less impairment in elimination in the elderly and in patients with renal insufficiency.

What other treatments should be given to hospitalized alcoholic patients?

Most patients will have magnesium deficiency and should receive IV magnesium. All should receive thiamine 100 mg IV daily for 3 doses, as well as a daily multiple vitamin with folate. Refer to social work.

When should I hospitalize a patient with complications of alcohol use?

Hospitalize patients with the following:

- Alcohol withdrawal with mental status changes or unstable vital signs
- Metabolic disturbances that are severe (hypokalemia, alcoholic ketoacidosis)
- Severe alcoholic hepatitis with recurrent emesis or signs of portal hypertension or encephalopathy
- Patients desiring inpatient alcohol treatment to facilitate transfer to an alcohol treatment program

Key Points

- Multiple mineral/electrolyte disorders occur with chronic alcohol use; hypomagnesemia is probably the most important and leads to hypokalemia and hypocalcemia.
- Alcoholic hepatitis can mimic acute cholecystitis with fever, leukocytosis, and right upper quadrant pain.
- Transaminases are usually only modestly elevated, with SGOT greater than SGPT, in alcoholic hepatitis.
- Alcohol use is an extremely common cause of secondary hypertension in the United States.

CASE 35-1

A 39-year-old man with a history of alcohol abuse presents with nausea, vomiting, and abdominal pain. He has had low-grade fevers as well and has been drinking 18 to 24 beers a day.
  A. What is your differential diagnosis for his abdominal pain?
  B. What laboratory tests would you order?
  C. His potassium is 2.9. What other electrolytes would you expect to be abnormal?

CASE 35-2

A 49-year-old man with a 20-year history of alcohol abuse is admitted with confusion and weakness. His last drink was 24 hours ago. He usually drinks 3 to 4 bottles of wine daily. On examination, he is tremulous with P of 128 and BP of 160/100. He is oriented only to person. Laboratory test results are as follows: Na 136, K 3.0, HCO₃ 13, BUN 20, Cr 1.0, Glu 60, Cl 98, and serum osmolality 280.
  A. What is the most likely cause for his metabolic acidosis? How would you treat it?
  B. What is appropriate therapy for his alcohol withdrawal?

COCAINE

ETIOLOGY

How and why do people use cocaine?

Cocaine is derived from the leaves of the coca plant and has been chewed as a stimulant for thousands of years. The user gains a euphoric sense of boundless energy and self-confidence. Users can be hypersexual, angry, or violent. The drug is metabolized quickly, and the high is followed by a "crash," during which the user feels depressed and irritable. Drug craving sets in during this period.

Powdered cocaine can be used intranasally (snorted), which gives a less intense high and is most expensive. Dissolved in water, cocaine can be injected intravenously, which gives an immediate and intense high. When no vein is available, cocaine can be injected subcutaneously ("skin-popping") or intramuscularly ("muscling"). "Crack" is a cheap, smokable form of cocaine that gives a very brief but intense high. Its introduction in the 1980s was associated with a surge in drug-related crime, violence, and social problems across the country.

EVALUATION

How do I know cocaine is causing a patient's problem?

Ask every patient about drug and alcohol use. People who do not offer information about their drug use at first will sometimes admit it if you tell them how important it is to treat their immediate problem. Urine drug screens detect cocaine for at least 48 hours after use.

What are the medical complications of cocaine?

Cocaine causes centrally mediated sympathetic overdrive, with tachycardia, hypertension, and vasospasm of coronary and cerebral arteries. Seizures, hypertensive encephalopathy, and ischemic and hemorrhagic strokes are common neurologic sequelae. Chest pain, MI, and dysrhythmias, such as supraventricular tachycardia, ventricular tachycardia, and ventricular fibrillation, are the most common cardiac complications. Rhabdomyolysis, acidosis, fever, and coma are additional results that can be rapidly fatal. Less serious are nonhealing scabs and shallow skin ulcers that result from uncontrollable picking and the sensation of bugs on the skin (formication) that occurs even in noninjection users, and epistaxis and septal necrosis in intranasal users.

If cocaine is a stimulant, why do users present with decreased consciousness?

At very high doses, cocaine's anesthetic effect predominates over its stimulant effect and causes life-threatening coma.

TREATMENT

How do I treat cocaine–related medical problems?

Intravenous diazepam is the primary treatment for most types of cocaine toxicity. By decreasing centrally mediated sympathetic overdrive, diazepam reduces agitation, seizures, hypertension, tachycardia, and vasospasm-mediated chest pain. Even ventricular tachycardia and ventricular fibrillation, if cocaine-induced, should be treated with diazepam in addition to the usual defibrillation. If diazepam alone does not control blood pressure, labetalol or nitroprusside are good choices. Pure β-blocker drugs, such as esmolol and metoprolol, cause unopposed α-adrenergic stimulation and may worsen the situation. A patient with chest pain that resolves with diazepam and shows no ischemic ECG changes can be safely discharged, but ischemic changes on ECG and/or elevated cardiac enzymes require admission and standard therapy for acute MI. Rhabdomyolysis, confirmed by a high serum CPK and positive urine myoglobin, is frequently fatal and requires IV diazepam, IV bicarbonate, and aggressive hydration.

HEROIN

ETIOLOGY

How and why are opioid drugs abused?

Opioids are naturally derived or synthetic drugs that mimic the effects of opium, producing pain relief, relaxation, sleep, and a powerful sense of well-being. These are also called *narcotics*. Oral narcotics, extensively used for medical pain relief, can be abused. A much more potent "high" comes from IV use. Heroin is the most commonly injected narcotic, but morphine, meperidine, and fentanyl are also available. Heroin may also be smoked or snorted. A "speedball" refers to injecting heroin and cocaine together.

EVALUATION

What are the toxic effects of heroin?

A heroin overdose occurs when the user takes enough heroin to suppress the respiratory drive. He is found unconscious and apneic with pinpoint pupils. Prolonged apnea leads to hypoxic brain injury and may be complicated by aspiration, hypothermia, and/or rhabdomyolysis from prolonged immobility. With frequent use, tolerance develops to the respiratory depressant effect of opioids. A common situation for heroin overdose is a user who has been abstinent for a period of time, then uses the same amount to which he was previously accustomed. Noncardiogenic pulmonary edema can occur after IV narcotic use in both new and experienced users. Its etiology is unknown.

How can I identify heroin overdose?

Most overdose patients are treated by prehospital personnel with naloxone, an opioid antagonist, and are therefore alert when they reach the hospital. Naloxone can be safely used on any unconscious patient as a diagnostic maneuver; a response proves opioid intoxication.

How can I identify heroin withdrawal?

Narcotic withdrawal begins as soon as a chronic user misses an expected dose. The longest-acting opioids, such as methadone, produce the longest-lasting withdrawal syndrome. Along with dysphoria and drug craving, physical symptoms include some or all of the following: nausea, vomiting, diarrhea, abdominal cramping and pain, lacrimation, rhinorrhea, yawning, chills, diaphoresis, myalgias, piloerection (goose flesh, thus "quitting cold turkey"), and involuntary muscle jerks ("kicking the habit"). Fever is not part of narcotic withdrawal, and any heroin user with a fever needs an aggressive search for an infection.

TREATMENT

When should I treat heroin overdose?

A patient who has hypoxia resulting from slow or ineffective respirations needs naloxone (IV or IM). If the patient does not immediately recover normal mental status, consider intubation to protect the airway and provide adequate air exchange. It is essential to consider other causes of depressed mental status in this case. Patients successfully treated with naloxone may become sleepy as the drug wears off, but if they are successfully oxygenating 1 hour after naloxone was given, are fully arousable, and have no infectious complications of their IV drug use, they may be safely discharged. Overdose of long-acting narcotics, usually methadone, requires frequent redosing of naloxone, and therefore the patient should be admitted.

How can I treat heroin withdrawal in a hospitalized patient?

The symptoms of heroin withdrawal are alleviated by substituting with a longer-acting narcotic, such as methadone. Withdrawal from methadone also occurs, but a hospitalization can be a transition to a structured detoxification program or a long-term methadone maintenance program. Although heroin withdrawal is intensely uncomfortable, unlike alcohol or benzodiazepine withdrawal, the syndrome is not physically dangerous. Clonidine is an alternative to methadone that lessens narcotic withdrawal symptoms.

INFECTIOUS COMPLICATIONS OF PARENTERAL DRUG ABUSE

ETIOLOGY

What types of infections affect IV drug users?

Shared needles transmit viral infections from user to user, including hepatitis B, hepatitis C (present in about 80% of IV drug users), and HIV. Nonsterile injection also causes local bacterial infections, including open ulcers from "skin popping"; deeper skin abscesses and cellulitis from intravenous use; and large, deep intramuscular abscesses from "muscling." Injected cocaine causes local vasoconstriction and thus tissue necrosis, so cocaine-related abscesses are generally larger and more difficult to heal. Bacterial cultures reveal *Staphylococcus, Streptococcus, Pseudomonas,* and oral flora, including anaerobes (in users who lick their needles). Tetanus may be present. Every injection can cause a transient bacteremia, with the potential for developing endocarditis, meningitis, septic pulmonary emboli, and lumbar osteomyelitis or epidural abscess. A depressed gag reflex during heroin use makes aspiration pneumonia common. Socioeconomic factors and poor immune function increase the risk of TB.

EVALUATION

How do bacterial infections differ in drug users?

Because of impaired immunity, elevated WBC and fever are often absent in drug users with a serious infection. Cellulitis, abscesses, and osteomyelitis are best diagnosed by examination. Chest x-ray is essential in diagnosing pneumonia, although individuals with AIDS may have pneumonia with a normal film. If fever is present in an IV drug user, it strongly suggests infection.

What primary care might specifically benefit patients who use intravenous drugs?

Primary care for the IV drug user is an emerging concept currently lacking supporting data; these patients' high risk of acquiring and transmitting a variety of infections makes the following steps sound reasonable. Screen for HIV, hepatitis A, B, and C and TB (by PPD plus controls). Patients who have not been exposed to hepatitis A or B should be vaccinated. Pneumococcal and tetanus vaccines are warranted. Because up to 50% of female IV drug users participate in prostitution, regular screening for gonorrhea, *Chlamydia,* and cervical cancer is also wise.

TREATMENT

Who needs to be hospitalized for a drug-associated bacterial infection?

Any IV drug user with a temperature greater than 38.5° C should be hospitalized and treated presumptively for endocarditis with nafcillin and gentamicin. If another infection is present that could account for the fever, such as pneumonia or cellulitis, it is appropriate to tailor antibiotics to that illness while ruling out endocarditis with blood cultures. Cellulitis alone or an abscess that can be drained in the clinic can be treated on an outpatient basis with oral antibiotics, such as cephalexin or dicloxacillin. Abscesses should be packed once or twice a day.

Key Points ···

- Cocaine has many potentially fatal toxic effects, most mediated by sympathetic overdrive.
- Heroin overdose causes respiratory depression and is reversible with naloxone.
- Heroin, cocaine, and methamphetamines do not have physically dangerous withdrawal syndromes, unlike alcohol or benzodiazepines.

CASE 35-3

A 30-year-old man calls 911 because of chest pain. He describes the pain as 10 out of 10 in severity, substernal, and crushing in nature. The pain has been present for 45 minutes and continues unabated. When you ask what he was doing when the pain started, he is vague, but the medics report "crack" paraphernalia at the scene. He has no prior cardiac history. His pulse is 110 and his blood pressure is 200/110. He appears anxious and sweaty.
- A. What will help you evaluate this problem?
- B. What therapies are appropriate?
- C. What will be this patient's disposition: home, medical ward, or cardiac care unit?

CASE 35-4

A 50-year-old woman is brought to the emergency department by her family. They found her snoring in her bed and they were unable to wake her up. They tell you that she has used drugs for many years, but they do not know what kind. On examination, you find a woman who has shallow, ineffectual respirations, small pupils, dry mucous membranes, and many sclerosed veins. Fresh needle tracks are evident. You cannot arouse her.
- A. What are your first steps?
- B. If your first attempts at treating the problem are not successful, what are some other diagnoses to consider?

Women's Health

ABNORMAL PAP SMEARS

ETIOLOGY

What causes abnormal Pap smears?

The Papanicolaou test, or Pap smear, is the most widely available screening test for cervical cancer. Atypical Pap smears, also known as *cervical dysplasia,* have been linked to a variety of risk factors, including multiple sexual partners, early age of sexual intercourse, and tobacco use. There is increasing evidence that human papilloma virus (HPV) plays a key role in most cases of cervical dysplasia. Other reasons for abnormal Pap smears include hormonal changes, inflammation related to vaginitis, and problems with Pap smear collection; these are generally easily identified by the cytopathologist.

EVALUATION

How often should Pap smears be obtained?

Annual Pap testing has been the rule, although recent data suggest that a 3-year interval may be just as effective in women at low risk of acquiring HPV (monogamous, multiple prior negative Paps).

How is the Pap smear result interpreted?

Most cytopathologists use the Bethesda classification system for reporting Pap smear findings. This system reports "epithelial cell abnormalities" (cervical dysplastic changes) separately from "specimen adequacy" and "benign cellular changes." Cervical dysplasia implies a precancerous condition. The goal for followup is to prevent progression to invasive cancer (Figure 36-1). Patients with high-grade dysplasia, or those with repeated findings of low-grade cellular abnormalities, should undergo colposcopic examination. Colposcopy allows the clinician to view the cervix under low-power magnifica-

tion and to biopsy cervical tissue to confirm cytologic findings of the Pap smear.

TREATMENT

How is cervical dysplasia treated?

Treatment options depend on the extent of disease and invasive potential. Conservative outpatient approaches include cryotherapy, laser vaporization, and the loop electrical excision procedure (LEEP). Surgical conization is indicated when patients have more severe dysplastic changes or when the transformation zone is not well visualized.

Key Points ··

- Risk factors associated with cervical dysplasia include HPV infection, early first intercourse, multiple sexual partners, and tobacco use.
- Refer for colposcopy when high-grade squamous intraepithelial lesion (SIL) is identified.
- Refer for colposcopy when repeated atypia or low-grade squamous intraepithelial changes on multiple Pap smears.

CASE 36-1

A 39-year-old women has a Pap smear result reading low-grade SIL, condylomatous changes present. Her history is significant for previous atypical Pap smears 4 years ago. She had been treated for HPV infection using cryotherapy. When you call her to discuss the results, she seems very anxious. She has read that HPV causes cervical cancer. She insists on being referred to an oncologist.

A. What will you recommend to her?
B. What is the relationship between HPV and cervical dysplasia?

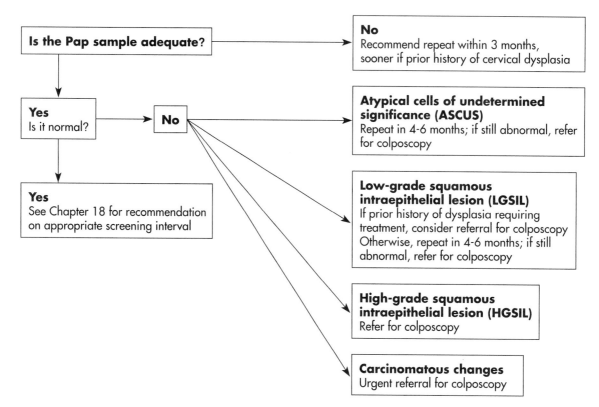

Figure 36-1 Algorithm for management of abnormal Pap smears.

ABNORMAL UTERINE BLEEDING

ETIOLOGY

How do we define abnormal bleeding?

Menstrual irregularities are one of the most frequent presenting complaints seen in women. Normal menarche generally occurs before the age of 16, with normal ovulatory cycle approximately every 23 to 39 days and menstrual flow lasting from 2 to 7 days. Abnormalities in menstrual cycle bleeding are characterized using specific terminology (Table 36-1); any combination of these is possible.

What are common causes of abnormal uterine bleeding?

Differential diagnosis depends on age and bleeding pattern. Always consider pregnancy first with any abnormal bleeding pattern. Aside from pregnancy, other causes are structural, hormonal, infectious, and neoplastic (Table 36-2). Irregular and infrequent bleeding that has persisted ever since onset of menses is likely due to polycystic ovary syndrome (PCOS). Intermen-

TABLE 36-1	
Terminology Used to Describe Abnormal Patterns of Menstrual Bleeding	
TERMINOLOGY	**PATTERN**
Amenorrhea	Lack of menses
Menorrhagia	Excessive bleeding at regular intervals, with menstrual cycle
Metrorrhagia	Irregular bleeding (can be too frequent or too infrequent)
Oligomenorrhea	Infrequent bleeding
Dysfunctional uterine bleeding (DUB)	Uterine bleeding in the absence of identifiable organic pathology, not in usual cyclic pattern

strual spotting can occur with pelvic infection or normal ovulation, or it may be due to ectopic pregnancy, especially if a period has been missed. Vaginal bleeding out of phase in postmenopausal women is suspicious for endometrial cancer. Cyclic bleeding can be normal with hormone replacement therapy, especially if hormones are cycled, but bleeding that does not follow typical withdrawal pattern must be evaluated.

TABLE 36-2

Common Causes of Abnormal Vaginal Bleeding Based on Bleeding Pattern

	TYPE OF BLEEDING			
	MENORRHAGIA*	METRORRHAGIA*	POSTCOITAL	POSTMENOPAUSAL
Structural causes	Fibroid Threatened abortion Coagulation disorder IUD		Cervical polyp	
Hormonal causes	Hypothyroidism DUB	PCOS Hypothalamic hypopituitarism Oral contraceptives Hyperprolactinemia		HRT
Neoplastic causes	Cervical cancer Endometrial cancer	Cervical cancer Endometrial cancer	Cervical cancer	Endometrial cancer
Infectious causes		Endometritis	PID	

IUD, Intrauterine device; *DUB*, dysfunctional uterine bleeding; *PCOS*, polycystic ovary syndrome; *HRT*, hormone replacement therapy; *PID*, pelvic inflammatory disease.
*Menorrhagia and metrorrhagia may coexist.

EVALUATION

How do I evaluate patients with abnormal uterine bleeding?

The pattern of abnormality helps guide diagnostic workup. Patients presenting with changes over 1 to 2 cycles with an otherwise unremarkable history and examination can keep a menstrual log. Ask about duration of the problem; pattern of bleeding; amount of bleeding; use of birth control; and associated symptoms, such as pain or fever. Quantifying vaginal bleeding can be a challenge. It may help to ask how many pads or tampons the patient has required in the past 24 hours. History of medications is also key. For example, birth control pills or Depo-Provera shots frequently cause menstrual abnormalities. Include orthostatics if bleeding is brisk and a pelvic examination to look for anatomic causes, such as fibroids or ectopic pregnancy. Verify normal secondary sexual characteristics, and look for virilization or hirsutism.

What laboratory tests or studies should I order?

Order tests sequentially on the basis of history and examination findings. Urine pregnancy test and TSH can almost always be justified because pregnancy and thyroid abnormalities are among the most common causes for atypical menses. Order hematocrit to detect anemia especially if excessive bleeding is reported; platelets and coagulation studies may be indicated if underlying medical conditions or the clinical picture suggest a clotting problem. If ectopic pregnancy is suspected, send a β-HCG level. In addition, prolactin, luteinizing hormone (LH), and follicle-stimulating hormone (FSH) can be helpful if an un-

derlying endocrine problem is suspected. Hyperprolactinemia can cause either amenorrhea or anovulatory bleeding. Hypothalamic dysfunction or hypopituitarism may be suggested on the basis of amenorrhea with low body weight. PCO syndrome may be a consideration in patients with hirsutism and a long-standing menstrual irregularity. Cervical culture may be taken during the pelvic examination if PID or endometritis is suspected. Ultrasound and/or endometrial biopsy may be required on occasion to evaluate for endometrial hyperplasia or tumor.

When should I hospitalize or refer?

Indications for urgent referral and hospitalization include excessive vaginal bleeding causing hemodynamic changes, a significant drop in blood count, and suspicion of ectopic pregnancy.

TREATMENT

What is the treatment for abnormal uterine bleeding?

Management of abnormal uterine bleeding should be directed at resolution of the underlying problem, for example, endometrial polyps, pregnancy, or infection. Urgent cessation of bleeding with surgical intervention is rarely indicated. Urgent medical treatment to stop prolonged bleeding is often desirable on the basis of low blood count or patient request. If contraindications to such therapy are excluded, short-term and rapid cessation of bleeding can often be achieved with a short course of progesterone (medroxyprogesterone 10 mg qd × 10 days). Oral contraceptive pills are used commonly for treatment of chronic anovulatory states with abnormal bleeding, such as PCO syndrome and hypothalamic dysfunction.

CASE 36-2

A nulliparous 22-year-old woman presents for routine annual examination. She reached menarche at the age of 11 and has always had irregular periods, which generally come 2 to 4 times a year. She was told in high school that this was "normal." She does not recall ever having testing for this in the past. She is not interested in birth control; she assumes that since she has irregular periods, she cannot get pregnant. She uses topical isotretinoin for acne. On examination, height is 64 inches, weight is 180 pounds, mild hirsutism, acanthosis nigricans, and normal secondary sex characteristics are present, and there is no evidence of virilization.

A. How will you evaluate this patient for her irregular menses?
B. What other conditions would you wish to exclude?
C. How will you counsel her regarding treatment?

BREAST HEALTH

ETIOLOGY

What normal and pathologic changes are seen in breast tissue?

Benign causes of lumps are simple cysts and fibroadenomas. Atypical hyperplasia, although benign, is a risk factor for subsequent development of cancer. Carcinoma in situ and invasive carcinoma of the ducts and/or lobules are malignant lesions.

What causes breast pain?

Prevalence studies show that 20% of women experience moderate to severe breast pain. Bilateral tenderness is most commonly caused by cyclic hormonal changes and does not require further evaluation. Although only 6% of cancers result in pain, persistent focal pain requires careful evaluation.

What are risk factors for breast cancer?

Breast cancer kills more than 40,000 annually in the United States, but women may live many years with breast cancer. Approximately 75% of breast cancer patients over age 50 have no risk factors aside from age. Women at particularly high risk have early menarche, late menopause, nulliparity, previous cancer, and, above all, first-degree relatives with breast cancer. Obesity, alcohol, and estrogen use increase risk slightly.

EVALUATION

What screening is recommended for breast cancer?

Screening patients over age 50 with annual examination and mammogram decreases mortality from breast cancer by 30%. Mammography for women ages 40 to 50 is reasonable, but benefits are smaller. Screen earlier with worrisome risk factors (BRCA1 or BRCA2 gene mutation, first-degree relative atypia on breast biopsy).

What clinical presentations are worrisome for underlying cancer?

Any palpable breast lump, asymmetric thickening, or focal pain should be regarded with suspicion. Breast cancer risk factors do not substantially alter pretest probabilities of cancer and so should not play a role in the decision to evaluate further. Workup is indicated for any focal finding or complaint. It is not possible to distinguish benign from malignant conditions on physical examination, but the presence of any of the following raises concern for malignancy (most breast cancers show none of these):

- A mass fixed to the chest wall
- Dimpling of the skin overlying the breast
- Recent-onset unilateral nipple inversion
- Spontaneous nipple discharge, especially if clear or bloody
- Scaly lesions of the nipple
- Failure of breast inflammation to respond promptly to antibiotics
- Persistent, focal breast pain

How do I perform a good breast examination?

Inspect and palpate both breasts systematically. Be certain to include the axillae and subareolar areas. Document location, size, and quality of breast examination findings.

What are the first steps in the workup of a breast lump, thickening, or focal pain?

Order a diagnostic mammogram in all patients age 25 and older. This differs from a screening mammogram in that it requires more time, additional views, and direct supervision by a mammographer. Breast ultrasound, an important adjunct to the evaluation of breast masses, reliably identifies benign simple cysts and helps to characterize solid lesions and to direct biopsy. Begin with ultrasound in women younger than age 25 because more dense tissue makes mammogram less accurate. When mammogram or ultrasound demonstrate a clearly benign finding (simple cyst or calcified fibroadenoma), no further evaluation is needed.

When should a biopsy be obtained?

Refer highly clinically suspicious lesions, such as fixed mass with dimpling, for biopsy regardless of mammogram and ultrasound findings. Similarly, lesions suggestive of cancer on imaging should undergo core needle biopsy under ultrasound or stereotactic guidance. Fine-needle aspiration (FNA), a cell sampling procedure (not a true biopsy), is useful when clinical and radiographic suspicion for malignancy is low. An abnormal FNA mandates biopsy. A mass with a negative FNA combined with negative mammogram and low-suspicion examination (the "triple test") has a chance of a missed cancer of less than 3% and can be followed clinically without biopsy.

What is appropriate followup for focal breast problems with normal mammogram?

Because 10% of breast cancers are not detectable on mammography, plan close clinical followup. Have a low threshold for consultation with a breast specialist.

How does staging determine prognosis in breast cancer patients?

Many prognostic factors help you choose therapy. Your patient will do better if her tumor is small, if it has estrogen receptors (ER), and if it has few S (synthesis) phase cells (the pathologist will determine this). The most important prognostic factor is the absolute number of positive axillary lymph nodes, so node dissection is part of every lumpectomy or mastectomy.

TREATMENT

What alleviates breast pain?

Well-fitting bra, low-fat diet, and reduced caffeine may be effective, but data are limited. Treat infection with antibiotics and abscess with drainage.

How are simple cysts and fibroadenomas managed?

For ultrasound-demonstrated simple cyst, no further followup is necessary. If the cyst is bothersome or interferes with examination, it can be aspirated. Remove fi-

broadenomas because of size over 2 cm, rapid growth, or pain.

What is the best treatment for a breast cancer lump?

Lumpectomy with radiation is as good as modified radical mastectomy. Patient preference, diffuse cancer, or large tumors may call for mastectomy. Most women are cured. Patients with negative nodes, tumor smaller than 1 cm, and favorable histology have excellent prognosis and are usually not given adjuvant chemotherapy. Hormonal therapy (tamoxifen) is used for ER-positive tumors of low risk. Chemotherapy is substituted or added for ER-negative tumors, high-risk histology, or older age.

How is metastatic breast cancer treated?

Most metastases are to bone, brain, or liver. Chemotherapy is the only option for ER-negative disease. Use hormonal manipulation in ER-positive patients: oophorectomy for premenopausal women and tamoxifen for postmenopausal women. If the disease progresses, try progestins and androgens.

How effective is therapy?

The 10-year disease-free survival is nearly 75% for node-negative cancer and 30% for invasive tumors or many positive nodes. Many people live with cancer that needs to be managed, if not cured.

Key Points ·······································

- Most breast cancer occurs in the absence of risk factors aside from age.
- Physical examination cannot reliably distinguish benign from malignant conditions.
- Screening mammography and breast examinations save lives.
- Begin with diagnostic mammography for evaluation of most breast complaints.
- Clinical followup is needed even if imaging studies are normal.

CASE 36-3

A 48-year-old woman presents to you with a month-long history of a sensation of fullness in the upper outer quadrant of her left breast. You detect a 2-cm lump with indistinct margins that is mobile and without overlying skin dimpling.
  A. What is the first step in the evaluation?
  B. If the diagnostic evaluation is negative, what followup should be planned?
  C. What should prompt a referral to a breast surgeon?

CASE 36-4

A 28-year-old woman presents with a 2.5-cm mobile, slightly tender mass in the inferior left breast. Mammogram is negative, although breast tissue is very dense.
  A. What other tests are indicated?
  B. What is appropriate followup if studies suggest a fibroadenoma?
  C. What is appropriate followup if studies suggest a simple cyst?

MENOPAUSE

ETIOLOGY

What is menopause?

Natural menopause is the permanent cessation of menses and marks a woman's entry into the postreproductive phase of life. The final menstrual period (FMP) is defined retrospectively after 12 consecutive months of amenorrhea. The menopause transition includes the years before the FMP when variability of the menstrual cycles increases. This transition period and the 12 months after the FMP are defined as the perimenopause. The perimenopause is a period of physiologic disruption due to fluctuating levels of hormones and symptoms. The incidence of both coronary artery disease and osteoporosis increase significantly following menopause.

What is a hot flash?

A hot flash is a symptom complex caused by the sudden downward resetting of the central core temperature set point. This results in a sensation of heat and the initiation of heat-dissipating mechanisms, such as vasodilation, sweating, and a reflex tachycardia. Hot flashes are more frequent and can be quite severe in the perimenopause and decline in following years. They are a common reason women seek care at perimenopause.

Can menopause cause depression?

Major depression and anxiety disorders are not associated with menopause and are in fact less prevalent than earlier in life. Mood swings may be associated with sleep problems, leading to daytime irritability, forgetfulness, and fatigue. Perimenopause is also a time of profound social and psychologic change for women: children leave home, elderly parents need assistance, and work roles and relationships with spouses may change. The stresses and health effects of these life events may be falsely attributed to coincidental biological changes associated with menopause. Major depression, if present, requires treatment and will not respond to hormone therapy alone.

Why is osteoporosis particularly prevalent in postmenopausal women?

Although both men and women show age-related decline in bone mineral density after age 40, most women have an accelerated phase of bone loss associated with the cessation of ovarian estrogen production in the 5 years after menopause. Men are protected against osteoporosis because they achieve higher peak bone mass, and they do not have an abrupt fall in sex hormones.

What are the risk factors associated with the development of osteoporosis?

Caucasian or Asian ethnic descent and slender build are risk factors. Personal history of prior fracture and family history of fracture are independent risk factors. Lifestyle issues also play an important role, including inadequate vitamin D and calcium intake; tobacco, alcohol, and caffeine use; and sedentary habits. Osteoporosis is also associated with hyperthyroidism; hyperparathyroidism; and chronic inflammatory conditions, such as collagen vascular diseases. Medications, such as corticosteroids, heparin, anticonvulsants, and methotrexate, will also predispose towards the development of osteoporosis.

EVALUATION

How does one determine if a woman is perimenopausal?

Perimenopause can be identified clinically by a combination of age and characteristic symptoms. The median age of onset of the menopausal transition occurs at 47.5, and the FMP at 51 years. The characteristic symptoms of hot flashes, sleep disturbance, and mood swings peak in perimenopause and diminish in the years following. Vaginal dryness and urinary frequency manifest later in the transition and in the postmenopausal years. Classic symptoms do not occur in every woman, may precede the transition by years, and may be caused by other conditions.

Are blood tests helpful in defining perimenopause?

Blood tests such as FSH have no place in defining this phase of life in nonhysterectomized women. FSH levels fluctuate markedly during this time and do not reliably correlate with stage of perimenopause or predict transition events. By contrast, women who have undergone hysterectomy will not manifest menstrual changes, so an elevated FSH is helpful in deciding when to begin hormone replacement. Unusual patterns, such as cycle irregularity at an early age, warrant further testing for unexpected pregnancy, thyroid disease, or hyperprolactinemia with β-HCG, TSH, and prolactin levels, respectively.

What are the expected bleeding patterns in the transition phase?

Most commonly, menstrual cycles become further apart and the volume of menstrual blood flow is reduced, reflecting the waning production of estrogen by the ovaries and the increasing frequency of anovulatory cycles. In 10% of women, menses cease abruptly.

What bleeding patterns should prompt further evaluation?

Heavy menstrual bleeding, prolonged menses (>7 days), and more than two cycles in a 1-month period should prompt investigation for endocrine (hypothyroidism) or structural abnormalities. Endovaginal ultrasound detects uterine fibroids and uterine polyps, which may cause heavy bleeding. In addition, ultrasound is useful for ruling out endometrial carcinoma: an endometrial stripe of less than 5 mm makes endometrial cancer very unlikely. Endometrial sampling using a Pipelle catheter can also detect endometrial hyperplasia or carcinoma.

How is osteoporosis diagnosed?

Dual electron x-ray absorptiometry (DEXA) is currently the most widely accepted modality for measurement of bone mineral density (BMD). Results are reported in terms of the T-score, which compares the individual patient's BMD with that of a young normal population, and the Z-score, which compares it with an age-matched control population. The World Health Organization defines osteoporosis as a T-score greater than 2.5 standard deviations below the young-normal mean. Disadvantages to this technique are that BMD is not equivalent to bone strength and that adjacent calcium deposits may cause an artifactual increase in the reading. DEXA is not currently used for screening. A number of other emerging modalities, such as ultrasound and metabolic bone markers, show promise in this regard.

TREATMENT

What are the options for treatment of perimenopausal symptoms?

Hot flashes, mood swings, and sleep disturbances are most effectively treated with hormone replacement therapy (HRT). The relatively new selective estrogen receptor modulators (SERMs), such as raloxifine, do not prevent hot flashes. Other treatment modalities are less effective but may be useful in women who cannot or do not wish to take HRT. These include clonidine, soy products, vitamin E, and environmental control, such as maintenance of cool ambient temperature and cotton clothing. A number of alternative medicines have been touted as effective, but to date none has demonstrated effectiveness.

What are the currently available replacement hormones?

For women with an intact uterus, HRT should consist of an estrogen and a progestin, the latter to protect against endometrial proliferation and uterine cancer. The most commonly used estrogens in the United States are conjugated equine estrogen (oral), micronized estradiol (oral), estradiol-17β (transdermal patches and vaginal creams), and piperazine estrone sulfate (oral). The available progestins are medroxyprogesterone acetate and micronized progesterone.

What replacement therapy regimens are currently used?

One of the estrogens described above is usually taken daily. Progestins may be given cyclically (e.g., medroxyprogesterone acetate 5 mg days 1-14) or continuously (e.g., 2.5 mg daily). The cyclic regimens should result in regular bleeding starting day 9 or later and are particularly useful in the early perimenopausal patient to regulate cycles. The daily continuous regimen should, after the first 6 to 12 months of therapy, lead to amenorrhea. Out-of-phase bleeding should result in adjustment of the regimen and/or evaluation of the endometrium by ultrasound or endometrial biopsy to rule out hyperplasia or cancer.

What options exist for treatment of osteoporosis?

Table 36-3 lists the pharmacologic options available for treatment of osteoporosis. Significant controversy exists in choosing therapy. Although estrogen has clearly demonstrated benefit in terms of both improving bone mass and fracture risk reduction, its effects on the endometrium, breast, and cardiovascular systems must be taken into consideration. Clinical decision-making should factor in the individual patient's risk factors for, and attitudes towards, conditions associated with menopause and estrogen replacement therapy. In women at high risk for osteoporosis, estrogen is the first choice if no contraindications exist. SERMs are useful in women intolerant of estrogen or with a history of breast cancer. Bisphosphonates are another excellent option either as treatment in women who cannot take estrogen or in addition to estrogen in women with symptomatic osteoporotic fractures.

Is there any way to prevent osteoporosis?

It is becoming increasingly clear that prevention of osteoporosis is a far more effective intervention, in reducing morbidity and mortality, than treatment of established disease. It is critical that conditions that may predispose towards inadequate bone mass development be identified in adolescence and early adulthood. These conditions include eating disorders, hypothalamic con-

TABLE 36-3
Drug Therapy for Osteoporosis

CHOICE	REDUCES FRACTURE	COST	COMMENTS
Calcium and vitamin D	+/−	$	Should be recommended to all women with inadequate dietary calcium. 1 g for premenopausal and 1.5 g for postmenopausal women.
Estrogen	+++	$$	Requires concurrent use of progestins unless posthysterectomy. May have beneficial effects on cardiovascular system. Increased risk for breast cancer.
Calcitonin	+	$$$	Must be administered parenterally. Analgesic effect helpful in fracture management.
Bisphosphonates	++	$$$$	Effects of sustained bisphosphonate use unclear. Increased risk for esophageal ulceration. FDA approved for prevention.
Selective estrogen receptor modulators	++	$$$$	Act on estrogen receptors in bone, and perhaps on cardiovascular system by lowering cholesterol, but have no effect on breast or endometrium.

ditions leading to amenorrhea, tobacco use, sedentary lifestyle, and intolerance of dairy products. In addition, it is important to recognize that low bone mass alone is not predictive of fracture. Fall risk is a major contributing factor to the development of fractures, particularly in the elderly. Providers should be aware that gait instability, poor vision, unsafe home environment, and medications that alter consciousness are potentially avoidable causes for falls in this population.

What are the benefits and risks of hormone replacement therapy?

HRT is believed to be protective against cardiovascular disease through a variety of mechanisms. However, it is unclear whether these benefits are limited to certain women, and whether they outweigh the risks of estrogen administration when relative contraindications to HRT exist, such as family history of breast cancer. Large-scale randomized clinical trials are ongoing to examine these issues.

Key Points ······················

- The symptoms of perimenopause are hot flashes, sleep disturbances, mood swings, and irregular menses, although not all women require or desire treatment.
- Evaluate heavy or frequent bleeding out of phase in the perimenopause for uterine pathology by endovaginal ultrasound or endometrial biopsy.
- Prevention is a far more effective intervention in reducing morbidity and mortality from osteoporosis than is treatment of established disease.

CASE 36-5

A 48-year-old woman seeks care for a 6-month history for bothersome hot flashes and infrequent menses. She is otherwise in good health and has a normal physical examination.
A. What tests are required to ensure that she is in the menopause transition?
B. What type of hormone replacement therapy would you prescribe?
C. Three months later, she reports prolonged menses lasting 14 days. What should you do next?
D. What other regimen might you prescribe?

CASE 36-6

A 48-year-old woman presents reporting multiple muscle and joint pains lasting more than 5 years, which she believes may be secondary to osteoporosis. Her menstrual cycles have been somewhat sporadic over the past year, but they seem to have normalized again over the last four cycles. She denies hot flashes. Her 70-year-old mother had been hospitalized for a hip fracture 10 years ago. She is currently on no medications. She has a 40 pack-year smoking history. Her height is 61 inches (she states she was previously 63 inches tall), and weight is 110 pounds. She has multiple paired tender points over the muscles, but no evidence for a fracture.
A. Are her muscle pains and loss in height secondary to osteoporosis?
B. What will you recommend as far as diagnostic testing?
C. Her bone density is 1.5 standard deviations below her age-matched mean. What do you recommend?

Case Answers

5-1. **A-B. Learning objective: Recognize what actions the duty of confidentiality requires.** The duty to maintain confidentiality remains strong in this case because information about the patient does not directly concern others' health, welfare, or safety. There is no imminent danger to others here. However, the wife is certainly affected by her husband's health and prognosis. Every effort should be made to encourage sharing of information, although it remains his right to do so or not.

5-2. **A-B. Learning objective: Identify key features of decision-making capacity and the appropriate steps to take should the patient be incapacitated.** This patient's underlying disease is impairing her decision-making capacity. If her wishes persist during lucid periods, this choice may be considered her real preference and followed accordingly. However, because her decision-making capacity is questionable, getting a surrogate decision-maker involved can help determine what her real wishes are.

5-3. **A-B. Learning objective: Define futility and discuss the appropriate decision-making process for writing a DNR order.** Medical futility means that an intervention, in this case CPR, offers no chance of meaningful benefit to the patient. Interventions can be considered futile if the probability of success (discharged alive from the hospital) is less than 1%, and/or if the quality of life after successful CPR is below the minimum acceptable to the patient. In this case, Mr. H would have a somewhat lower-than-normal chance of survival from CPR, based on his quadriplegia (homebound lifestyle is a poor prognostic factor) and his mild pneumonia (in cases of severe pneumonia and respiratory failure, survival is less than 1%). However, his quality of life, although not enviable, is not without value. Because he is fully awake and alert, you could talk with Mr. H about his view of the quality of his life. You could share with him the likely scenarios should he have an arrest and need CPR. After this discussion, Mr. H can tell you if he would like to have CPR or not. You cannot say on the basis of the current situation that CPR is futile. A decision about resuscitation should occur only after talking with the patient about his situation and reaching a joint decision.

6-1. **A. Learning objective: Calculate PPV.** Assume 1000 patients. Using a pretest probability of 25%, 250 will have disease and 750 will have no disease. Then, working backwards, use the sensitivity and specificity of 98% to calculate the number of true positives (A = 98% of 250 = 245) and true negatives (D = 98% of 750 = 735). Quadrant B is total disease absent − true negatives (750 − 735 = 15). Quadrant C is total disease present − true positives (250 − 245 = 5). With all quadrants filled in, you can calculate PPV and NPV. With a calculated PPV of 94%, we can say that with a positive test, this high-risk patient is 94% certain to have HIV infection (see table below).

Predictive Value Calculations for HIV Test in a High-Risk Patient		
Pretest probability = 25% Assume N = 1000		
	DISEASE	
TEST	*Present in 250*	*Absent in 750*
Positive	A 245	B 15
Negative	C 5	D 735

$$\mathbf{PPV} = \frac{245}{(245 + 15)} = \mathbf{94\%}$$

$$\mathbf{NPV} = \frac{735}{(735 + 5)} = \mathbf{99\%}$$

B. *Learning objective: Recognize that a low pretest probability markedly decreases positive predictive value.* When applied to high-risk patients, the HIV test has excellent positive and negative predictive value; the results are quite different when applied to low-risk populations. Assume 1000 patients, now using a pretest probability (or disease prevalence in this population) of 1/1000. Disease is present in 1 and absent in 999. Using sensitivity and specificity of 98%, estimate true positive (0.98) and true negative (979) and then subtract as above for quadrants B and C. Then calculate PPV and NPV. What is striking is that although this test is highly sensitive and specific, a positive test result in this population has only a 5% likelihood of reflecting true disease (see table below).

Predictive Value Calculations for HIV Test in Low-Risk Patient

Pretest probability = 1/1000
Assume N = 1000

TEST	DISEASE	
	Present in 1	*Absent in 999*
Positive	A 0.98	B 20
Negative	C 0.02	D 979

$$\text{PPV} = \frac{0.98}{(20 + 0.98)} = 5\%$$

$$\text{NPV} = \frac{979}{(979 + 0.02)} = 99.9\%$$

ABDOMINAL PAIN

7-1. **A. *Learning objective: Use clinical information to make a differential diagnosis for right lower quadrant pain in a young woman.*** Appendicitis, inflammatory bowel disease, irritable bowel disease, PID, ectopic pregnancy, or other pelvic pathology are possible causes of right lower quadrant pain in a young woman. Recent antibiotic use may have made oral contraceptives less potent or may have led to *C. difficile* colitis.

B. *Learning objective: Identify key questions that help narrow the differential diagnosis in a young woman with right lower quadrant pain.* Describe how the pain has progressed over time (appendicitis classically starts diffusely then intensifies and migrates in hours to the RLQ; torsed ovary starts and stays in a lower quadrant and is maximal at onset). Have there been recurrent episodes (suggests inflammatory, irritable bowel)? Have menses been missed (ectopic pregnancy)? Is there any diarrhea (usually accompanies *C. difficile* colitis, inflammatory bowel or irritable bowel)? Is there anorexia or nausea (appendicitis causes anorexia, pregnancy might cause nausea)? Is there pain with defecating (ulcerative colitis causes tenesmus)? Is there fever (appendicitis, IBD)?

C. *Learning objective: Design appropriate workup for right lower quadrant pain in a young woman.* Her history of bloody stool points away from a pelvic source. Without such a history, pelvic examination and pregnancy test are mandatory. In this patient, a stool guaiac test and complete blood count are a good starting point. Pursue testing for invasive bacterial infection, and if negative, get colonoscopy to look for inflammatory bowel disease.

7-2. **A. *Learning objective: Make a differential list for an elderly person with diffuse, severe abdominal pain.*** The differential list includes ischemic bowel disease, aortic aneurysm rupture, perforated bowel, pancreatitis, obstipation, colon cancer, bladder outlet obstruction, and pyelonephritis. Ischemic bowel is most likely, given his age, the prior history of postprandial abdominal pain and the soft abdomen despite severe pain. Aortic dissection seems less likely without radiation to the back or specific signs of poor perfusion to the lower extremities, but examination should seek to rule this out—check for asymmetric pulses or blood pressure, or pulsatile abdominal mass. Perforated bowel is also less likely without peritoneal signs. Pancreatitis is less likely because it should radiate to the back and should cause more focal tenderness on examination. It is unlikely he has obstipation with recent passage of stool. Colon cancer is rarely a cause of abdominal pain unless it causes perforation or obstruction, both of which seem unlikely, given his soft abdomen. Bladder outlet obstruction is possible given the large prostate. Pyelonephritis is possible, especially in light of the enlarged prostate and possible bladder outlet obstruction.

B. *Learning objective: Obtain appropriate studies to assist in diagnosis in elderly patients with diffuse, severe abdominal pain.* Obtain an abdominal series to rule out perforation or obstipation, a complete blood count to assess for infection or anemia, chemistry panel to assess for acidosis or renal insufficiency, arterial blood gas, and urinalysis to rule out urinary tract infection. Foley catheter may reveal the large urine volume of a bladder outlet obstruction. Perform serial examinations to follow clinical course. To confirm your suspicion of ischemic bowel, order abdominal CT, which should demonstrate edematous bowel if ischemic bowel is present. Acidosis suggest infarcted bowel and usually requires urgent surgical resection of the dead bowel.

ANEMIA

8-1.   **A. *Learning objective: State thalassemia as the most likely cause of a microcytosis out of proportion to the reduction in hematocrit, and list the common blood smear finding of thalassemia.*** The degree of microcytosis out of proportion to her anemia and her ethnic background, she most certainly has α-thalassemia or hemoglobin E disease. You expect to see a uniform population of small red cells, as well as target cells, on smear.

B. *Learning objective: Know the diagnostic workup in patients suspected of having thalassemia.* There is no specific test for α-thalassemia, and the diagnosis is made by clinical presentation. If the clinical presentation had been more compelling for iron deficiency (lower hematocrit, pregnancy, heavy periods), you could order iron studies.

C. *Learning objective: Avoid placing patients with microcytic anemia on empiric iron therapy.* No treatment is needed in this patient. She should receive genetic counseling. Patients with thalassemia are often placed on empiric iron because of their low MCV. This is a mistake and can result in iron overload.

8-2.   **A. *Learning objective: Know the differential diagnosis for macrocytic anemia.*** He has a decreased reticulocyte index and an elevated MCV. Possible causes for this anemia include dietary folate deficiency, phenytoin-related poor folate absorption, vitamin B_{12} deficiency, alcohol, or hypothyroidism. Given the megaloblastic changes of hypersegmented PMNs seen on peripheral smear, folate and B_{12} deficiency need to be excluded.

B. *Learning objective: Know the laboratory workup of megaloblastic anemia.* Order an erythrocyte folate level and a vitamin B_{12} level. If folate is low and B_{12} is normal, start folic acid. Hematocrit and blood smear should normalize in 6 to 8 weeks. Repeat hematocrit at that time to make sure that he does not have a second cause of his anemia or poor absorption of folate resulting from his medications.

CHEST PAIN

9-1.   **A. *Learning objective: List causes of pleuritic pain in a young person.*** The differential diagnosis is broad. Angina and aortic dissection are included for completeness sake, but both are very unlikely in this young patient, especially in light of the pleuritic nature of his pain. The pleuritic quality also argues against esophageal cause. More likely causes of pleuritic pain in young people are costochondritis (perhaps related to his recent cough), pneumonia, pleurisy, pneumothorax, and pericarditis.

B. *Learning objective: Recognize ECG findings of pericarditis.* ECG reveals diffuse ST elevation. Given the low likelihood of ischemia or infarction, the pleuritic quality of pain, and the diffuse ECG changes, pericarditis is most likely. Additional ECG findings with pericarditis include diffuse P-R depression or T-wave inversions. With significant pericardial effusion, ECG may show generalized low-voltage or electrical alternans (beat-to-beat variability in the size of the QRS complex resulting from the heart "swinging" back and forth in the pericardial space).

C. *Learning objective: State the pertinent examination findings of pericarditis.* On physical examination, the most useful finding is the presence of a pericardial friction rub. This creates a high-pitched scratching sound, often with three separate components, heard best during expiration, with the patient sitting up. With significant pericardial effusion, distant heart sounds, elevated neck veins, and pulsus paradoxus may be found (see Table 9-1).

D. *Learning objective: State the common causes of pericarditis.* Differential diagnosis of pericarditis is broad, with recent viral infection most likely in light of his viral upper respiratory infection; renal failure and pericardial bacterial infections are less likely. Viruses implicated in causing pericarditis include coxsackievirus A and B, echoviruses, adenovirus, and influenza, among others. The disease is usually self-limited, resolving in days to weeks, but recurrences can occur.

E. *Learning objective: State the treatment for viral pericarditis.* The usual treatment for viral pericarditis is a course of antiinflammatory therapy, either with NSAIDs or prednisone.

9-2.   **A.** *Learning objective: Identify cardiac risk factors.* Her independent risk factors include hypertension, diabetes, low HDL, postmenopausal status, and family history of CAD. Smoking status is not mentioned, so you need to ask. In addition, her examination reveals morbid obesity, which is associated with increased CAD risk, although this is not an independent risk factor.

B. *Learning objective: List a differential diagnosis for chest pain in patients with multiple cardiac risk factors.* Differential diagnosis includes myocardial ischemia or infarction at the top of the list. Aortic dissection is also possible with radiation to the back or her neck, although the description of her pain is not classic. Certainly, esophageal causes should be considered because these can exactly mimic myocardial infarction. Moreover, this patient has several risk factors for GERD, including morbid obesity and calcium channel blocker use. Other possibilities include pneumonia, pleurisy, PE, PUD, biliary colic, pancreatitis, and musculoskeletal causes, although her history is not particularly suggestive of these. The life-threatening causes noted above must be excluded before entertaining the rest.

C. *Learning objective: Recognize myocardial injury on ECG.* Anterolateral ST depression (leads V3-V6) suggests myocardial ischemia. Admitting diagnosis is "unstable angina, rule out myocardial infarction." The duration of her pain makes infarction a distinct possibility, although she may rule out for MI by serial enzymes. Without ST segment elevation or new left bundle branch block, she is not a candidate for thrombolysis. Nonetheless, she should be admitted to the CCU and given aspirin, intravenous nitrates, and heparin. A β-blocker is an excellent addition, especially in light of her resting tachycardia (see Chapter 23, Ischemic Heart Disease section).

D. *Learning objective: Discuss the likelihood of aortic dissection based on features of the clinical presentation.* As noted above, aortic dissection is possible because her pain, although not classic for dissection, does radiate to the back. In addition, she has long-standing hypertension. Pertinent negatives that help exclude dissection are symmetric arm pressures and pulses (all four extremities), and absence of a diastolic AI murmur at the left sternal border. On chest x-ray, lack of mediastinal widening is reassuring although by no means definitive. If her pain responds as expected to nitrates, dissection is less likely. On the other hand, ongoing pain despite apparently appropriate treatment for ischemia should provoke consideration of other diagnostic possibilities.

COUGH

10-1.   **A.** *Learning objective: List the likely causes of cough in patients with exercise-induced cough and allergies.* Most likely is exercise-induced cough-variant asthma worsened by cat allergy from residual cat hair left in her apartment (remains up to 6 months after cat is gone). Differential also includes postinfectious bronchospasm and PND.

B. *Learning objective: Identify helpful historical or examination clues in making a diagnosis of cough-variant asthma.* Helpful clues include family or personal history of asthma, history of reactions to NSAIDs or aspirin (associated with asthma), a cat in the home (even from previous occupant), and prior inhaler use. Helpful examination findings include posterior pharyngeal cobblestoning or nasal exudate suggesting associated allergic PND, wheezing, wheezing with rapid forced expiration, and eczema (atopy).

C. *Learning objective: Obtain spirometry to confirm airway obstruction.* Get office spirometry when exercise or allergies induce cough.

D. *Learning objective: Treat bronchospastic cough with a trial of empiric β-agonists, and suggest preventive measures.* Give a β-agonist inhaler. Suggest carpet cleaning if previous owner had a cat, and bathing cats weekly (helps allergic cat-owners).

10-2. **A.** *Learning objective: Recognize the presentation of cough resulting from post-nasal drip or medication side effects.* Her most likely cause of chronic cough is PND, as suggested by morning cough, scant sputum, and throat clearing, usually as a result of allergic rhinitis. Her ACE inhibitor, GERD, or allergies may also exacerbate the cough.

B. *Learning objective: Review the history and physical to rule out cancer and assess for common causes of cough in older patients.* Ask about constitutional symptoms and reflux symptoms (nocturnal epigastric pain, regurgitation of food). Look for cachexia or lymph nodes on examination, suggesting cancer or chronic infection. Look for cobblestoning in the posterior pharynx from PND.

C. *Learning objective: Use empiric trials to diagnose chronic cough.* Stop her ACE inhibitor for a week (substitute another drug, such as a β-blocker, in the meantime). If she still has a cough, an empiric trial of decongestants and/or nasal steroids is appropriate to diagnose PND.

D. *Learning objective: Recognize cough as a symptom of CHF in the appropriate clinical setting.* An S_3 and crackles are signs of heart failure, as are cough worse with exercise and when recumbent, and should prompt workup for CHF. If the S_3 is right-sided, consider interstitial lung disease (cough worse with exercise and deep inspiration).

DIARRHEA

11-1. **A.** *Learning objective: Ask pertinent questions in a patient with acute diarrhea to help determine the cause.* He has acute diarrhea with signs of an infectious or inflammatory process (low-grade fever, focal abdominal pain). Ask about exposure to chronic care facilities (visiting friends) or day care (playing with children), travel, recent egg or meat exposure, prior surgeries, or known diverticular disease. If he denies these, then viral infection, diverticulitis, or acute bacterial infection are most likely.

B. *Learning objective: Order appropriate initial laboratory workup for acute diarrhea.* For acute diarrhea of longer than 3 days' duration, order stool fecal leukocytes (follow up with stool culture if positive). Consider a complete blood count, especially in the elderly to evaluate the degree of systemic toxicity.

C. *Learning objective: Design initial treatment for acute diarrhea.* Because he has a low-grade temperature and is volume replete, you could send him home for bed rest and a clear liquid diet pending test results. Another option is to treat him empirically for diverticulitis with antibiotics. Diverticulitis is inflammation and probable bacterial overgrowth in diverticula (present in 70% of people over age 70; 15% will become symptomatic) and should be suspected in older patients with abdominal pain, fever, left lower quadrant pain, and diarrhea. Patients with mild disease (T < 38.5° C, mild-to-moderate pain, WBC < 13,000-15,000) can be managed as outpatients. If he develops worsening pain, fever, peritoneal signs, or rising white blood count, he should be hospitalized for observation and IV antibiotics.

DIZZNESS AND SYNCOPE

12-1. *Learning objective: Prioritize the evaluation and diagnosis of vertigo based on likely causes.* She almost certainly has vestibulitis/neuritis because of the sudden onset of symptoms, the duration of illness, the severity, the benign examination, and onset after an upper respiratory illness. She clearly describes vertigo rather than presyncope. It is more prolonged and severe than one would expect for benign positional vertigo, and she is too young for that disease (unless she has had head trauma). She has no other features of Meniere's disease (previous episodes, decreased hearing, tinnitus). She will need a brief course of powerful antidizziness medicines (perhaps diazepam given the severity) or hospital admission if she cannot keep pills down.

12-2. **A.** *Learning objective: Create a complete list of reversible causes of nonvertiginous dizziness in an elderly, complicated patient.* The list is as follows: poor vision, peripheral neuropathy (decreased proprioception), volume depletion resulting from diarrhea, gastrointestinal blood loss (guaiac positive), cardiac outflow obstruction (systolic murmur), significant tachyarrhythmia (such as PSVT), and atrial fibrillation.

B. *Learning objective: Recognize which maneuvers are necessary to assess for worrisome causes of dizziness.* Postural vital signs would be useful to assess the severity of blood loss. Although the systolic murmur may be due to a high flow state, check for sluggish carotid upstrokes and paradoxical splitting of the second heart sound to ensure that there is not a life-threatening cardiac outflow obstruction.

C. *Learning objective: Design an appropriate evaluation plan.* If he is postural, obtain a hemoglobin or hematocrit to assess blood loss. If his pulse is greater than 110 (more than expected as a response to decreased volume), obtain an ECG to look for significant tachyarrhythmia. Which to do first would depend on the results of further evaluation (see answer *B* above).

DYSPEPSIA

13-1. **A.** *Learning objective: Recognize history consistent with aspirin- or NSAID-associated PUD, and stop these medications.* Stop aspirin use immediately. Give H_2-blockers or proton pump inhibitors to allow healing of inflammation or ulceration.

B. *Learning objective: Recognize that aspirin use in the presence of H. pylori increases the likelihood of PUD.* If he does not respond after 2 weeks, draw *H. pylori* titers. Start presumptive treatment if positive.

C. *Learning objective: Recognize that patients with a history of ulcer formation secondary to aspirin or NSAID use are likely to form them again.* A lower dose will not prevent recurrence. Consider adding gastroprotective agents, such as misoprostol or proton pump inhibitors. Patients with a history of GI bleeding with NSAIDs should absolutely avoid further NSAID use.

13-2. *Learning objective: Identify key points of lifestyle modification for GERD.* Recommend lifestyle modifications. Advise her to cut back on her caffeine and tobacco use, eat low-fat foods, and avoid eating for 4 hours before going to sleep. Instruct her to raise the head of the bed by tilting up the whole frame (about 6 inches) rather than by the use of pillows, which exacerbate the problem by increasing intraabdominal pressure. If her symptoms do not resolve, begin a trial of proton pump inhibitor therapy.

DYSPNEA

14-1. **A. Learning objective: Recognize a typical presentation for exercise-induced asthma.** This patient has a history suggestive of exercise-induced asthma. Her past history of eczema is a risk factor for developing asthma. Her cough and worsening of symptoms with cold weather are also common in patients with asthma.

B. Learning objective: Design an appropriate evaluation for a patient with new-onset asthma. Spirometry provides information about airflow obstruction. Obstruction that reverses with bronchodilators confirms a diagnosis of asthma. Spirometry may be normal in patients with exercise-induced asthma. A therapeutic trial (see below), measurement of spirometry or a peak flow measurement after exercise, or a methacholine challenge test, if necessary, could be used to confirm a diagnosis of exercise-induced asthma.

C. Learning objective: Select appropriate treatment for asthma. Inhaled β_2-adrenergic agonists, such as albuterol or metaproterenol, can be used before exercise in patients with exercise-induced asthma. Cromolyn and nedocromil inhalers are alternative treatments for asthma. Patients with more severe asthma who require daily treatment with inhalers to control symptoms should be started on inhaled corticosteroids to reduce airway inflammation.

14-2. **A. Learning objective: Select and prioritize tests in evaluating a patient with dyspnea of unclear etiology.** A chest x-ray evaluates for an atypical pneumonia, ongoing significant congestive heart failure, neoplasm or other less common pulmonary problems. Other tests to consider include oximetry with exercise to establish whether her oxygen saturation drops significantly with exertion, spirometry to look for evidence of airway obstruction, CBC to look for anemia, and an ECG to look for ischemia or other heart disease.

B. Learning objective: Select appropriate evaluation for a patient with possible pulmonary emboli. This chest x-ray raises the question of a pulmonary embolus. A lower extremity ultrasound examination to look for a deep venous thrombosis is a good initial test. In this patient ultrasound is positive for clot and her dyspnea resolves after a course of anticoagulation. If this patient's ultrasound examination is negative for clot, proceed to a lung perfusion scan. If V/Q scan is negative, obtain pulmonary angiogram because clinical suspicion for PE is high.

FATIGUE

15-1. **A. Learning objective: Recognize red flags for physical disease in patients with fatigue.** Short duration of fatigue and associated symptoms of cough, subjective fever, and night sweats are concerning for physical disease.

B. Learning objective: Ask questions to focus your history on likely causes in patients with focal symptoms. The cough points to a pulmonary source for her fatigue, and the fevers and night sweats suggest infection or tumor. Ask other questions related to respiratory function, such as whether the cough is productive; what sputum looks like; and if there is shortness of breath, dyspnea on exertion, orthopnea, or chest pain (pleuritic, positional, or exertional). Also ask about infectious exposures, especially tuberculosis and HIV. Ask about other constitutional symptoms, such as weight loss.

C. Learning objective: Appropriately focus your workup in a patient with fatigue and risk factors for HIV and TB. Obtain chest x-ray, CBC, PPD (with controls if immunosuppressed), HIV, pregnancy test (if indicated), sputum Gram stain, AFB stain, and cultures.

15-2. **A. Learning objective: Identify concerning features from history and examination in patients with fatigue.** For physical disease, these factors are age, weight loss, and "aches and pains"; the longer duration of the fatigue and the symptoms of depression (poor sleep, listlessness, and anhedonia) are concerning for psychiatric disease.

B. Learning objective: Obtain pertinent history in patients with fatigue. Ask more about the aches and pains (swollen joints, fevers, rashes, headaches, jaw claudication to suggest temporal arteritis or other systemic rheumatologic disease) and depressive symptoms (recent upheavals in his life, other symptoms of depression, suicidal ideation). Ask more about his diabetes control, cardiac symptoms, and other end-organ damage.

C. Learning objective: Order appropriate laboratory tests to work up fatigue. Obtain chemistry panel, CBC with differential, LFTs, TSH, and ESR (somewhat controversial in younger patients).

GASTROINTESTINAL BLEEDING

16-1.   A. Learning objective: Recognize clues to the site of gastrointestinal bleeding. This patient's history suggests several possible sites for bleeding: colon from recurrent colon cancer, bleeding diverticula in the colon, or from the stomach resulting from NSAID-related gastropathy (piroxicam is an NSAID; look up all unknown medications). The BUN-to-creatinine ratio of 45 makes an upper GI tract source more likely than a colonic source. The BUN-to-creatinine ratio is almost always greater than 25 in upper GI bleeding. In rapid and severe upper gastrointestinal bleeding, the BUN level is usually greater than 40 because of absorbed nitrogen load from blood in the small intestine. Colonic bleeding does not usually lead to a rise in the BUN level. An NSAID-induced ulcer is most likely in this patient. They frequently are painless, with bleeding being the first sign of problems. The lack of pain is believed to be due to the antiinflammatory effects of the drug. The elderly are at much greater risk for development of NSAID-induced ulcers.

B. Learning objective: State the most common causes of lower GI bleeding. Diverticulosis is the most common cause of lower GI bleeding. Note that it is diverticulosis and not diverticulitis that is associated with acute bleeding. Other causes include angiodysplasia, ischemic colitis, inflammatory bowel disease, and colorectal malignancy.

C. Learning objective: State the treatment options to prevent NSAID induced ulcers. NSAIDs vary in their risk of causing bleeding—salsalate (Disalcid), a nonacetylated salicylate, has the lowest risk. Ibuprofen has less risk than drugs such as piroxicam (Feldene) and ketorolac (Toradol), which have the greatest risk. Proton pump inhibitors offer the most protection with the best tolerability. Misoprostol also offers protection but is limited by the side effect of diarrhea. High-dose H_2-blockers offer some benefit but not as a proton pump inhibitor.

16-2.   A. Learning objective: List and recognize the physical findings suggestive of liver disease. The physical findings of gynecomastia, palmar erythema, and spider angiomata are signs of liver disease likely resulting from increased peripheral conversion of testosterone and other androgens to estrogen. Signs of portal hypertension can also be seen on examination: caput medusa and enlarged hemorrhoidal veins. Ascites develop because of perturbation in Starling forces throughout the hepatic sinusoids and splanchnic capillary bed. On physical examination, ascites will lead to shifting dullness to percussion or the presence of a fluid wave. Examination findings suggestive of alcoholism (but not necessarily liver disease) include Dupuytren's contractures, testicular atrophy, and parotid gland swelling. Terry's nails (pale proximal nail, with a 2- to 3-mm, dark red or brown distal band) are seen in patients with liver disease. The pathophysiology is not known.

B. Learning objective: State the appropriate resuscitation steps in a patient with a large GI bleed. Immediately assess the patient for signs of a large bleed. Particular attention should be given to the pulse and blood pressure. If the blood pressure and pulse are normal, check orthostatic blood pressures and evaluate for symptoms when the patient sits up. Two large-bore catheters (16-gauge) should be placed peripherally or, if impossible, a central catheter should be placed (internal jugular approach is safer for coagulopathic patients). Give intravenous normal saline. Type and cross the patient for blood (packed RBCs). If the initial hematocrit is less than 30 or the patient is actively bleeding large volumes, begin urgent transfusion. A Foley catheter is helpful to monitor urine output. Watch closely for worsening coagulopathy. If coagulopathy is present, replace platelets and other blood components.

C. Learning objective: Use somatostatin as the first-choice pharmacologic intervention for esophageal variceal bleeding. This patient has an acute variceal bleed. The pharmacologic agent of choice is somatostatin, or its synthetic analog octreotide, which reduces splanchnic blood flow and has no systemic side effects. Vasopressin also reduces splanchnic blood flow, but up to half of treated patients may develop cardiovascular side effects. β-Blockers do not stop acute bleeding but are effective at preventing first-time variceal bleeds and rebleeding.

D. *Learning objective: Know when to use the appropriate interventions for variceal bleeding.* Endoscopic variceal ligation of bleeding varices has become the first-line endoscopic treatment for varices because of its good success rate (86% hemostasis) and low complication rate (2% to 3%). Sclerotherapy is also effective but has a higher complication rate (10% to 15%). In a recent meta-analysis comparing sclerotherapy with variceal ligation, ligation reduces rebleeding, mortality from bleeding, and overall mortality more than sclerotherapy. Balloon tamponade (Sengstaken-Blakemore tube or Minnesota tube) is not as effective as sclerotherapy or variceal ligation at controlling acute bleeding. Transjugular intrahepatic portosystemic shunt (TIPS) is effective at controlling bleeding but with a higher complication rate than variceal ligation.

HEADACHE

17-1.   **A.** *Learning objective: Diagnose migraine headaches based on history.* This young woman's unilateral throbbing headache, accompanied by nausea and phonophobia, is classic for migraine. No red flags are present.
B. *Learning objective: Imaging is not required for headache with benign history and examination.* Studies have shown that with a normal neurologic examination, and no red flags for an ominous cause, imaging (CT or MRI) is not necessary.
C. *Learning objective: Identify abortive treatment for migraine.* Given her infrequent symptoms, a nonsteroidal, such as naproxen (Naprosyn), is a reasonable choice at the first sign of headache. There may be gastroparesis, so consider adding a promotility agent, such as metoclopramide or cisapride. Warn the patient of overuse of analgesics and the propensity to cause withdrawal headaches. If she develops more severe symptoms that do not respond to the naproxen (e.g., unable to work for more than a day, vomiting,) consider a triptan. Before you prescribe a triptan, review risk for cardiovascular disease. In a young person, cardiovascular disease is unlikely.
D. *Learning objective: Recognize the importance of prophylactic treatment for frequent headaches.* With the increased frequency of her headaches, consider prophylactic treatment. Choices include β-blockers, low-dose tricyclic antidepressants, or calcium channel blockers.

17-2.   **A-B.** *Learning objective: Recognize and appropriately evaluate for SAH.* This man has a subarachnoid hemorrhage until completely proven otherwise. The sudden onset, association with weight lifting, and severity all point to this diagnosis. Although his CT scan is negative, there is still a 5% chance of a missed bleed. You must perform an LP to calculate for blood in the CSF.

HEALTHY PATIENTS

18-1.   **A.** *Learning objective: Know what preventive health counseling is appropriate for young healthy males.* The leading causes of death in this age-group are motor vehicle accidents and other unintentional injuries, homicide, suicide, malignant neoplasms, and heart disease. General screening considerations are height, weight, activity level, blood pressure, and assessment for substance abuse. Counseling is directed at injury prevention, such as seat belt use, motorcycle helmets, safe use of firearms; avoidance of the use of tobacco, excessive alcohol intake, and illicit drug use; safe sex practices; healthy diet and adequate physical activity; use of sunscreen protection; and good dental health.
B. *Learning objective: Identify key immunizations for this age-group.* Immunizations include tetanus, hepatitis B, and measles-mumps-rubella (MMR) if not previously immunized. Other interventions may be indicated if, by history, he is in a high-risk population.
C. *Learning objective: Recognize that prostate screening has no role in young men.* There is no indication for prostate cancer screening in this age-group.

18-2.   **A.** *Learning objective: Apply the model for change to this patient's process.* This young man is in stage 2, contemplation. Although he is discouraged, he is still contemplating trying again.

B. *Learning objective: Design an approach to help patient move through stages of change.* Focus questions on what barriers interfered with success on his last attempts. Work to increase motivation by helping him identify personal benefits of weight loss.

C. *Learning objective: Recognize and support the determination stage.* Now that he has determined to lose weight again, work on specific plans of action. Explore what medical and social supports are available to him. Readdress barriers and motivations. Make explicit plans for date to start and next followup appointments.

JOINT AND MUSCULAR PAIN

19-1.   **A.** *Learning objective: List common causes of diffuse muscle pain.* This is a classic presentation for fibromyalgia with sleep disruption and multiple tender points. It is important to rule out thyroid disease, which can cause myalgias and depression. PMR is unlikely in a woman her age. Myositis is a rare cause of muscle pain associated with weakness. Drugs (e.g., gemfibrozil and HMG-CoA reductase inhibitors) can cause myositis.

B. *Learning objective: Identify appropriate tests for workup of diffuse muscular pain.* Nothing in this patient's history or examination indicate an autoimmune process. Her examination and history are consistent with fibromyalgia. It is reasonable to obtain a TSH and, if she demonstrated muscle weakness, a CPK. An ANA is a very nonspecific test and would not be helpful in this clinical setting.

C. *Learning objective: Appropriately treat fibromyalgia.* Provided thyroid disease is adequately treated, prescribe exercise and low-dose tricyclic antidepressants for improved sleep.

19-2.   **A.** *Learning objective: Identify the main causes of shoulder pain.* Most likely this represents rotator cuff tendinitis with accompanying bursitis. Other causes to consider are thyroid disease, PMR, myositis, and malignancy, given weight loss and age.

B. *Learning objective: List appropriate workup for a patient with weight loss and shoulder pain.* Given her age and weight loss, obtain an x-ray to look for lytic lesions, an ESR to screen for atypical presentation of PMR, and a TSH. If weakness is present, obtain CPK as workup for myositis.

C. *Learning objective: List signs and symptoms of rotator cuff tear.* This patient's decreased active range of motion could indicate a tear. However, pain may limit her, so an injection of lidocaine for acute pain control with subsequent repeat strength testing is indicated. With the limitation of both active and passive ranges of motion, frozen shoulder is a possibility, as well.

LOW BACK PAIN

20-1.   **A.** *Learning objective: Design appropriate initial workup for acute back pain without red flags.* No further testing is required here. There are no red flags. His positive straight leg raise indicates nerve root involvement, such as mild disk herniation. Because the rest of his examination is normal, you can watch and wait.

B. *Learning objective: Design an appropriate conservative management plan for acute low back pain.* He should rest for a maximum of 3 days. He will be more comfortable with a pillow beneath his knees if he lies on his back. High-dose ibuprofen (800 mg tid) will decrease acute pain and inflammation. Physical therapy or chiropractic manipulation can also be offered but is not necessary.

C. *Learning objective: State the importance of early return to work, with restrictions.* He should return to work as soon as possible; however, he will need light duty. By the guidelines in the chapter, he should not lift anything heavier than 20 pounds. He needs instruction in proper lifting techniques.

D. *Learning objective: State the expected recovery time for low back pain.* He should be back to normal in 4 weeks if he responds appropriately to conservative management measures.

20-2.   **A.** *Learning objective: Identify red flags for pathologic causes of low back pain.* Her red flags are age, diabetes, and UTIs (recurrent bacterial infections put her at risk for osteomyelitis). Her gardening probably does not qualify as mild trauma.

B. *Learning objective: Order appropriate tests for patients at risk for serious causes of low back pain.* Start with an x-ray of her lumbosacral spine and an ESR. This will screen for cancer, osteomyelitis, and fracture. If she has symptoms of urinary tract infection or fevers or chills, you could add a urinalysis and CBC.

C. *Learning objective: Distinguish peripheral neuropathy examination findings from radicular findings.* Her distal numbness is consistent with diabetic neuropathy—this is stocking-glove in distribution, not dermatomal. Her straight leg test does not cause radicular pain; it only causes low back pain and so is not positive (does not indicate nerve root tension/disk disease). If her x-ray and ESR are normal, her diagnosis is acute low back pain.

LOWER EXTREMITY PAIN, SWELLING, AND ULCERS

21-1.   **A.** *Learning objective: Recognize that a palpable peripheral pulse rules out significant peripheral vascular disease.* Her ABI is greater than 0.9 (= 130/140). The ABI does not usually need to be measured in someone with a palpable peripheral pulse. It will not provide you with any more information. The dorsalis pedis pulse is nonpalpable in 8% of people without clinical disease.

B. *Learning objective: Recognize a neuropathic ulcer in a diabetic patient.* She has a neuropathic ulcer at a pressure point on an insensate foot. Her ulcer will never heal as long as she is ambulating, regardless of other topical therapies. Her examination does not support venous insufficiency (location of ulcer and the absence of edema, superficial varicosities, or dermatitis). It is not an ischemic ulcer given her palpable peripheral pulse, ABI greater than 0.9, and lack of physical findings (no dependent rubor, delayed capillary refill, or loss of hair growth).

C. *Learning objective: State the appropriate treatment and prevention for a neuropathic ulcer.* Refer to a foot clinic or orthopedic surgeon who has experience with total-contact casts. The cast is removed weekly to monitor ulcer healing. The other option is a trial of non–weight bearing with crutches; most people are unable to do this consistently enough for healing to occur. Even with only very occasional weight bearing, the ulcer is unlikely to heal. She also needs education about proper foot care: inspect feet daily, wear shoes that are well cushioned and have a wide toe box, lubricate feet to prevent fissures/cracks, recognize and treat tinea, avoid going barefoot, and trim toenails properly. Regular foot clinic visits may help.

21-2.   A. *Learning objective: List and differenti-ate the presentation of common causes of acute unilateral lower extremity swelling.* She has either a DVT or a ruptured Baker's cyst. Cellulitis is unlikely, given the lack of erythema. A superficial thrombophlebitis is more localized and does not cause extensive edema. She has no history of trauma, making a hematoma an unlikely cause.

B. *Learning objective: Exclude a DVT with appropriate testing in patients with acute unilateral lower extremity edema.* Because the potential consequence of not treating a DVT can be catastrophic, rule this out first. The test of choice is a duplex ultrasound. Though her history and knee effusion suggest Baker's cyst, it is possible that she has both a DVT and a Baker's cyst.

LYMPHADENOPATHY

22-1.   A. *Learning objective: Recognize that atypical presentations of common diseases are more likely than rare diseases.* Differential diagnosis includes infectious mononucleosis, resolving pharyngitis, branchial cleft cyst, sarcoidosis, Hodgkin's disease, non-Hodgkin's lymphoma, scrofula, and toxoplasmosis. Remember that in a healthy young patient with no other symptoms or signs, cervical adenopathy is most often EBV mononucleosis or pharyngitis. A single large node can also be a cluster of several smaller nodes that become apparent as they shrink.

B. *Learning objective: Order the appropriate test for cervical adenopathy in a young patient.* Initial testing should include CBC with differential, Monospot, and chest radiograph. If the chest film shows hilar adenopathy, then sarcoidosis or Hodgkin's becomes the likely diagnosis.

C. *Learning objective: Provide appropriate followup for cervical lymphadenopathy.* The Monospot is negative in approximately 10% of adults with infectious mononucleosis. His few days out of work support the diagnosis of mononucleosis or another viral illness. If the CBC and chest film are normal and the Monospot is negative, call the patient. If the patient is still sick, have him return to recheck the Monospot, review HIV risk factors, and consider HIV viral load. Have him return in 1 month to reexamine him. If his nodes are resolving, he may follow up as needed. Some physicians would include PPD testing, even in those with no risk factors for TB.

22-2.   A. *Learning objective: Always consider cancer in an older adult with lymph-adenopathy and refer appropriately.* The differential is very different in an older adult patient: cancers of the head and neck are far more likely. In the absence of an alternative cause and with the history of tobacco and alcohol, both strong risk factors for head and neck malignancies, this patient has cancer until proven otherwise. Early referral to an otolaryngologist would be wise.

B. *Learning objective: Select appropriate biopsy technique for cervical lymph-adenopathy.* Excisional biopsy of nodes in the neck is not appropriate if cancer is suspected. FNA or needle biopsy is preferred. Excisional biopsy may cause tumor contamination of local tissue.

COMMON CARDIAC ARRHYTHMIAS

23-1.   A-B. *Learning objective: Recognize and treat atrial fibrillation.* Rhythm strip shows atrial fibrillation, a common arrhythmia especially in the setting of congestive heart failure. Because of rapid rate and absence of atrial contraction, the left ventricle does not fill well during diastole. This results in a decreased cardiac output, which may cause fatigue and shortness of breath with activity. Treat rapid ventricular rate with a β-blocker or calcium channel blocker. Anticoagulate patients without contraindications.

23-2.   A-B. *Learning objective: Recognize and treat ventricular tachycardia.* ECG rhythm is fast and QRS is wide, that is, a ventricular tachycardia. This is potentially lethal and often occurs in the setting of myocardial infarction. Treat with immediate cardioversion and an antiarrhythmic drug, such as lidocaine or amiodarone. Quick treatment is the key to patient survival. EXTRA CREDIT: This rhythm strip demonstrates a particular type of VT called torsades de pointes, wide QRS complexes of changing amplitude that twist about the isoelectric line. This type of VT is often treated with IV magnesium.

CONGESTIVE HEART FAILURE

23-3. **A.** *Learning objective: State common symptoms and signs of CHF.* His presentation is explained by an MI during his "bad episode" of angina with ensuing CHF. Ask about orthopnea (how many pillows he needs, and if this has changed recently), PND, and prior edema. Quantify exercise capacity and ask about other reasons for shortness of breath. Has he had heart failure before? Ask about weight, diet, and cardiac risk factors. Check vital signs; weight; JVP; PMI; heaves; heart sounds; lung examination for rales, wheezes, or dullness (effusions), abdominal bruits or abdominojugular reflux; and extremities for cyanosis, clubbing, edema, and perfusion.

B. *Learning objective: Design appropriate workup for new-onset CHF.* He should have a CBC, chemistry panel, ECG, oxygen saturation, chest x-ray, and an echocardiogram. Enzymes are unlikely to be helpful, given his history of symptoms 2 weeks ago. He likely will need LV catheterization to assess his need for intervention, such as angioplasty or CABG.

C. *Learning objective: Start therapy for mild CHF.* This patient has mild CHF with new-onset edema, indicating volume overload. Start an ACEI (e.g., enalapril 5 mg PO bid) and furosemide 10 to 20 mg PO qam. Check creatinine and potassium in 3 to 7 days and see him weekly until stable or asymptomatic. He may be able to stop furosemide when stable. A β-blocker is indicated for ischemic heart disease and CHF once he is stable.

23-4. **A.** *Learning objective: Recognize right-sided CHF.* He has RV heart failure based on an elevated JVP, RV S_3 gallop, positive abdominojugular reflux, and peripheral edema.

B. *Learning objective: State common causes of right heart failure.* Although the most common cause of RV failure is LV failure, his daytime somnolence and excessive weight suggest sleep apnea. Hypoxemia during apneic periods in sleep apnea causes pulmonary hypertension, cor pulmonale (RV enlargement), and eventual RV failure. Other causes of RV failure include severe pulmonary disease, as from COPD.

ISCHEMIC HEART DISEASE

23-5. **A.** *Learning objective: Identify a history suggestive of chronic angina.* Exertional chest pain, relieved by rest, is typical for angina. Making angina more likely are his risk factors: age, gender, smoking history, hypertension, and hyperlipidemia. Finally, stress test reproduced symptoms and demonstrated inferior ST depression, consistent with ischemia.

B. *Learning objective: Design and interpret work-up for ischemic heart disease.* Not much additional testing is necessary. History, risk factors, and ETT all strongly support a clinical diagnosis of angina. It is worthwhile reviewing his ETT to look for poor BP response, early ECG changes, ECG changes involving more than 5 leads, and changes lasting longer than 5 minutes into recovery to indicate multivessel disease or LV dysfunction. A fasting lipid panel will guide drug therapy for hyperlipidemia.

C. *Learning objective: Design appropriate medical management for angina.* Medical therapy without further invasive workup is appropriate. A reasonable regimen is to start a long-acting nitrate (e.g., nitroglycerin patch) and sublingual nitroglycerin for use during episodes of pain. Treat hypertension. Although the long-acting nitrate may improve hypertension, this alone is unlikely to provide adequate control. A reasonable antihypertensive agent is a β-blocker, especially because his resting heart rate is moderately elevated. Finally, depending on his lipid profile, lipid-lowering therapy may be appropriate.

D. *Learning objective: Counsel patients who have ischemic heart disease about risk factor modification.* Counsel about smoking cessation and encourage him to enroll in a program. In addition, explore dietary habits and counsel about a low-fat, low-cholesterol diet.

23-6.   **A. *Learning objective: Recognize unstable angina.*** Although her chest pain could have a benign cause (such as esophageal pain), her known CAD, the response to nitrates, and the anterior ischemic changes on ECG all suggest myocardial ischemia. Anginal pain occurring at increased frequency and at rest gives her a diagnosis of unstable angina.

B. *Learning objective: Design appropriate and immediate intervention for unstable angina.* Immediate interventions are directed at improving myocardial oxygen delivery and inhibiting thrombosis. Give supplemental oxygen by nasal cannula. Nitrates to improve coronary artery blood flow could be administered topically but in this case are probably best given IV to rapidly titrate up to the desired effect. Antithrombotic therapy should include aspirin 160 to 325 mg, chewed, and heparin, either standard unfractionated IV heparin with PTT monitoring or low-molecular-weight heparin administered subcutaneously. Morphine is also useful acutely in alleviating pain, because of both its central effects and its venodilating effects, which reduce preload.

C. *Learning objective: Appropriately use stress-testing to risk-stratify patients with ischemic symptoms.* She needs a risk-stratifying test with her recent episode of unstable angina. The question is whether this should be an invasive or noninvasive test. In the current case, most people would probably recommend coronary angiography because this patient appears to have a large area of myocardium at risk. Four years ago she had an inferior area of ischemia. Now she presents with an unstable anterior area of ischemia, suggesting at least two-vessel disease. If her coronary anatomy shows three-vessel disease, revascularization is indicated for its survival benefit. Having said this, not all patients with unstable angina require angiography. Lower-risk patients who respond appropriately to medical therapy may be risk-stratified noninvasively.

23-7.   **A. *Learning objective: Recognize MI with associated poor LV function.*** Acute crushing substernal pain associated with large anterior ST elevations suggests acute anterior MI. Moreover, his vital signs, examination, and chest x-ray suggest significant compromise of LV function.

B. *Learning objective: Design appropriate treatment for acute MI.* As with the second case, immediately give oxygen and aspirin. Give nitrates and morphine to relieve pain, but be careful to avoid hypotension because BP is marginally low already. Quickly assess for contraindications to thrombolytics. If no contraindications are present, this patient is a candidate for thrombolysis with chest pain for less than 12 hours and ST segment elevation in 2 or more contiguous leads. If streptokinase is used, heparin is not necessary because of the prolonged lytic state associated with this drug. Use heparin if TPA is used for thrombolysis.

C. *Learning objective: State the differential for acute pulmonary edema after MI.* The patient now has acute pulmonary edema 4 days after anterior MI, as well as a new systolic murmur. In this case, the differential diagnosis includes arrhythmia, extension of his myocardial infarction, contained cardiac rupture, acute mitral regurgitation (MR), or ventricular septal defect (VSD). ECG rules out arrhythmia. The lack of new ECG changes, lack of pain, and new murmur make extension of infarction less likely, although it is reasonable to draw repeat cardiac enzyme. Contained rupture is a possibility but is unlikely simply because most people with this condition present with hypotension and cardiac arrest. More likely with acute pulmonary edema and systolic murmur after large anterior MI is either acute MR or VSD. Acute MR can be due either to papillary muscle ischemia or rupture. Although acute MR is more common after inferior MI, anterior MI is also associated with this condition. Acute VSD occurs with septal MI and full-thickness necrosis of an area of septum, creating an opening between the left and right ventricles.

D. Learning objective: Design appropriate testing for a patient with new murmur and pulmonary edema after MI. Based on the differential diagnosis listed above, indicated tests include ECG, chest x-ray (confirm pulmonary edema), and echocardiogram to look for VSD or acute MR. If echo is not immediately available, pulmonary artery (PA) catheterization is a useful alternative. Specifically, in the setting of acute MR, large V waves seen in the wedge pressure tracing are suggestive. In addition, PA catheter reveals an "oxygen step-up" in mixed venous blood with VSD. To do this test, draw simultaneous blood gases from the distal and proximal ports of the PA catheter. If oxygenated, LV blood is passing directly through the VSD into the RV, the distal blood gas from the pulmonary artery will reveal a significant increase in oxygen saturation compared with the proximal gas from the superior vena cava. In the current case, ECG reveals no changes, chest x-ray reveals acute pulmonary edema, and echocardiogram shows acute mitral regurgitation.

E. Learning objective: Treat acute mitral regurgitation in the setting of MI. The treatment of acute MR includes medical stabilization followed by either revascularization and/or surgical repair of the valve. Lower both preload with IV nitroglycerin and afterload with IV nitroprusside. Decreasing afterload directs more of the cardiac output toward the aortic outflow tract and lowers regurgitant volume. Diuretics are useful if BP allows. In centers with the capability, intraaortic balloon counterpulsation pumping is useful. This balloon inflates during diastole and deflates during systole, decreasing afterload and improving coronary blood flow during diastole. If MR is due to papillary muscle ischemia, revascularization is usually attempted with PTCA. Although this can be successful, many patients still require surgical repair of the valve, even if good coronary flow is reestablished.

VALVULAR HEART DISEASE

23-8. **A. Learning objective: Recognize rheumatic fever as the main cause of multiple valvular disease.** Rheumatic heart disease causes AS, AR, and MS, all consistent with this patient's examination findings.

B. Learning objective: Design an appropriate initial workup for a patient with symptoms of valvular disease. Use an aggressive diagnostic approach because she is symptomatic and has a diastolic murmur. Obtain ECG to document atrial fibrillation, chest x-ray to look for pulmonary congestion, and echo to visualize valves; grade severity of disease by valve area and gradient; and estimate LV function.

C. Learning objective: Appropriately treat the complications of valvular disease, and refer to a cardiologist. Treat atrial fibrillation with rate control agents (e.g., digoxin or β-blocker), and anticoagulate with warfarin. Treat orthopnea and heart failure with gentle diuresis (e.g., furosemide). Do not use an ACE inhibitor because she has aortic stenosis. Refer to cardiology for consideration of valve replacement and/or valvuloplasty.

D. Learning objective: Remember to offer antibiotic prophylaxis for dental procedures. She should receive 2 g of amoxicillin PO 1 hour before the extraction. Her dentist should be involved in the management of her anticoagulation.

23-9.   **A. *Learning objective: Recognize aortic dissection, a life-threatening cause of valvular disease.*** Ask him *not* to infuse the streptokinase! This patient may meet the criteria for thrombolytics, but he also has a contraindication: possible aortic dissection. Patients with dissection may look like they are having a heart attack and may even have ST elevations on ECG. However, thrombolytics will cause potentially fatal hemorrhage in patients with aortic dissection, making this condition an absolute contraindication to thrombolytic therapy. Patients with chest or throat pain and diastolic murmur require rapid assessment to look for aortic dissection, causing acute aortic regurgitation.

B. *Learning objective: Appropriately manage acute aortic regurgitation caused by aortic dissection.* Assess the ABCs (airway, breathing, circulation). Start cardiac monitoring and oxygen, and place 2 large-bore IV lines. Get a chest x-ray, and support vital signs as needed. Give fluids or blood products for hypotension. The IV β-blocker esmolol and IV vasodilator sodium nitroprusside are useful short-acting agents to treat hypertension and tachycardia because they can be quickly turned off if conditions change. Consult cardiology and cardiothoracic surgery to decide on the preferred imaging study (transesophageal echocardiogram, aortography, or chest CT). Use morphine for pain and anxiety.

DERMATOLOGY

24-1.   **A. *Learning objective: Recognize eczema and its typical distribution pattern.*** This is a typical presentation of eczema. Some clues: young age, history of another "atopic" condition such as asthma, and distribution of the rash on the flexor surfaces of her arms.

B. *Learning objective: Recognize secondary infection of an excoriated rash.* The yellow crusting is concerning for secondary bacterial infection. The appearance is similar to the "honey-crusting" seen with impetigo. Impetigo is usually caused by common skin flora, such as staphylococcal or streptococcal species.

C. *Learning objective: Design treatment for eczema with secondary bacterial infection.* The patient should first receive an antibiotic with activity against skin flora, such as cephalexin. Antihistamines may be added, especially at night, to minimize scratching. Keep fingernails short. Once the infection has cleared, treat with a medium-potency topical steroid with liberal application of a lanolin-free moisturizer.

24-2.   **A. *Learning objective: Recognize the typical presentation of herpes zoster.*** This is a very typical presentation of herpes zoster. Clues are the patient's older age, the painful prodrome of the rash, and the rash's characteristic dermatomal distribution.

B. *Learning objective: Recognize the efficacy of antiviral therapy in the acute treatment of zoster.* Start oral acyclovir, famciclovir, or valacyclovir to speed healing and to shorten the course of postherpetic neuralgia should it occur. Antivirals are more effective the sooner they are given. Efficacy if given more than 72 hours after the onset of symptoms has never been proven.

C. *Learning objective: Recognize the risk of corneal involvement in facial zoster.* Because he has forehead lesions, get an urgent ophthalmology evaluation to rule out corneal involvement. If there are early signs of corneal lesions on careful examination, start immediate high-dose IV acyclovir to prevent corneal scarring and blindness.

24-3.   **A. *Learning objective: State the features of a suspicious mole.*** In addition to noting the lesion's asymmetry, flatness, and size, ask whether the lesion has been itching or bleeding, and note color variation. Examine the rest of the skin and regional lymph nodes.

B. *Learning objective: Recognize a mole highly suspicious for melanoma.* The primary concern is for malignant melanoma. Whenever a patient notes growth of a pigmented lesion, especially with asymmetric borders, suspicion for melanoma should be high.

C. *Learning objective: Design appropriate diagnostic evaluation of a highly suspicious mole.* Given the high clinical suspicion for melanoma, the most appropriate initial procedure should be definitive excision because there is a theoretic risk that a punch biopsy through the lesion might increase the risk of metastasis.

ADRENAL DISORDERS

25-1.   **A.** *Learning objective: Recognize the presentation of acute adrenal crisis.* Differential diagnosis includes adrenal crisis, hypoxia, bleeding, myocardial infarction, and sepsis. History of COPD suggests steroid dependence with resulting adrenal suppression. He may not have received stress-dose steroids before surgery. Hypotension unresponsive to saline challenge is a common finding in adrenal crisis. This patient is in adrenal crisis.

B. *Learning objective: Design a workup that includes screening for adrenal insufficiency in hypotensive patients with risk factors for adrenal insufficiency.* Obtain serum cortisol immediately, before treatment. Do not wait for results to begin treatment. A single dose of steroids will not worsen outcome if the patient turns out to have sepsis instead. A cortisol less than 20 μg/dl is diagnostic. To rule out hypoxia, infection, acute MI, and bleeding, obtain ABG, blood cultures, CBC, serial hematocrits, urinalysis, basic chemistry, chest film, and ECG.

C. *Learning objective: Appropriately treat adrenal crisis with high-dose hydrocortisone.* Treat emergently with hydrocortisone 100 mg IV q6h, volume repletion with glucose and IV saline, and other supportive measures as needed. Empiric antibiotics may be warranted while culture results and cortisol level are pending.

DIABETES

25-2.   **A.** *Learning objective: Recognize the presentation of type 1 diabetes.* His random glucose of greater than 200 with symptoms of polydipsia, polyuria, and weight loss confirms diabetes. Based on age, normal weight, and urine ketones, he has type 1 diabetes. Although more common in persons under age 30, type 1 diabetes can occur at any age. His family history (obesity, type 2 diabetes) does *not* increase his risk for type 1 diabetes. For older patients, islet cell antibodies confirm the diagnosis of type 1 diabetes.

B. *Learning objective: Design initial insulin therapy.* Start insulin dose at the lower end of the dosing range (0.5 U/kg/day) because he is slender, young, and has type 1 diabetes. Convert 150 pounds to 70 kg. Then multiply 70 kg by 0.5 U/kg/day to get a total daily dose of 35 U—round up to 36 for a number easily divisible by 3. Give two thirds of this dose in the morning (24 U) and one third in the evening (12 U). To further break down this morning dose, you will want to give NPH and regular in a ratio of 2:1, i.e., 16 NPH and 8 regular. For the evening insulin, give equal parts NPH and regular i.e., 6 U of each. The evening dose of regular should be given before dinner to cover the meal, and the NPH should be given at bedtime so its peak coincides with morning cortisol and glucose surges. Occasionally, even the lower range of dosing is too much insulin for slender patients with type 1 diabetes, so monitor these patients closely. Have patients check glucose 4 times daily, qac and qhs (i.e., before meals and at bedtime). Goals are a fasting glucose of 80 to 120 and a glycated hemoglobin of 7%. Consider extra insulin dosing before lunch and snacks in patients with type 1 diabetes to mimic physiologic insulin secretion and futher delay end-organ complications.

C. *Learning objective: Order appropriate screening tests in a patient newly diagnosed with type 1 diabetes.* Order fasting lipid panel and TSH. Start annual urine microalbumin testing after 5 years. He does not need eye examination for 5 years because he has type 1 diabetes and is younger than age 30.

25-3. **A.** *Learning objective: List the diagnostic criteria for type 2 diabetes.* He probably has type 2 diabetes based on a random glucose greater than 200 plus symptoms of nocturia and fatigue, obesity, and acanthosis nigricans (consistent with insulin resistance). He also has an elevated blood pressure. His paresthesias and sensory loss, consistent with diabetic neuropathy, suggest that he has had diabetes for some time. His neuropathy and foot deformity (hammertoes resulting from sensory loss) place him at moderate risk for foot ulcers.

B. *Learning objective: Counsel a patient with type 2 diabetes about treatment and order appropriate initial screening tests.* Initial treatment is with diet, referral to a nutritionist, and exercise; consider an exercise treadmill before he embarks on exercise, given family history. He should return with serial blood pressure and glucose measurements after a 4- to 6-week trial. Given random glucose of 240 plus symptoms, he may need an oral agent (250 mg/dl is a reasonable cutoff for diet and exercise alone). If he has significant microalbuminuria or hypertension, start an ACEI (e.g., benazepril 5 mg PO qd). Counsel about risk of foot problems and the need for well-fitted shoes. Capsaicin cream, applied bid or tid, may relieve paresthesias. Obtain glycated hemoglobin, fasting lipid panel, TSH, ECG, microalbuminuria, and a dilated eye examination.

C. *Learning objective: Choose an appropriate oral agent for a patient with type 2 diabetes.* Because of his obesity and evidence of insulin resistance, metformin is the drug of choice. Start with 500 mg PO bid and titrate up to good control or maximum dose of 850 mg PO tid over several weeks. Warn about GI side effects, which can affect compliance.

HYPERLIPIDEMIA

25-4. **A.** *Learning objective: Identify goal cholesterol.* This woman has a single cardiovascular risk factor, hypertension. Her goal LDL cholesterol is less than 160. This is primary prevention.

B. *Learning objective: Treat secondary causes of high cholesterol before starting lipid-lowering medication.* LDL of 215 is above 190, the threshold for starting drug therapy. She has appropriately had a diet trial. However, her hypothyroidism may be elevating cholesterol and triglycerides. Try thyroid replacement therapy, and recheck a fasting lipid panel in 3 to 4 months. At that point, if LDL is still greater than 190, estrogen is a good choice.

25-5. **A-B.** *Learning objective: Design cholesterol management for a patient with known CAD.* She has known coronary heart disease, so treatment goal is less than 100. Any statin is a good choice for lowering LDL. First increase the dose of her pravastatin to 40 mg and ask her to take it at night because it is more effective then. Recheck fasting lipid panel in 3 months. If she needs a second cholesterol-lowering medicine, niacin is reasonable. Also review diet and exercise.

25-6. *Learning objective: Manage cholesterol in known CAD.* He has coronary heart disease. Although at first glance his fasting lipid panel values do not seem too bad, the goal is LDL lower than 100. He has demonstrated significant lifestyle changes with smoking cessation and exercise. Instruct him in a Step 1 diet and refer to a nutritionist. Recheck fasting lipid panel in 3 to 6 months. Although high-dose β-blockers can increase cholesterol, post-MI patients benefit from this class of drugs substantially; there is no need to change his low-dose β-blocker.

THYROID DISEASE

25-7.

A. Learning objective: Recognize apathetic hyperthyroidism in an elderly patient. Weight loss with anorexia, proximal muscle weakness (as evidenced by his difficulty with stairs), and an atrial arrhythmia are classic signs of apathetic hyperthyroidism in an older person. If TFTs are normal, rule out depression or occult malignancy. He also needs treatment for atrial fibrillation.

B. Learning objective: Interpret thyroid function tests and identify the most likely cause of hyperthyroidism based on features of the clinical setting. This patient has a suppressed TSH and elevated free T_4, consistent with his clinical hyperthyroidism. Toxic multinodular goiter is suggested by his lumpy thyroid examination and is common in the elderly. Acute thyroiditis is unlikely because the thyroid is not tender. Graves' disease usually presents in younger women so is less likely here.

C. Learning objective: Describe treatment of toxic multinodular goiter. Initially, start methimazole or propylthiouracil (PTU). Once he is euthyroid, radioactive iodine ablation can be performed. Propranolol may control his heart rate while antithyroid medication takes effect. Propranolol should be used during radioactive iodine ablation to avoid thyrotoxicosis from gland destruction.

25-8.

A. Learning objective: Recognize myxedema coma and list other common problems in the differential. Differential includes MI, infection, hypothyroid myxedema coma, stroke, metabolic derangement (hyponatremia or hypernatremia, hypercalcemia), depressant drug overdose, and alcohol ingestion.

B. Learning objective: Recognize and name seven features of myxedema coma. Elevated TSH, low free T_4, depressed mental status, hypothermia, bradycardia, hypoventilation, macroglossia, cool dry doughy skin, constipation, congestive heart failure, and pericardial effusion are all classic for myxedema coma, a potentially fatal condition.

C. Learning objective: Describe medications and supportive therapies for myxedema coma. Give IV levothyroxine and high-dose glucocorticoids for life-threatening myxedema coma. Additionally, she needs intensive supportive care. Her respiratory status is in jeopardy: hypoventilation and aspiration risk resulting from somnolence warrants ABG and intubation. Even with clinical response to medical therapy, some patients require prolonged ventilatory support, presumably because of accompanying, slow-to-resolve respiratory muscle weakness. Cardiac status is also worrisome (bradycardia, CHF, and probable pericardial effusion). Pericardial effusion in hypothyroidism usually develops slowly, does not lead to tamponade, and often responds to medical therapy without requiring urgent pericardiocentesis. For hypothermia, gentle rewarming is usually sufficient. Myxedema coma is often precipitated by infection, so look for this with examination, blood, urine, and sputum cultures and begin antibiotics if indicated.

D. Learning objective: Describe laboratory abnormalities associated with hypothyroidism. CPK, SGOT, LDH, and cholesterol can all be elevated and usually normalize with levothyroxine. Hematocrit and sodium may be low.

E. Learning objective: List the likely causes of hypothyroidism. Radioiodine ablation for Graves' disease is the most common cause of hypothyroidism. In this case, she may not have been taking prescribed thyroxine. Hashimoto's thyroiditis is also common. If this is the case, her symptoms could have developed insidiously or perhaps were attributed to old age. Because she lives in the United States, where salt is supplemented with iodine, and there was no mention of a goiter on her examination, iodine insufficiency is unlikely.

BILIARY TRACT DISEASE

26-1.   A. *Learning objective: Identify key history, examination, and laboratory tests that help narrow your differential diagnosis in a woman with right upper quadrant pain.* Has she had this before (gallstones, peptic ulcer)? How much alcohol does she use (pancreatitis)? Is she having unprotected sex, traveling, or using IV drugs (hepatitis)? Has she had recent dysuria, hematuria, frequency, or flank or back pain (pyelonephritis)? Has she had any changes in her bowel habits (gastroenteritis, bowel obstruction)? Has the stool been abnormally colored (melena suggests peptic ulcer, pale stools suggest common bile duct obstruction)? Examine for signs of sepsis with orthostatic vital signs, for signs of retroperitoneal hemorrhage suggesting pancreatitis, for jaundice suggesting hepatitis or cholangitis, and for peritoneal signs (perforated viscus). CBC looks for signs of infection. Electrolytes may show an acidosis from sepsis or bowel perforation. Bilirubin and alkaline phosphatase look for biliary obstruction. SGOT and SGPT look for hepatocyte inflammation. Amylase and lipase evaluate for pancreatitis. Abdominal films look for free air or bowel obstruction. Urgent abdominal ultrasound or CT scan looks for evidence of biliary tree obstruction, cholecystitis, or gallstones. In her case, CBC, alkaline phosphatase, and bilirubin are high.

B. *Learning objective: Identify three potentially life-threatening conditions that cause right upper quadrant pain.* You would not want to miss a perforated ulcer, ascending cholangitis, or pancreatitis because these can rapidly worsen and are potentially fatal.

C. *Learning objective: Appropriately triage a patient with possible ascending cholangitis and sepsis to intensive care.* This patient is very ill. High pulse and low blood pressure (especially low relative to her usual hypertension) are worrisome indicators of sepsis. Respiratory rate is high, increasing concern for sepsis, acidosis, and a compensatory respiratory alkalosis. She needs inpatient intensive care for resuscitation, rapid diagnosis, and treatment.

D. *Learning objective: Recognize potentially lethal cholangitis, and appropriately treat with urgent ERCP and empiric antibiotics.* RUQ pain and signs of early sepsis make cholangitis possible. She needs urgent GI consult for ERCP. Start empiric IV antibiotics. Ampicillin/sulbactam or other β-lactam/β-lactamase inhibitor is more cost-effective than any three-drug therapy. Give IV fluids and monitor closely because her condition may quickly deteriorate.

LIVER DISEASE

26-2.   A. *Learning objective: State the differential diagnosis for jaundice.* The differential includes viral, alcoholic, autoimmune, and drug-induced hepatitis. Biliary obstruction resulting from gallstones or neoplasm is also possible. Hereditary causes of liver disease are not likely in this patient because of the acute onset and the patient's older age.

B. *Learning objective: Order appropriate laboratory studies in a jaundiced patient.* Given jaundice, order ALT, AST, bilirubin, albumin, PTT, PT INR, and alkaline phosphatase. If transaminases are elevated to a greater degree than bilirubin and alkaline phosphatase, order hepatitis A, B, and C serologies. If bilirubin and alkaline phosphatase are more elevated, consider imaging to rule out biliary obstruction.

C. *Learning objective: Ask a thorough history to look for potential exposures as the cause of an acute hepatitis.* Quantitate alcohol intake. Ask about potential toxic exposures and medications, including over-the-counter remedies. This patient had elevated aminotransferases and a bilirubin of 10.2. Hepatitis serology studies were normal except for HAV IgG (indicating old infection). A careful review of his medical history revealed that he had been recently hospitalized with an inferior myocardial infarction and had been discharged on trazodone to help with sleep, a possible cause of drug-induced hepatitis. Withdrawal of trazodone resulted in resolution of his symptoms and normalization of bilirubin and aminotransferases.

26-3. **A. Learning objective: Recognize potential chronic hepatitis, and order appropriate laboratory tests.** This patient has risk factors for hepatitis C with IV drug and alcohol use. Liver function tests are warranted. With elevated transaminases and a normal bilirubin, viral serologies are also appropriate. In her case, HCV antibody and PCR are positive, albumin is 3, and PT INR is 1.8.

B. Learning objective: Recognize the importance of liver biopsy in the evaluation of a person with hepatitis C infection. This patient has evidence of chronic hepatitis C and borderline hepatic synthetic function with a decreased albumin and an elevated INR. Liver biopsy is the gold standard for assessing the severity of her disease. Aminotransferase levels do not reflect the severity of hepatic injury. Biopsy shows bridging and multilobular necrosis.

C. Learning objective: State the treatment options for severe hepatic injury from hepatitis C. This patient has evidence of severe liver injury with bridging and multilobular necrosis. The injury is probably accelerated because of her alcohol ingestion. Advise her to abstain from all alcohol. Not only will this slow progression of her disease but it will help to provide her with treatment options. This patient has all three criteria for α-interferon treatment: elevated ALT, detectable HCV RNA, and evidence of bridging or portal necrosis. However, most hepatologists will not give interferon if patients continue to drink alcohol, and she will not be considered for liver transplant until she abstains from drinking alcohol for 6 months.

PANCREATITIS

26-4. **A. Learning objective: List three disorders in which abdominal pain can radiate to the back.** Pancreatitis, abdominal aortic aneurysm, pyelonephritis, osteomyelitis, and epidural abscess all can cause back pain in association with abdominal pain.

B. Learning objective: Identify key features of the clinical presentation that help differentiate causes of abdominal pain radiating to the back. Pancreatitis is likely with long-standing use of alcohol. Young age makes abdominal aortic aneurysm (AAA) unlikely even though he smokes. Check for other risk factors of AAA, including hypercholesterolemia, hypertension, or signs of other vascular disease, such as carotid bruits or diminished pulses. He does not have a chronic bladder catheter, prostatic enlargement with bladder obstruction, or history of urinary tract stones or symptoms to put him at risk for pyelonephritis. He lacks TB exposure or IV drug use to place him at risk for vertebral or epidural infection.

C. Learning objective: Order appropriate laboratory tests to diagnose pancreatitis and assess prognosis. Amylase and lipase are sensitive and specific for pancreatitis. Assess prognosis using Ranson's criteria. He has three criteria: WBC greater than 16,000, SGOT greater than 250, and glucose greater than 200. Follow hematocrit, fluid requirement, calcium, BUN, and PaO_2 in the first 48 hours to assess all criteria.

D. Learning objective: Design appropriate therapy for acute pancreatitis. Order bowel rest, pain control, and NG tube suction to decrease emesis. IV meperidine may be better for pain control than morphine to avoid sphincter of Oddi spasm, although no evidence suggests a difference in outcome. If orthostatic, give normal saline boluses and recheck. Add dextrose to IV fluids for basal energy needs because he is not eating. If his illness persists, requiring prolonged bowel rest, start parenteral nutrition. He needs close monitoring for complications.

GERIATRICS

27-1. **A. *Learning objective: Recognize a drug-related cognitive impairment, and adjust medications to confirm diagnosis.*** Drugs and depression are the most common causes of reversible cognitive impairment, and although this patient may well have coexisting dementia, the next step in her evaluation should be to adjust her medications and reassess. All three of her medications are potentially implicated: clonidine is a centrally acting agent that can affect mentation, NSAIDs (ibuprofen) and Tylenol PM (a common over-the-counter sleeping pill containing diphenhydramine) both can impair cognition.

B. *Learning objective: Obtain full dementia workup when impairments only partially reverse with medication adjustments.* Patient age and history are most consistent with Alzheimer's, but proper evaluation includes appropriate laboratory work and imaging studies as per text.

C. *Learning objective: Recognize the likely diagnosis of Alzheimer's disease, and state available treatments.* Consider pharmacologic treatment with acetylcholinesterase inhibitors ± vitamin E and/or *Ginkgo biloba* along with support and education for the patient and family.

27-2. **A. *Learning objective: Recognize history consistent with urge incontinence, and design appropriate workup.*** History is most consistent with urge incontinence. Causes are either due to local processes (detrusor instability) or failure of CNS inhibition (detrusor hyperreflexia). He has no history or examination findings to suggest the latter. Proper evaluation should proceed with urinalysis, laboratory tests, and PVR as per text and Figure 27-2.

B. *Learning objective: Recognize BPH as a likely cause of this patient's urge incontinence.* The patient has no signs of prostate infection or cancer, urinary tract infection, or hematuria to suggest bladder tumor or stones. His constellation of symptoms (urgency, frequency, decreased stream) and findings (soft, enlarged nontender prostate) is most likely due to BPH.

C. *Learning objective: State that in the absence of surgical indications, patient preferences should drive treatment for BPH symptoms.* The patient could reasonably prefer watchful waiting, although given his incontinence, this seems unlikely. In this man with an enlarged prostate a trial of either an α-blocker or finasteride is reasonable. Although the former will improve his symptoms more quickly, the latter will decrease his long-term chances of developing retention or needing surgery. If urge incontinence persists, low doses of anticholinergic antispasmodics may be helpful, but because of the risk of retention, a PVR must be checked if these drugs are used in patients with BPH. If medical therapy is ineffective or not tolerated, or if the patient prefers surgical options to chronic medical therapy, surgery should be pursued.

BLEEDING DISORDERS

28-1.   **A. Learning objective: Recognize a history consistent with disorders of primary hemostasis (platelet problems).** His single past episode of gum hemorrhage is a clue to a mild problem with primary hemostasis. This history is entirely consistent with either mild von Willebrand's disease, which can present later in life, or antiplatelet agent ingestion.

B. Learning objective: Design appropriate workup when history suggests a problem with primary hemostasis. The most useful test in this patient is a bleeding time, performed when the patient has not recently bled, and has had no antiplatelet agent use for the prior 10 days. Although a normal bleeding time in this situation will not give you a definitive diagnosis, an abnormal bleeding time indicates an underlying problem with primary hemostasis. The diagnosis of von Willebrand's disease may then be confirmed with platelet aggregation studies. If the bleeding time is normal, it may be that his underlying disorder is so mild that he only has bleeding problems when challenged with antiplatelet agents.

C. Learning objective: Use low MCV to identify possible iron deficiency anemia. This middle-aged man has anemia with a low MCV, suggesting iron deficiency. Rule out other causes of blood loss, especially occult GI cancer.

D. Learning objective: Design appropriate therapy for a mild bleeding disorder. Your patient has iron-deficiency anemia and excessive bleeding. The most important thing to do is recommend that he stop aspirin and NSAIDs. This alone may prevent further epistaxis. If his nosebleeds have been exclusively from the right side, you may want to rule out the possibility of a vascular abnormality. If the bleeding time is prolonged and the diagnosis of von Willebrand's disease is established, be sure to inform him of the use of preoperative DDAVP for any elective surgical procedure in the future.

28-2.   **A. Learning objective: Recognize the warning signs of DIC.** Your patient has a baseline acquired bleeding tendency resulting from his chronic liver disease and associated vitamin K–dependent clotting factor deficiency. However, he has also developed tense ascites and may have spontaneous bacterial peritonitis (SBP) from which he has become septic. DIC may progress very quickly in this patient with diminished reserve.

B. Learning objective: Identify the clues in the physical examination that help diagnosis of DIC. Check mucosa and venipuncture sites for oozing because spontaneous hemorrhage from mucosal surfaces and wounds is the hallmark of DIC. The presence of new ecchymoses and/or petechiae in dependent areas point to thrombocytopenia as a contributing factor.

C. Learning objective: Design a workup that helps you manage the patient with DIC. Obtain a full coagulation panel in addition to a CBC and platelets. The only way to distinguish a consumptive coagulopathy resulting from underlying liver disease from DIC will be the ability to regain control of the bleeding and improve his coagulation picture. The most important thing you can do is to identify and treat any underlying infection.

CLOTTING DISORDERS

28-3.   **A. *Learning objective: Recognize a history suggesting hypercoagulable state, and design appropriate workup.*** The most likely diagnosis is antiphospholipid antibody syndrome (APAS). Look for a prolonged PTT. Addition of normal plasma in a 1:1 mix confirms the diagnosis when the PTT does not normalize, indicating presence of an inhibitor. Obtain an assay for anticardiolipin antibodies. Because she is young, you may wish to screen for protein C, protein S (obtain before starting warfarin), and antithrombin III (obtain before starting heparin) deficiencies. Results may be difficult to interpret because she is postpartum. Her Hispanic background makes factor V Leiden mutation unlikely.

B. *Learning objective: Individualize anticoagulation.* She is at a very high risk for recurrent thrombosis, so maintain INR at 3 to 4. If she wants more children, she needs very close monitoring on high-dose LMW heparin before and throughout pregnancy. She may also benefit from low-dose aspirin or steroids during pregnancy because these reduce spontaneous abortion in women with anticardiolipin antibodies. Consider referral to a rheumatologist for assistance in managing her underlying autoimmune disorder.

ONCOLOGY

28-4.   **A. *Learning objective: Design appropriate workup for a solitary pulmonary nodule.*** Perform complete history and examination to identify other causes of this nodule besides lung cancer (perhaps an aspergilloma or metastatic gastric cancer). Review old chest x-rays to establish the history of the lesion. Characterize the lesion by chest CT, and look for enlarged chest nodes. Bone scan may reveal bony metastases causing back pain. Chance of cancer is high; an early-stage non–small-cell lung cancer that might be cured by excision is the best possible tumor you could find.

B. *Learning objective: List chest x-ray features of pulmonary nodules that suggest malignancy.* Malignant nodules are more likely to double in volume (not diameter) between 7 and 465 days. Nodules unchanged for 2 years are unlikely to be cancer. Eccentric or stippled calcifications, irregular shape, and poorly defined borders all suggest malignancy. The "pretest probability" is also important: a nodule in a 25-year-old nonsmoker is unlikely to be lung cancer.

C. *Learning objective: List potential causes of hypercalcemia in a man with a pulmonary nodule.* A squamous cell lung cancer might produce parathyroid-like hormones or, less likely, bony metastases (remember his sore back), causing elevated calcium. Other potential causes unrelated to lung cancer include hyperparathyroidism, immobility, and multiple myeloma. Chest x-ray showed an eccentrically calcified nodule, work-up for nodes and metastases was negative, FEV_1 was high enough to allow lobectomy that showed adenocarcinoma with negative regional nodes. High calcium persisted, and eventually a parathyroid adenoma was removed. He knew it was a close call, and this helped him quit smoking!

28-5.   **A.** *Learning objective: Think of leukemia when someone has dyspnea, fatigue, and bleeding.* Common causes of "low energy," such as depression and CHF, do not cause bleeding. The nosebleed may be coincidental; consider other diagnoses, such as pneumonia, TB, anemia, and lung cancer. History of other bleeding really helps distinguish incidental from worrisome cause; she also reports bleeding from her gums.

B. *Learning objective: Learn how to diagnose acute leukemia.* Look for gum infiltration, adenopathy, petechiae, lung consolidation, meningitis, and focal neurologic deficits. Peripheral smear with blasts is a strong hint, but a bone marrow biopsy showing greater than 30% blasts defines leukemia. Auer rods—those red cigars in the cytoplasm—clinch the diagnosis of AML. Next, you need the cytoimmunologist to subtype the AML with membrane antigens.

C. *Learning objective: Anticipate common complications of AML.* Look for sepsis (fever, tachycardia, hypotension), and check coagulation studies to rule out DIC. Because the WBC is greater than 150,000, anticipate sludging and tumor lysis with renal failure. CNS involvement is not common in adults. However, if she develops a cranial nerve deficit such as a 7th nerve palsy, she needs head CT and LP.

28-6.   **A.** *Learning objective: List cancers that can cause nodes in the supraclavicular fossa.* Virchow's node is a left supraclavicular node usually from metastatic intestinal cancers (stomach, colon). He is at risk for colon cancer because of his brother's colon cancer. Testicular cancers can present in the neck, but he is a bit old for this tumor. Perform testicular examination to be sure. His 50 pack-years of smoking increases lung cancer risk. Fever could be due to postobstructive pneumonia, a "B" symptom of lymphoma, sarcoidosis, or tuberculosis.

B. *Learning objective: Describe the work-up for chest lymphadenopathy.* Although node biopsy is tempting, further imaging first helps you decide between a needle biopsy (to look for lung cancer or intestinal cancer) and excisional biopsy (needed for lymphomas). Chest and abdominal CT show no lung mass, but there is diffuse adenopathy and splenomegaly missed on examination. The biopsy shows an intermediate-grade lymphoma, which is stage IV-B.

C. *Learning objective: Learn the long-term effects of some cancer treatments.* He undergoes intensive chemotherapy with CHOP (cyclophosphamide, doxorubicin, vincristine, prednisone). He is alive at 5 years but is sterile and has an increased risk for a second primary cancer at any site.

GENITAL INFECTIONS

29-1. **A. *Learning objective: Assess risk factors for concerning causes of dyspareunia and vaginal discharge.*** In any woman of reproductive age, inquire as to the date of last menstrual period. Assess for systemic signs of infection, such as fever, chills, or malaise. Recent antibiotic use makes candidal vaginitis more likely.

B. *Learning objective: Identify appropriate evaluation in a woman with discharge.* Start with external examination to look for herpes ulceration or warts. Regardless of what you see on examination (which is neither sensitive nor specific), obtain *Chlamydia* and *Gonorrhoeae* cultures from the cervix. Evaluate the vaginal fluid for white blood cells, clue cells, *Trichomonas*, and pH. Even if she is due for a Pap smear, do not perform one at this time. If she has infection, her results may be abnormal because of inflammation. Have her return for Pap smear after treatment for a diagnosed condition or after negative workup. Also, given that she is at some risk, offer HIV and RPR testing. If she is late for her period, get a urine pregnancy test.

C. *Learning objective: Counsel patients on implications of HPV exposure.* Educate this patient about the high prevalence of this virus, the lack of protection with condoms, and that her most important task is to have routine Pap smears. Her partner may want treatment with topical preparations or cryotherapy to shrink the lesions, but these treatments are not curative.

29-2. **A. *Learning objective: Generate a differential for fever, vaginal pain, and dysuria.*** As per the Urinary Tract Infections section in Chapter 29, 10% of women not responding to initial short-course therapy may have upper tract disease. Vaginal mucosal tenderness could be due to candidal vaginitis after antibiotic therapy. Any woman with fever and pelvic pain is at risk for PID. This is also be a good history for primary HSV infection. Although it does not explain the fever, she could be entering menopause, with associated vaginal atrophy from estrogen deficiency. Finally, sulfa drugs can be associated with toxic epidermal necrolysis, so look in her mouth for evidence of other mucosal sites of involvement.

B. *Learning objective: Design appropriate workup for fever, vaginal pain, and dysuria.* Obtain GC/CT culture and LCR, respectively, urine dip, and culture. If vesicles are visible, send HSV culture. CBC is necessary for possible pyelonephritis and PID. Vaginal fluid KOH and saline wet mount will evaluate for candidal or atrophic vaginitis. Don't forget a pregnancy test because she has missed two cycles.

C. *Learning objective: Recognize likely candidal colonization.* The absence of white blood cells indicates that the candidal hyphae are likely colonizers. The likelihood of candidal infection is increased, however, because of her antibiotic use. If no other cause is found, a trial of fluconazole is reasonable.

HIV INFECTION PRIMARY CARE

29-3.   **A. *Learning objective: Understand when to start antiretroviral therapy and what agents to use.*** This patient has a CD4 count of 405 but a high viral load of 30,000. He has been on AZT + ddI, so he may be resistant to these. When CD4 is less than 500, all authorities strongly encourage starting antiretroviral therapy. Combination therapy is the rule with at least three drugs. The goal is to use at least two drugs that the patient has not seen before. Given this patient's high viral load of 30,000, a protease inhibitor is a cornerstone for combination treatment. One option is a protease inhibitor (indinavir or nelfinavir) + AZT + 3TC, giving the patient two new drugs (a protease inhibitor plus 3TC) and a combination of AZT + 3TC because 3TC often restores AZT sensitivity. Another option is to include a nonnucleoside drug: d4T + 3TC + efavirenz. Efavirenz is a nonnucleoside analogue that works well with nucleoside analogues. Never use single-drug therapy. Also, it is not wise to use another two-drug nucleoside combination. One very important thing to evaluate before starting therapy is if the patient is going to be compliant. If there are problems with compliance, intermittent antiretroviral therapy quickly leads to resistance; noncompliance is a good reason to defer therapy.

B. *Learning objective: Order appropriate routine testing for HIV-infected individuals.* This patient needs a PPD, VDRL, toxoplasmosis titers, LFTs, hepatitis serologies, cholesterol panel, CBC, and platelet count. VDRL is important because of the increased incidence of syphilis (especially in those with a history of male-male sexual contact or IV drug use). Toxoplasmosis titers assess risk for developing toxoplasmosis in the future. LFTs and hepatitis serologies provide a baseline and assist in determining if hepatitis B vaccine is needed. Cholesterol panel provides a baseline for evaluating the effect of protease inhibitors. CBC provides an important baseline, particularly if zidovudine is restarted (causes anemia and neutropenia). Platelet count is important because of a fairly high incidence of immune-mediated thrombocytopenia (ITP) in patients with HIV. Vaccines against *Pneumococcus* and hepatitis B (if nonimmune) are warranted.

HIV INFECTION COMPLICATIONS

29-4.   **A. *Learning objective: Recognize that the severity of seborrheic dermatitis correlates with immune function and CNS disease.*** Seborrheic dermatitis is extremely common in patients with HIV (80% have it at some point). Severity worsens with declining immune function or CNS disease. Interestingly, this holds true even for non–HIV-infected patients in whom seborrheic dermatitis is commonly seen, such as in patients with Parkinson's disease.

B. *Learning objective: Recognize that molluscum suggests declining immunity, and HL suggests more rapid disease progression.* Molluscum contagiosum is seen usually when CD4 is less than 100 and is a sign of declining immunity, especially with giant molluscum. OHL is specific for HIV disease and may be a marker for increased risk of disease progression.

C. *Learning objective: Discuss the differential diagnosis for headache in an AIDS patient.* This patient presents with headache, encephalopathy, and fever. On physical examination he has focal findings on the left side. The most likely diagnosis is cerebral toxoplasmosis. This is made even more likely because the patient was not on toxoplasmosis prophylaxis (trimethoprim/sulfamethoxazole is the best prophylactic drug). Other possibilities include CNS lymphoma and progressive multifocal leukoencephalopathy (PML); both cause focal motor findings and can cause encephalopathy but usually not fever.

D. *Learning objective: Order CNS imaging for AIDS patients with headache and fever.* Because of the focal neurologic examination, CNS imaging is key. Options are contrast CT scan and MRI. MRI is more sensitive (and about 2½ times as expensive). PML usually does not show up on CT scans but does on MRI. Serum IgG for toxoplasma is an important part of the workup. If the MRI scan is negative (which is very unlikely), LP would be appropriate.

MENINGITIS

29-5. **A.** *Learning objective: Design workup for mental status change in an elderly patient.* This patient needs urinalysis and urine culture, blood cultures, and a chest x-ray. Based on results of these tests, you will decide if he needs more invasive testing (lumbar puncture).

B. *Learning objective: State the most common causes for delirium in the elderly.* This patient has had a sudden change in mental status in the setting of fever and an elevated WBC. Mental status change may be the only symptom of infection in the elderly. The most common causes of acute delirium in the elderly are urinary tract infection and pneumonia. Meningitis is a very rare cause. Another very important cause of delirium is medication side effects. This patient probably has a UTI. If urinalysis and x-ray are normal, an LP would be appropriate.

29-6. **A.** *Learning objective: Use appropriate tests to evaluate for meningitis.* This patient presents with high fever, seizures, evidence of pneumonia, and alcoholism, important risk factors for pneumococcal disease. Order blood cultures, arterial blood gas, and head CT scan. A CT scan should be obtained here before LP because patient is obtunded and cannot give history and he has seized (increases likelihood of a mass lesion). The risk of herniation is low (6%) even in the setting of increased intracranial pressure but is a complication worth avoiding. If contrast CT does not show shift, perform an LP. Order CSF protein, glucose, WBC count, Gram stain, and culture. Give antibiotics before the patient goes to the CT scanner.

B. *Learning objective: Recognize pneumococcal meningitis.* Most pneumococcal meningitis is seeded from a pneumonia, as in this case. *Listeria* and meningococcus are less likely to have concurrent pulmonary infection. This patient could have a brain abscess causing the seizure, seeded from the lung (usually occurs in the setting of a pulmonary shunt or right-to-left cardiac shunt).

C. *Learning objective: Design appropriate empiric therapy for patients with probable pneumococcal meningitis.* This patient should have empiric therapy to cover pneumococcus, meningococcus, and *Listeria.* Vancomycin + ceftriaxone + ampicillin is appropriate. Vancomycin is given because of increasing penicillin-resistant pneumococcus. Vancomycin only controls bacteremia but does not penetrate the CNS well. Ceftriaxone will penetrate the CNS well and is effective against intermediate PCN-resistant pneumococcus. Ampicillin is added to cover for *Listeria.* As soon as CSF Gram stain or culture is positive, simplify therapy.

PNEUMONIA

29-7. **A. *Learning objective: List likely organisms causing pneumonia in an older smoker.*** Abrupt-onset cough with rusty sputum and shaking chill suggest community-acquired pneumonia. Pneumococcus is most likely. *Haemophilus, Moraxella,* and, much less likely, *Legionella* are also possible because of her smoking history. Because she does not live in an institution, TB, *Staphylococcus,* and *Pseudomonas* are unlikely. There is no history of alcohol, sedating medications, or neurologic disease to suggest aspiration. Her pulse is unexpectedly low for the degree of fever, a finding called *pulse-temperature dissociation* and sometimes associated with *Legionella,* although this can occur with any pneumonia.

B. *Learning objective: Design appropriate workup for a patient who likely has pneumonia.* Check vital signs, pulse oxymetry, and orthostatic changes in pulse or pressure to determine IV requirements and detect early sepsis. Perform lung examination looking for signs of consolidation or effusion (dullness, fremitus, egophony, bronchial breath sounds). Send for CBC, chemistry panel, blood culture, blood gas, and sputum Gram stain and culture. Order chest film.

C. *Learning objective: Choose appropriate empiric antibiotic coverage based on details of the clinical setting.* A second- or third-generation cephalosporin (e.g., cefuroxime, cefotetan, ceftriaxone) is adequate to cover potentially β-lactam–resistant *Pneumococcus, Haemophilus,* or *Moraxella.* Although *Legionella* is not as likely, it is potentially life-threatening. Add high-dose erythromycin or use single drug therapy with IV levofloxacin or trovafloxacin to cover *Legionella* in light of her smoking (likely lung disease) and pulse-temperature dissociation.

D. *Learning objective: Recognize the usual course of response to therapy in patients with pneumonia.* Patients may spike fevers 2 to 4 days into therapy, although in general, the peak temperature gradually drops over that time. Leukocytosis may not resolve until up to 4 days of therapy. Continue current therapy and monitor for any signs of deterioration. Generally, empiric antibiotics are broad and left unaltered over the first 72 hours of therapy unless an organism is found or patients get rapidly worse.

E. *Learning objective: Recognize deviation from the usual course of response to therapy, and design appropriate workup to detect complications.* Fever should be abating at this point. Look for a resistant organism, an empyema or other complication, drug fever, or a noninfectious cause of fever. Order repeat chest x-ray and blood and sputum cultures. If x-ray shows fluid, obtain bilateral decubitus films to see if the fluid is free-flowing (amenable to pleural tap) and tap the fluid immediately.

29-8. **A. *Learning objective: Recognize altered mental status as a presentation of pneumonia in an elderly patient, and generate a broad differential diagnosis.*** Differential includes pneumonia, PE, MI, electrolyte disturbance (hyponatremia, hypercalcemia), sepsis (from a UTI, ischemic bowel, meningitis, cholecystitis), or pancreatitis.

B. *Learning objective: Design workup in an older patient with altered mental status.* Aside from careful history and examination, obtain chemistry panel, calcium, amylase, liver function tests, chest x-ray, oxygen saturation, ABG, ECG, and urinalysis to start with, looking for the entities in answer 8A. Consider lumbar puncture if fever or elevated WBC are found with no apparent source of infection. Stiff neck or other meningeal signs mandate head CT and LP.

C. *Learning objective: List most likely organisms causing pneumonia in an elderly patient who resides in a nursing home.* Pneumococcus, Staphylococcus aureus, Pseudomonas aeruginosa, other gram-negative rods, TB, and anaerobes are all possible causes of infection in this nursing home resident with altered mental status. Alcohol use, poor dentition, or impaired swallowing resulting from underlying neurologic disease make aspiration even more likely.

D. *Learning objective: Describe factors making atypical presentations of pneumonia more likely.* Elderly patients may not have the vigorous immune response necessary to produce sputum, cough, or fever. Pain localization can be inaccurate, and lower lobe pneumonia can present as abdominal pain.

URINARY TRACT INFECTIONS

29-9. **A. *Learning objective: Order appropriate tests to evaluate possible pyelonephritis.*** This patient has a symptom complex and laboratory pattern consistent with pyelonephritis. Order urine culture and urine Gram stain. Urine cultures should not be done for simple cystitis but are recommended for pyelonephritis. Also, consider ordering blood cultures.

B. *Learning objective: State the rationale for hospital admission.* Admit this patient. She has vomiting, so oral antibiotic therapy will not be effective. Her blood pressure is borderline (systolic 90). She also has an anion gap acidosis, most likely caused by lactic acid from hypoperfusion. She needs IV fluids, IV antibiotics, and monitoring.

C. *Learning objective: State the most common organisms causing pyelonephritis in young women.* *Escherichia coli* is most frequent. Other gram-negative rods, such as *Klebsiella,* can occasionally be seen. *Enterococcus* and *Staphylococcus saprophyticus* are almost never seen in young women with pyelonephritis. *Enterococcus* is a cause of pyelonephritis in patients with history of multiple courses of antibiotics and with history of catheterization. *S. saprophyticus* is seen in young women with cystitis but usually not pyelonephritis.

D. *Learning objective: Choose appropriate IV antibiotics for pyelonephritis.* Several options are available to cover *E. coli* in a simple, cost-effective manner. A once-per-day third-generation cephalosporin (ceftriaxone) is an excellent choice. Other options include a quinolone or aminoglycoside. Trimethoprim/sulfamethoxazole works but must be dosed every 6 hours, making it a more costly option. The cost of administering each dose is about $20, so a qid drug costs $80 just to administer. Switch the patient to trimethoprim/sulfamethoxazole when she can take oral medicines (or a quinolone if allergic to sulfa drugs or if culture shows resistance to trimethoprim/sulfamethoxazole).

29-10. **A. *Learning objective: Recognize nosocomial infection of the urinary tract.*** This patient developed signs of infection in the hospital after broad-spectrum antibiotic therapy. In addition, he has a Foley catheter (in the bladder), which makes the urinary tract a likely site of infection. A high WBC and abnormal urinalysis supports this hypothesis. Another possibility is *Clostridium difficile* colitis (some patients may not initially have diarrhea). Previous antibiotic therapy is the most important risk factor for *C. difficile*. A final possibility is an infected IV site (a common problem in inpatients).

B. *Learning objective: Select empiric antibiotic therapy for the nosocomial infection.* This patient has nosocomial pyelonephritis. Because of the previous antibiotic therapy and Foley catheter, he is at risk for several hospital-acquired organisms—most importantly, *Enterococcus* and *Pseudomonas*. Prior cephalosporin therapy is a major risk factor for subsequent enterococcal infection. Appropriate empiric therapy is with a drug active against *Enterococcus* (ampicillin, mezlocillin, vancomycin) *plus* a drug that covers gram-negative rods, including *Pseudomonas* (aminoglycoside, aztreonam, ceftazidime or cefoperazone, quinolone).

ACID-BASE DISTURBANCES

30-1.   **A. *Learning objective: Identify the primary acid-base derangement.*** Alkalemia with a pH of 7.5 is a primary respiratory alkalosis because P_{CO_2} is low.

B. *Learning objective: Recognize that a compensatory metabolic acidosis should be a non–anion gap acidosis.* Low HCO_3^- is a metabolic acidosis. One might be tempted to call this compensatory. However, a compensatory metabolic acidosis should be a non–anion gap acidosis because it is generated by renal bicarbonate loss. His anion gap acidosis is instead a coexisting process.

C. *Learning objective: Identify all coexisting primary acid-base derangements by cal-culating anion gap, osmolar gap, and delta-delta.* Anion gap is elevated at 22 [140 −(103 + 15)], meaning anion gap acidosis is present. Calculated osms are 296 [2(140) + 28/2.8 + 108/18)]. Osm gap is 1 [296 − 295], essentially normal, rules out osmotically active ingestion. Subtract a normal anion gap (12) from the patient's elevated anion gap (22) to get the change in anion gap (22 − 12 = 10). When you add the change in anion gap to his bicarbonate of 15, you get 25, so close to 24 that you can declare there are no other simultaneous metabolic processes.

D. *Learning objective: Interpret acid-base abnormalities in the context of clinical information to develop a reasonable differential diagnosis.* He has been taking large doses of aspirin for back pain. Aspirin causes a respiratory alkalosis by stimulating CNS breathing centers to hyperventilate, as well as an anion gap acidosis caused by salicylic acid. His melena is likely from NSAID-induced gastritis. Other less likely explanations of his acid-base derangements would have to invoke two separate processes. Early sepsis could cause an anion gap acidosis with compensatory hyperventilation, although the pH should be less than 7.4, reflecting the primary acidosis.

30-2.   **A. *Learning objective: Identify the primary acid-base derangement.*** Acidemia with a low bicarbonate indicates a primary metabolic acidosis.

B. *Learning objective: Identify the compensatory acid-base derangement.* Low P_{CO_2} from hyperventilating creates a compensatory respiratory alkalosis.

C. *Learning objective: Identify all coexisting acid-base derangements by calculating anion gap and osmolar gap and comparing the change in anion gap to the change in bicarbonate (delta delta).* Anion gap is 32 [130 − (88 + 10)]. Calculated osms are 310 [2(130) + 28/2.8 + 720/18]. Osm gap is 5 [315 − 310]. Using "delta-delta," the rise in anion gap is 20 [32 − 12], and when you add this to the bicarbonate, you get 30 [20 + 10]. Because this is greater than 24, a metabolic alkalosis is also present.

D. *Learning objective: Interpret acid-base abnormalities in the context of clinical information.* She has diabetic ketoacidosis (polyuria, polydipsia, high glucose), causing an anion gap acidosis. She has some respiratory compensation, blowing off CO_2 to reduce her acidemia. Additionally, she has a coexisting primary metabolic alkalosis, probably from vomiting.

ACUTE RENAL FAILURE

30-3. **A. Learning objective: Diagnose prerenal ARF.** This patient is prerenal as a result of her upper GI bleed and probably has ATN. Her BUN/Cr ratio is greater than 20, suggesting volume depletion, and urine output is very low (oliguric) despite hydration and catheterization (rules out obstruction). FeNa and urine sediment examination are indicated. Urine sediment should show hyaline casts, unless hypovolemia has caused ATN, in which case there may be granular and "muddy brown" casts.

B. Learning objective: Calculate FeNa. FeNa is 0.6, consistent with prerenal ARF.

C. Learning objective: State complications of ARF, and design appropriate monitoring. She is likely to develop volume overload, peripheral and pulmonary edema, and even CHF. She will also develop electrolyte imbalances and acidemia. She may develop dysfunctional platelets. She should have strict measurement of daily intakes and outputs (I&O) and weights. Daily examination should include vitals, mental status examination, JVP, CV, lung examination, and examination for edema. Laboratory tests should include CBC, chemistries, Ca, Mg, Phos, chest x-ray, and ECG (if K^+ is elevated). Reestablishing urine output may simply be a matter of time, but diuretics may help. Dose all medications according to renal function. Adjust diet for renal failure (low Na, low K), and avoid medications containing K^+ and magnesium (antacids contain Mg).

D. Learning objective: State indications for dialysis. No indication currently (see text).

30-4. **A. Learning objective: Recognize postrenal azotemia, and place a Foley catheter.** This elderly man has acute urinary retention from anticholinergic medication superimposed on benign prostatic hypertrophy or possibly prostate cancer. The suprapubic mass is his bladder. Place a Foley catheter in the bladder to confirm your diagnosis.

B. Learning objective: Look for postobstructive diuresis. After catheter placement, high-volume diuresis may cause electrolyte wasting. Monitor and replace output and electrolytes.

30-5. **A. Learning objective: Recognize interstitial nephritis, and state possible causes.** The active urine sediment in this case, with protein and eosinophils (93% specific for acute interstitial nephritis [AIN]), indicates interstitial nephritis caused by cephalosporin. Patients with AIN have rash, fever, and peripheral eosinophilia approximately 30% of the time. If red blood cell casts or dysmorphic red cells were present, the differential would include poststreptococcal glomerulonephritis (arises 1 to 2 weeks after streptococcal infection of skin or pharynx) or IgA nephropathy (arises concurrent with URI or GI infection). His history of drug use suggests possible bacterial endocarditis, hepatitis B or C, or heroin-associated nephropathy. These do not cause eosinophils in the urine.

B. Learning objective: Manage acute interstitial nephritis. Most cases respond to cessation of the causative medication. For persistent renal failure, prednisone may be necessary.

30-6. **A. Learning objective: Recognize a pulmonary-renal syndrome.** He has renal failure with borderline anemia, a history of sinusitis and ongoing lung disease, elevated blood pressure of uncertain duration, and trimethoprim/sulfamethoxazole use. The differential for his azotemia includes Wegener's granulomatosis (sinus, lung, and renal involvement), elevation in creatinine caused by trimethoprim/sulfamethoxazole, or chronic renal impairment resulting from hypertension. Other diagnoses are less likely, although other causes of pulmonary and renal disease should be considered, for example, SLE and Goodpasture's syndrome. Postrenal obstruction caused by BPH is also possible in a middle-aged man.

B. Learning objective: Order appropriate tests in the workup of glomerulonephritis. Order ANA (SLE), c-ANCA (Wegener's), ESR, urinalysis (for RBC casts), and chest x-ray at a minimum. Prostate examination and bladder percussion help rule out postrenal obstruction, as does catheterization for a postvoid residual. The highest-yield diagnostic test for Wegener's granulomatosis is renal biopsy, but because he has sinus and lung disease, a transbronchial or sinus biopsy might be sufficient.

C. Learning objective: State urine findings in acute glomerulonephritis. Urine sediment might show crenated, dysmorphic red cells (exposed to a high osmotic gradient in the tubules vs. RBCs from the bladder that will not be dysmorphic) and red cell casts (look at a fresh sample yourself because casts decompose).

30-7. **A.** *Learning objective: Recognize nephrotic syndrome and its causes.* This patient has nephrotic syndrome (renal failure with edema, 24 hour protein > 3.5 g, and dyslipidemia). The most likely causes of his nephrotic syndrome include his heroin use, HIV nephropathy, polyarteritis nodosa (related to hepatitis B), ibuprofen use (interstitial nephritis usually has less protein, < 1.5 g/24 hours), and renal disease such as membranous nephropathy, or even minimal-change disease (more common in children).

B. *Learning objective: Order tests to work up nephrotic syndrome.* Obtain HIV test, CBC, hepatitis B and C serologies, p-ANCA, chest x-ray, and probably a renal biopsy. ANA reflexive panel and ESR might be helpful.

C. *Learning objective: State the urine abnormalities seen in nephrotic syndrome.* Oval fat bodies and Maltese crosses are found in the urine sediment in nephrotic syndrome. You might also see other clues to etiology (e.g., WBC casts and eosinophils in interstitial nephritis).

ELECTROLYTE DISTURBANCES AND FLUID MANAGEMENT

30-8. **A.** *Learning objective: Prioritize hyperkalemia as a life-threatening problem.* Hyperkalemia is most life-threatening. Hypertension is likely baseline and can be addressed over days to weeks as long as there is no end-organ damage. Dyspnea with elevated JVP, rales, and edema are signs of moderate fluid overload; address with diuretics or hemodialysis over hours to days. Metabolic non–anion-gap acidosis is likely chronic, resulting from renal failure.

B. *Learning objective: State the ECG findings of hyperkalemia.* Moderate hyperkalemia causes peaked T waves. More severe hyperkalemia widens the QRS, reflecting the increased time for ventricular depolarization. With severe hyperkalemia, ECG looks like a sine wave with peaked Ts and wide QRS indistinguishable from each other in an undulating wave.

C. *Learning objective: Identify interventions for acute hyperkalemia, and state the mechanism of each.* To avoid cardiac arrhythmia, first give IV calcium gluconate to rapidly stabilize cardiac membranes. Next, give IV glucose (amp of D50) and insulin (5 to 10 U) to carry potassium into the intracellular space. Be careful not to give so much insulin as to cause hypoglycemia. Alkalinize with bicarbonate for a transient intracellular potassium shift. Kayexalate can be initiated with the acute therapies but is too slow-acting to reverse severe hyperkalemia. Furosemide helps over hours if the patient is making urine. Use dialysis for severe hyperkalemia, although it takes some time to set up; administer calcium, glucose with insulin, and bicarbonate while waiting for dialysis to begin.

30-9. **A. *Learning objective: Use the details of a clinical situation to generate a list of probable causes of hyponatremia.*** Hydrochlorothiazide could be causing a hypovolemic or euvolemic hyponatremia. However, she is systemically ill with confusion, dyspnea, and cough, suggesting cardiac or pulmonary pathology. Cough and dyspnea could be heart failure, not unlikely in a woman with multiple risk factors for CHF (hypertension, smoking, and alcohol use). She also has risk factors for pneumonia and for lung tumor, either of which could lead to SIADH.

B. *Learning objective: Recognize the importance of volume status in the workup of hyponatremia.* Evaluate fluid status to direct further inquiry. Orthostatic vital signs, dry mucous membranes, and poor skin turgor may indicate decreased volume. Hypoxia, rales, jugular vein distention, or leg or sacral edema indicate fluid overload. The lack of either group of signs indicates euvolemia. Cachexia might make you suspicious for tumor. Focal signs of lung consolidation may make you think of pneumonia or tumor. Hoarse voice, dry skin, and coarse hair suggest hypothyroidism. Focal neurologic examination might make you worry about a CNS tumor.

C. *Learning objective: Design appropriate workup for euvolemic hyponatremia, and state options for management of SIADH.* Obtain chest x-ray to look for pneumonia or tumor. Without lung findings to explain hyponatremia, evaluate further with a head CT and consider LP. TSH is also reasonable. She most likely has SIADH resulting from pneumonia, although the possibility of a lung tumor has not been totally ruled out. Treat with free water restriction to about 500 to 1500 ml per day. Some people opt to use IV normal saline along with free water restriction over the first day for more rapid response, especially if sodium is very low (<120). Patients seizing from low sodium can be given 3% hypertonic IV saline. Whatever the approach, raise sodium by no more than 1 mEq/hr. Follow sodium levels hourly initially until rate of rise is stable. If hyponatremia does not resolve with treatment of pneumonia, think about diuretic or perhaps an occult lung or CNS process as a contributing cause.

HYPERTENSION

30-10. **A. *Learning objective: Identify factors contributing to hypertension.*** Oral contraceptives, NSAIDs, acute pain, and excessive alcohol use can all contribute to her hypertension.

B. *Learning objective: Design appropriate followup for patients in whom mild hypertension is found.* Recheck within the next 2 months or so, before she forgets to return.

C. *Learning objective: Counsel patients appropriately about lifestyle modifications to lower blood pressure.* With a single measurement under extenuating circumstances, her blood pressure will likely normalize, so she can continue her birth control pills. NSAIDs are also appropriate for short-term management of pain and inflammation. However, you need to address her alcohol use. Regardless of whether it has increased her blood pressure, she is drinking enough to cause significant medical and social sequelae. Intervention in a young woman is more likely to succeed than in more chronic alcohol users. Use your CAGE questions for further screening.

30-11.   **A.** *Learning objective: State three reasons to change nifedipine.* The three reasons are: (1) unacceptable side effects (constipation and lower extremity edema are common with calcium channel blockers); 2) increased mortality with short-acting calcium channel blockers; 3) she has to take a pill 3 times a day, which may make compliance difficult and may relate to why her blood pressure is still elevated.

B. *Learning objective: Perform appropriate initial evaluation for hypertension in patients with unclear prior evaluation.* With a patient who is new to you, you need to begin at the beginning. If she has not had diet and exercise counseling, review this with her. Examine her for end-organ damage: perform a careful eye and heart examination, and at minimum obtain a laboratory panel of electrolytes and renal function. Next, consider whether she could have secondary causes for her hypertension. Because her hypertension has been long-standing, further testing is probably not indicated. On the other hand, her age alone puts her at risk for renal artery stenosis, so if three medications do not control her pressure, consider a renal artery duplex.

C. *Learning objective: Choose appropriate antihypertensive therapy in a patient with gout and bradycardia.* Although her lower-extremity edema invites a low-dose diuretic, the increase in uric acid may cause her gout to flare. A β-blocker may also be a poor choice because her pulse is bradycardic. Many elderly patients have bradycardia or borderline heart block from impaired electrical conduction in the heart (as a consequence of degeneration/aging, not ischemia per se). In patients with a low pulse (<60), check an ECG before starting a β-blocker. A calcium channel blocker, such as diltiazem or verapamil, may delay conduction at the AV node and worsen heart block. An α-blocker is a cheap alternative, but orthostatic hypotension puts older patients at risk for falls. An ACEI may be the best choice—check renal function after a week of therapy. If her lower-extremity edema is from CHF (from long-standing hypertension), an ACEI is the first choice for afterload reduction.

30-12.   **A.** *Learning objective: Identify features on history and examination that suggest reasons for hypertension.* Potential factors include family history, obesity, Cushing's disease (depression, obesity, diabetes, stretch marks, and low potassium), hyperaldosteronism, and sleep apnea (fatigue, falling asleep while driving, obesity).

B. *Learning objective: Order appropriate tests for suspected secondary causes of hypertension in an obese patient with hypokalemia.* Perform serial workup beginning with a 24-hour cortisol because she has several stigmata of Cushing's. Other tests to do in serial fashion include a renal vascular duplex (diabetes puts her at risk for vascular disease), an aldosterone/renin ratio (low potassium occurs both with Cushing's hyperaldosteronism), and a sleep study looking for sleep apnea (prevalent in up to 40% of obese women).

C. *Learning objective: Begin treatment for hypertension with lifestyle modification.* Lifestyle modification is imperative in this patient. Weight loss and exercise will help not only her hypertension but also her diabetes. Just 10 pounds can make a big change in medication requirements. If no other cause for hypertension is found, she likely also needs antihypertensive therapy because her blood pressure is quite high and lifestyle changes alone will not correct it. Control other risk factors for coronary heart disease by checking cholesterol, treating diabetes, and starting estrogen replacement (unless contraindicated).

NEUROLOGY

31-1. **A. Learning objective: Recognize delirium and distinguish it from dementia.** This patient has waxing and waning mental status with inattention, classic for delirium. The cognitive deficits of dementia, in contrast, usually develop slowly over months to years and attention remains intact until very late.

B. Learning objective: List a differential diagnosis for delirium. Differential includes infection (meningitis, pyelonephritis, cholangitis), electrolyte abnormality (hyponatremia, hypercalcemia most likely), seizures, stroke, myocardial infarction, and medication effect.

C. Learning objective: Plan appropriate workup for a patient with delirium. Obtain CBC, chemistry panel, calcium, liver function tests, oxygen saturation, ECG, and chest film. If a cause is not readily apparent, consider head CT and lumbar puncture. Results show Na 140; Cl 110; HCO_3^- 27; Ca 14 (normal < 10.5); and normal LFTs, ECG (aside from a shortened Q-T interval), and chest x-ray.

D. Learning objective: Identify hypercalcemia as a cause of delirium. Bonus: Recognize that a low anion gap in a patient with hypercalcemia suggests multiple myeloma. Hypercalcemia explains the patient's dehydrated volume status and delirium. The low anion gap is a clue that perhaps multiple myeloma is the culprit.

E. Learning objective: Design further tests to confirm the cause of hypercalcemia. In this patient with the low anion gap a focused workup for myeloma is appropriate, to include serum and urine protein electrophoresis; if positive, check bone survey to look for the characteristic punched-out lesions. In other patients in whom the diagnosis of myeloma is not suspected, it is best to start with an intact parathyroid hormone measurement because hyperparathyroidism is most common. If this is negative, review history and examination for signs of malignancy, update all overdue cancer screening, and pursue any other suggestive findings with further workup for malignancy. Also consider granulomatous disease, such as TB and sarcoid—chest film is a good place to start for these. See the Electrolyte Disturbance: Calcium section in Chapter 30 for more suggestions.

32-2. **A. Learning objective: List a differential diagnosis for first-time seizure.** Differential includes new-onset true epilepsy, cocaine, alcohol withdrawal, electrolyte disorder (especially hyponatremia or hypocalcemia), focal CNS infection (i.e., toxoplasmosis in the setting of advanced HIV infection), primary or metastatic brain tumor, and stroke (unlikely based on his age).

B. Learning objective: Ask a pertinent history to reveal potential causes of seizure. Ask about history of epilepsy, substance use (including alcohol and cocaine), HIV risk factors, and signs of tumor (weight loss, headache).

C. Learning objective: Design a workup to rule out structural and metabolic causes of first-time seizure. Obtain CBC, chemistry panel, calcium, magnesium, toxicology screen, head CT scan, and LP. Testing reveals a mildly elevated WBC, slightly low calcium and magnesium, a mild anion gap acidosis, negative toxicology screen, and normal head CT scan. LP reveals a mild pleocytosis. After all the tests, the patient's girlfriend reveals to you that he usually drinks very heavily but stopped abruptly 2 days ago.

D. Learning objective: State appropriate treatment for alcohol withdrawal seizures. With the further history, he likely is having an alcohol withdrawal seizure. Treatment is supportive with observation, seizure precautions (padded bed rails), hydration, thiamine, folate, and electrolyte replacement as needed. Most alcohol withdrawal seizures are single seizures. If seizing recurs, an IV benzodiazepine, such as lorazepam, can be given. Do not give phenytoin for alcohol withdrawal seizures. Advise the patient to abstain from alcohol in the future.

DEPRESSION

32-1.

A. *Learning objective: State criteria for depression.* Question him more specifically regarding sleep pattern, concentration, and anhedonia. Also inquire into mood, suicidal ideation, and thoughts of worthlessness and guilt.

B. *Learning objective: Include medical causes for symptoms in the differential.* If you determine that this patient meets criteria for depression, begin treatment. However, he has several medical issues that should be addressed. His agitation and weight loss may be due to hyperthyroidism, so check TSH. Nocturnal urination and back pain raise the question of prostatic malignancy and diabetes. If these symptoms are new, he requires an LS spine x-ray, an ESR, a PSA, and electrolytes.

C-D. *Learning objective: Design therapy for depression in the elderly, including treatment for coexisting insomnia.* If this patient is willing, psychotherapy has the benefit of avoiding polypharmacy, always a problem in the elderly. If therapy is not an option, an SSRI is a good choice. Because of his age, begin at half the usual starting dose. For his insomnia, avoid anticholinergics because this will worsen his prostatic symptoms and may cause confusion. Likewise, avoid benzodiazepines in the elderly, which contribute to confusion and falls. A better solution is nefazodone (Serzone) at night for 1 to 2 weeks. Finally, his isolation and sensory impairments make him a setup for depression. An adult day care program, as well as reading and hearing aids, would be beneficial.

32-2.

A. *Learning objective: Recognize contributing factors to depression.* This woman has several potential risk factors for depression. These include unresolved grief surrounding her husband's death, ongoing alcohol use, and recent addition of progesterone and estrogen.

B. *Learning objective: Design an appropriate treatment plan for a suicidal patient.* This patient has specific plans for suicide and has access to a lethal weapon. In addition, her alcohol use is aggravating her depression and will make her more susceptible to impulsive actions. The most appropriate action is to have her evaluated immediately by either a psychiatrist or a psychiatric social worker for possible hospitalization. Do not leave the patient unsupervised until she is safely transferred to their care.

ASTHMA

33-1. **A.** *Learning objective: Recognize common symptoms of asthma, and take a good asthma history.* This is a patient with previously undiagnosed asthma with wheezing and dyspnea on exertion, limiting activity. Get a detailed description of symptoms to learn if she has symptoms *not* associated with exercise. Does she wake up feeling short of breath? Ask about childhood illnesses; often children who "get bronchitis a lot" actually have asthma. Ask about seasonal allergies. Did she just get a new pet? Did she move into a new dorm room? Ask about family history of asthma and atopy. Is she using aspirin for sore joints after hard basketball workouts? Has she started smoking or experimenting with other inhaled drugs? Her answers give you a better understanding of her disease so that you can begin to classify severity and treat appropriately.

B. *Learning objective: Perform a proper evaluation to diagnose asthma.* History and examination are the best tools for making the diagnosis of asthma and excluding other diagnoses. In addition, obtain spirometry. Repeat the spirometry 10 minutes after an albuterol dose. If spirometry is normal, or less than 12% reversibility is seen with albuterol, repeat these tests right after a practice or on any day when she is feeling poorly. You can also teach her how to use a peak expiratory flow meter and record her morning, prepractice, postpractice, and evening flow rates over a week's time. She can also record symptoms such as nighttime awakenings. Review the diary together.

C. *Learning objective: Choose appropriate asthma therapy.* Appropriate evaluation allows you to classify asthma severity. Even if she only has exercise-induced asthma, if she is working out more than 2 times a week, she will be classified as having persistent asthma. Modify precipitants as the first treatment step, although it would be difficult to tell her to stop exercising. Counsel about stopping aspirin or other NSAIDs. Suggest 2 to 4 puffs of albuterol before working out. Also, prescribe albuterol to be used as needed. Begin a "controller" therapy, such as inhaled triamcinolone at a dose of 4 puffs bid. Reevaluate her in a few weeks and make adjustments as necessary. Also, make sure she learns correct technique in using her inhalers.

33-2. **A.** *Learning objective: Recognize that asthma can be fatal and design immediate intervention.* This is a patient with an acute asthma exacerbation. Her ability to speak only in short sentences is an early sign of impending respiratory failure. Instruct her to take 60 mg of prednisone at home if she has some and to go to an ER immediately. She should not drive herself, and an emergency medical technician can be called if necessary.

B. *Learning objective: State the evaluation and treatment for acute asthma exacerbation.* Check vital signs, and give prednisone or methylprednisolone and continuous albuterol via nebulizer. Follow serial vital signs, including pulsus paradoxus. Look for use of accessory muscles of respiration and paradoxical abdominal motion. Listen to the lungs for air movement, wheezing, and the inspiratory-to-expiratory (I:E) ratio. Although it sounds like a URI is the most likely precipitant, consider getting a chest x-ray to look for signs of pneumonia. Sputum can be thick and greenish even in the absence of infection, but a sputum culture can be helpful. ABG may also be helpful. Watch for trends in vital signs and examination. Any sign of worsening is an indication for immediate hospitalization, preferably to an ICU.

C. *Learning objective: Recognize respiratory failure as an indication for hospitalization in severe asthma exacerbations.* Common signs of impending respiratory failure include presence of a widening pulsus paradoxus, decrease in respiratory rate or use of accessory muscles, which suggests fatigue, and prolongation of the expiratory phase. Wheezing is often a difficult sign to interpret because a patient who has compromised air movement may have no wheezing but as she improves, diffuse wheezing may appear. If hypoxemia or hypercarbia is found on the ABG, hospitalization is prudent. It is important to recognize early respiratory failure and intubate with mechanical ventilation in a controlled setting, not after the patient exhibits hemodynamic compromise. Signs of respiratory failure are clear indications for immediate hospitalization. Otherwise, observe for 3 to 4 hours. If no improvement is seen, hospitalization is indicated. If improvement is observed, continued observation for a few more hours may be warranted.

CHRONIC OBSTRUCTIVE PULMONARY DISEASE

33-3. **A. Learning objective: Recognize that emphysema is a tissue diagnosis, and use PFTs to assess degree of functional obstructive pulmonary disease.** Emphysema is a pathologic diagnosis that requires a tissue biopsy, which is invasive and unnecessary in most patients. The tissue changes seen with emphysema cause loss of lung elasticity with loss of airway tethering. These changes lead to chronic airway obstruction by allowing collapse of medium airways (worse with expiration), trapping of air in distal airways, and lung hyperinflation. A diagnosis of COPD can be suggested by symptoms of dyspnea and chronic cough. Pulmonary function tests confirm the diagnosis of airway obstruction if FEV_1 and FEV_1/FVC ratio are less than 80% predicted. PFTs also reflect air trapping by showing increased total and residual lung volumes.

B. Learning objective: Obtain a history to diagnose chronic bronchitis. Determine if chronic productive cough occurs on most days for at least 3 months per year over at least 2 successive years to confirm a clinical diagnosis of chronic bronchitis.

C. Learning objective: State a differential diagnosis of clubbing, and recognize that emphysema does not cause clubbing. Emphysema does not cause clubbing. Clubbing usually accompanies inflammatory lung processes, such as chronic bronchitis, bronchiectasis (dilation and thickening of airways caused by chronic infection), pulmonary fibrosis, and lung cancer. Other systemic diseases that can cause clubbing include inflammatory bowel disease, thyroid disease, and congenital cyanotic heart disease. We may find that this patient has chronic bronchitis if we probe more carefully for historical information. However, with his 40 years of heavy smoking, his clubbing raises concern about a possible lung cancer.

D. Learning objective: Describe chest x-ray findings suggesting emphysema. Chest x-ray findings suggestive (but not diagnostic) of emphysema include hyperinflated lungs, flattened diaphragms, increased retrosternal air (seen on AP film), and bullous disease (pockets of dark air representing space in the lung tissue resulting from parenchymal loss).

E. Learning objective: Design a workup to establish severity of disease and rule out lung cancer in a heavy smoker with clubbing and back pain. O_2 saturation cannot assess degree of CO_2 retention. ABG is required to determine pH and degree of CO_2 retention to see how far he is from a baseline compensated state. With back pain and clubbing, obtain a chest x-ray to look for tumor. PFTs help assess severity of obstruction. Obtain spine imaging to investigate back pain. Order CBC: elevated hematocrit is expected because of rise in erythropoietin from chronic hypoxia; normal or low hematocrit raises concern for cancer. Electrolytes, BUN, creatinine, magnesium, calcium, and LFTs might all provide useful baseline information. His workup reveals an O_2 saturation of 89% on room air, ABG = 7.39, P_{CO_2} = 50, P_{O_2} = 60, bicarbonate = 30, FEV_1 = 1 L, and $FEV1/FVC$ = 60% predicted. Chest x-ray shows hyperinflation, flattened diaphragms, multiple bulla, and a right upper lobe 2-cm nodule.

F. Learning objective: List therapies for chronic COPD. Because pH is essentially normal, he is likely at baseline without exacerbation of severe COPD. Treat with smoking cessation efforts, ipratropium bromide, and albuterol, and consider steroids and theophylline. Home oxygen is warranted once PaO_2 is less than 55. Lung reduction surgery or transplantation may be beneficial, although they are unlikely to be offered before the cause of his lung nodule is resolved.

PULMONARY EMBOLISM

33-4.   **A. *Learning objective: Recognize the clinical picture of PE, and list other plausible diagnoses.*** This woman's case is classic for PE. She has at least one of the three risk factors (stasis from a recent long plane ride), classic symptoms of dyspnea, pleuritic CP, hemoptysis, physical examination with evidence of elevated right heart pressures (elevated JVP and accentuated S_2), a swollen lower extremity, and atrial fibrillation. Your differential should include PE, pneumonia, TB, CHF (especially right-sided with elevated JVP and clear lungs), cardiac ischemia, pneumothorax, pericarditis, and tamponade.

B. *Learning objective: Design an appropriate workup for a patient with suspected PE.* Obtain chest x-ray, ABG with calculation of A-a gradient, V/Q scan, and leg Doppler (document site, extent, rule out extravascular compressing lesion), and consider workup for hypercoagulability, including a careful review of symptoms for signs of tumor. Confirm that she is up to date with primary care screening. Draw blood tests before initiating anticoagulation: hematocrit and platelet count to establish a baseline for subsequent problems on anticoagulation, PT, PTT, chemistry panel, pregnancy test, and levels of endogenous anticoagulants AT-III, protein C, protein S, and factor V Leiden. Stool guaiacs should be obtained to rule out an occult GI hemorrhage before starting anticoagulation. If the V/Q scan is low probability and your clinical suspicion is high, these patients still have a 40% likelihood of having a PE. Doppler may confirm clot and allow you to avoid angiogram. Otherwise, pulmonary angiogram may be required to nail down the diagnosis of PE. This patient has a high-probability V/Q scan, allowing you to anticoagulate without an angiogram.

C. *Learning objective: Outline appropriate therapy for PE in a hemodynamically stable patient.* Give oxygen, and monitor O_2 saturation frequently. Start IV heparin as soon as possible to prevent clot propagation with a bolus of 80 U/kg (based on ideal body weight) and continuous infusion of 18 U/kg/hr. Ideally, this regimen should give her a therapeutic PTT of 2 to 2½ times normal after 6 hours. Follow PTT every 6 hours until stable with adjustments to the heparin infusion rate to keep PTT therapeutic. She will need oral warfarin therapy for 6 months, starting as soon PTT is therapeutic. Patients have a widely varying response to warfarin, and clinicians vary on how aggressively they load the drug. An aggressive schedule for loading warfarin is 10 mg a day for 1 to 2 days, then 5 mg a day with adjustments made to keep the PT INR between 2.0 and 3.0. A less aggressive regimen may start with 5 mg qd. Aggressive regimens may overshoot your INR goal, whereas less aggressive regimens may take longer. Heparin and warfarin should overlap, even if a therapeutic PT is attained sooner, because warfarin can cause an imbalance of procoagulant and anticoagulant factors resulting from the different half-lives, potentially increasing coagulability during the its first 5 days. She needs frequent PT checks, initially daily until her INR is therapeutic, then at decreasing intervals. She needs nutrition counseling about how to manage vitamin K–containing foods and education about potential drug interactions. She should wear a medical bracelet stating that she takes warfarin.

D. *Learning objective: Evaluate and treat a patient with hemodynamically unstable PE.* Her symptoms are worrisome for hemodynamically unstable, massive PE. Quickly obtain vital signs, which in her case are BP 80/50, HR 160, JVP > 10 cm, and oxygen saturation of 70% on 6 L of oxygen. Secure ABCs (airway, breathing, and circulation), and call for help! Give 100% oxygen and resuscitate with normal saline bolus to raise blood pressure. Add dopamine if necessary to support blood pressure. Discuss with consultants whether to use thrombolytics or refer for surgical embolectomy.

GOUT

34-1. ***Learning objective: Choose appropriate therapy for acute gout with attention to risk factors.*** This patient has an acute attack of gout. The therapy choices are complicated by his renal insufficiency and diabetes. He should not receive NSAIDs or high-dose colchicine because of his renal insufficiency. Steroid treatment would likely markedly raise his blood sugars, which appear under poor control (Hgb$_{alc}$ 10 + random glucose 350). An intraarticular injection of corticosteroids is the best option.

RHEUMATOID ARTHRITIS

34-2. **A.** ***Learning objective: Recognize early manifestations of rheumatoid arthritis, and list other disorders that might mimic RA.*** Rheumatoid arthritis is the most likely diagnosis, but patients with systemic lupus erythematosus may have similar presentation. Presence of objective joint swelling rules out fibromyalgia alone as the cause of her symptoms. Duration of symptoms rules out viral disorders associated with arthritis, such as parvovirus B19.

B. ***Learning objective: Order appropriate laboratory tests in a patient newly diagnosed with rheumatoid arthritis.*** A CBC is indicated because some patients may manifest anemia as part of rheumatoid arthritis. The sedimentation rate may be elevated, but a normal ESR does not rule out RA. Rheumatoid factor is indicated. This test is more for prognostic value than diagnosis because many other disorders can have rheumatoid factor. High titers of rheumatoid factor are associated with a worse prognosis; in particular, worse joint disease and risk of extra articular features, such as vasculitis. A high titer of ANA with a negative or slightly positive RF would point more to the diagnosis of SLE. X-rays of the hands in early rheumatoid arthritis are usually normal except for juxtaarticular osteopenia. In early more aggressive disease, marginal joint erosions may be present.

C. ***Learning objective: Recognize the importance of early treatment of rheumatoid arthritis.*** In a patient with active synovitis and positive rheumatoid factor, early treatment is important. Patients are usually initially placed on hydroxychloroquine followed immediately by methotrexate given once per week. An NSAID may give symptomatic relief but will not halt joint destruction.

34-3. **A.** ***Learning objective: Recognize extraarticular manifestations of rheumatoid arthritis.*** Patients with rheumatoid arthritis may develop extraarticular manifestations, such as rheumatoid vasculitis; peripheral neuropathy often secondary to vasculitis; compression neuropathies, such as carpal tunnel syndrome; rheumatoid nodules, including pulmonary nodules; or Felty's syndrome, characterized by leukopenia and splenomegaly. This patient has a neuropathy secondary to rheumatoid vasculitis. Extraarticular manifestations including vasculitis are usually associated with high titers of rheumatoid factor. In the differential diagnosis, footdrop is a peroneal nerve compression caused by prolonged crossing of the legs or radiculopathy.

B. ***Learning objective: Order appropriate tests for a new, significant neuropathy.*** Nerve conduction test distinguishes a vasculitic neuropathy from a compression syndrome neuropathy. ESR is usually elevated in these patients, and the rheumatoid factor is generally strongly positive.

C. ***Learning objective: Choose appropriate treatment for this disorder.*** Treat patients with neuropathy secondary to rheumatoid vasculitis with prednisone 50 mg/day and cyclophosphamide 1 to 2 mg/kg/day. Prednisone is gradually reduced. After 3 months of cyclophosphamide treatment, azathioprine can be substituted.

SYSTEMIC LUPUS ERYTHEMATOSUS

34-4. **A. *Learning objective: State the common causes of polyarticular symmetric inflammatory arthritis, and recognize other features suggestive of lupus.*** Possible causes of her polyarticular symmetric joint inflammation include postviral, SLE, RA, or psoriatic or reactive arthritis. Other features of her presentation (oral ulcers, photosensitivity, pleuritis, spontaneous abortion) are suggestive of lupus and are not characteristic of the other conditions on this list.

B. *Learning objective: State the diagnostic criteria for lupus.* This patient meets five criteria for lupus: oral ulcers, arthritis, photosensitivity, malar rash, and probable serositis (episodes of chest pain). If ANA is positive, lupus is a nearly certain diagnosis.

C. *Learning objective: Order appropriate laboratory tests to evaluate a patient with probable lupus.* Order ANA with autoantibody reflexive panel, CBC with differential, PTT, ESR, complement levels (C3, C4, and CH50), RPR or VDRL, BUN, creatinine, and urinalysis. A positive ANA and anti–double-stranded DNA, in combination with her symptoms, make lupus nearly certain. Low complement levels and an elevated ESR suggest disease activity. Elevated BUN and creatinine or active urine sediment indicate renal involvement. Prolonged PTT or falsely positive VDRL or RPR suggests antiphospholipid antibody syndrome. Complete blood count is important to detect thrombocytopenia, anemia, and leukopenia (treatable complications of lupus). She has a positive ANA and anti–double-stranded DNA, ESR of 50, and low complement level.

D. *Learning objective: Design appropriate therapy for mild lupus.* In choosing therapy, you must balance the risks and benefits of each medication. Because this patient has relatively mild disease (i.e., no serious or life-threatening organ involvement, such as rapidly progressing renal disease or CNS involvement), start with an NSAID and hydroxychloroquine (the least toxic medications). If she does not improve, consider adding low-dose steroids.

VASCULITIS

34-5. **A. *Learning objective: Recognize the presentation of giant cell arteritis.*** The most likely diagnosis is giant cell arteritis, given the patient's age, morning shoulder stiffness and pain, (likely temporal) headache, and jaw claudication.

B. *Learning objective: Order appropriate diagnostic tests for temporal arteritis.* She needs an ESR to confirm the inflammatory nature of her symptoms and a temporal artery biopsy.

C. *Learning objective: Appropriately treat giant cell arteritis.* Prednisone in a dose of 40 to 60 mg/day is the usual therapy given to prevent blindness. People with jaw claudication are at increased risk of visual changes that can be permanent; some physicians add low-dose aspirin to the regimen at least initially.

ALCOHOL

35-1. **A. *Learning objective: State the common causes of abdominal pain associated with alcohol use.*** Nausea, vomiting, low-grade fevers, and abdominal pain are likely caused by alcoholic hepatitis. Pancreatitis is also possible. Gastritis from alcohol use is less likely.

B. *Learning objective: Order appropriate tests for evaluating abdominal pain in a patient with history of alcohol abuse.* Order transaminases, bilirubin, amylase, alkaline phosphatase, and a CBC. If he has alcoholic hepatitis, expect his AST to be 2 to 3 times greater than his ALT. Pancreatic amylase would be elevated if he has pancreatitis. Checking a CBC looks for a low hematocrit (GI tract bleeding) and an elevated WBC (seen with alcoholic hepatitis and pancreatitis). Consider a chest x-ray to look for aspiration pneumonia.

C. *Learning objective: State the common electrolyte disorders associated with heavy alcohol use.* Low magnesium, calcium, potassium, and phosphate levels are likely in the setting of chronic alcohol use.

35-2.   **A.** *Learning objective: Recognize alcoholic ketoacidosis.* This patient has an anion gap acidosis in the setting of heavy alcohol use. Consider an ingestion of methanol or ethylene glycol in addition to alcoholic ketoacidosis in your differential. The lack of an osmolal gap makes those ingestions unlikely. Treat alcoholic ketoacidosis with fluid resuscitation containing glucose. Remember to check a magnesium level, replace electrolytes, and give thiamine and a multivitamin with folate.

B. *Learning objective: Treat alcohol withdrawal appropriately.* He should receive benzodiazepines in adequate doses, which may require dosing every 2 to 4 hours initially. He would probably also benefit from a β-blocker because he is tachycardic and hypertensive.

COCAINE, HEROIN, AND PARENTERAL DRUG USE

35-3.   **A.** *Learning objective: Evaluate chest pain in the setting of cocaine ingestion.* Confirming the history of cocaine use, either by the patient's account or by urine drug testing, is essential. The usual cardiac risk factors should be sought. You should obtain an electrocardiogram and cardiac enzymes. Cocaine-associated chest pain may be due to hypertension and vasospasm, and when these are relieved, the chest pain resolves. However, there may also be myocardial damage and coronary thrombosis, which need to be aggressively treated.

B. *Learning objective: Treat myocardial infarction in the setting of cocaine use.* IV diazepam alone may decrease blood pressure, tachycardia, vasospasm, and anxiety enough to relieve cocaine-associated chest pain. However, if the pain cannot be relieved, the electrocardiogram shows ischemic changes, or the cardiac enzymes are positive, the patient must be treated like any patient with unstable angina or acute myocardial infarction. This treatment includes oxygen, aspirin, heparin, nitrates, morphine, blood pressure control (although pure β-blockers should be avoided when cocaine is present due to unopposed alpha effects), and consideration of thrombolytics or urgent revascularization.

C. *Learning objective: Triage a patient with transient chest pain vs. ongoing myocardial ischemia.* Patients with cocaine-associated chest pain or hypertension with symptoms that resolve with diazepam and who do not have electrocardiogram changes or cardiac enzyme elevations may be safely discharged. Patients who require the interventions described above need admission to a coronary care unit.

35-4.   **A. *Learning objective: Assess an unconscious patient.*** The small pupils and known drug abuse suggest heroin overdose in this case. Provide oxygen and make sure the airway is open while you prepare to administer naloxone, 0.4 mg IV. A bedside glucose measurement can be done at the same time because hypoglycemia presents the same way and can be reversed immediately with glucose. Continue to monitor the patient's respirations; if she is not breathing effectively, she may need to be intubated.

B. *Learning objective: Recognize problems other than overdose that may cause unconsciousness in drug users.* A patient who does not regain consciousness after naloxone may have a myriad of other problems. First reassess the airway and vital signs. Multiple doses of naloxone can be safely tried because larger doses of narcotic need larger doses of naloxone to reverse them. Consider a head CT because brain injury, stroke, hemorrhage, septic brain emboli, and brain abscess can present with obtundation. The patient may have had a seizure and now may be in a postictal state; past history from the family could point in this direction. Intoxication with alcohol, benzodiazepines, barbiturates, tricyclic antidepressants, or carbon monoxide should be considered. The patient may be septic or suffering a massive myocardial infarction. Finally, the patient may be in the "crash" phase of cocaine or methamphetamine use, but this is a difficult diagnosis to confirm and thus the more serious causes of obtundation need to be considered.

ABNORMAL PAP SMEARS

36-1.   **A. *Learning objective: Correctly interpret Pap results, and refer any patient with dysplasia for colposcopy.*** Because the Pap test is a cytologic examination of the cells on the surface of the cervix, signs of dysplasia on Pap testing must be confirmed by tissue biopsy; this is performed during colposcopy. Although this patient may consult a gynecologic oncologist if she wishes, her management would still consist of colposcopy first.

B. *Learning objective: State the association between HPV and cervical dysplasia.* HPV is strongly associated with high-grade SIL or cervical cancer in up to 90% of cases. Certain strains of HPV, such as HPV-16 and HPV-18, have been associated with development of invasive cervical cancer. HPV subtyping is not currently widely used in clinical practice. Cervical atypia is considered precancerous, and thus it is advisable to treat the recurrence of this patient's HPV. However, it is important to recognize that complete eradication is seldom sustained, and that in the future, prognostic information based on HPV subtyping may become available to guide management in such patients.

ABNORMAL UTERINE BLEEDING

36-2.   **A. *Learning objective: Identify and diagnose polycystic ovarian syndrome.*** This patient's primary oligomenorrhea, hirsutism, obesity, and acanthosis nigricans are strongly suggestive of polycystic ovarian syndrome (PCOS). This is a poorly understood condition with heterogenous presentation. Despite the suggestive name, the anatomic finding of polycystic ovaries is variably present. There is a significant degree of controversy regarding the basic pathophysiologic mechanism of disease. Most experts agree that there is inappropriate feedback involving the ovarian-pituitary axis, leading to relative hyperandrogenism. An LH-to-FSH ratio of greater than 2:1 can be confirmatory; however, its absence would not rule it out. It is not necessary to perform a pelvic ultrasound. A TSH and prolactin level should also be done to rule out thyroid and pituitary diseases.

B. *Learning objective: Recognize the association of insulin resistance and endometrial cancer in patients with PCOS.* Polycystic ovarian syndrome has been associated with insulin resistance and endometrial cancer. Exclude these by fasting glucose and endometrial monitoring by ultrasound or biopsy (guidelines for frequency or mode of screening do not currently exist).

C. *Learning objective: Prescribe oral contraceptives to prevent unwanted pregnancy, regulate cycles, and prevent atypical endometrial changes.* Amenorrhea or oligomenorrhea can lead to endometrial hyperplasia and atypia. Patients with PCOS should receive oral contraceptive pills to help regulate endometrial shedding; this also protects against pregnancy because infertility cannot be assumed. Patients who do not desire contraception may choose instead to use cyclic medroxyprogesterone to induce menstruation every 3 months.

BREAST HEALTH

36-3.   **A. *Learning objective: Design appropriate workup for a breast lump.*** Order diagnostic mammogram. Unless a clearly benign finding is noted, perform ultrasound and FNA.

B. *Learning objective: Plan followup when workup for a breast lump is negative.* A negative "triple test"—physical examination without suspicious features, negative mammogram, and benign FNA—reduces but does not eliminate the possibility of cancer. Perform followup examinations every 3 to 6 months for at least 1 year to ensure stability.

C. *Learning objective: Recognize indications for referral of patients with abnormal breast findings.* Suspicious mammogram, ultrasound, or FNA should prompt early referral. Referral is also indicated if the mass enlarges over time.

36-4.   **A. *Learning objective: Identify the role of ultrasound in workup of abnormal breast lesions.*** Ultrasound is useful, especially when mammogram is difficult to interpret because of high breast density. Alternately, FNA may reveal a cyst or fibroadenoma.

B. *Learning objective: Appropriately manage a fibroadenoma.* Fibroadenomas are benign, disorganized breast tissue. Indications for removal are size greater than 2 cm, rapid growth, and discomfort.

C. *Learning objective: Appropriately manage a simple breast cyst.* If ultrasound of the mass clearly demonstrates a simple cyst, no further followup is necessary. If the mass is bothersome to the patient or interferes with mammography or physical examination, aspirate under ultrasound guidance.

MENOPAUSE

36-5. **A. Learning objective: Recognize that menopause is a clinical diagnosis.** No further testing is required.

B. Learning objective: Design hormone replacement therapy for a perimenopausal woman. A cyclic regimen might be preferred in women in the transition whose ovaries continue to produce some sex hormones at irregular intervals. It may be possible to regulate cycles with this regimen.

C. Learning objective: Evaluate out-of-phase or prolonged bleeding in a woman on HRT longer than 6 months. Consider an endometrial biopsy or pelvic ultrasound to evaluate the endometrial lining and rule out hyperplasia; malignancy; or structural abnormality, such as polyp or fibroid.

D. Learning objective: Use progestin to stabilize endometrium. If the endometrial biopsy and uterine ultrasound are normal, the next step is to increase progestin to foster transformation of the proliferating endometrium. Alternatively, very-low-dose birth control pills can be used to completely capture cycles and provide regular bleeding.

36-6. **A. Learning objective: Recognize that osteoporosis is generally asymptomatic.** In early osteoporosis, there are no history or examination findings. Advanced disease may be diagnosed on the basis of painful atraumatic fractures or radiologic evidence of vertebral compression fractures. This patient's symptoms are likely attributable to fibromyalgia. A woman's height will normally be reduced over time based on loss of hydration in the vertebral disks.

B. Learning objective: Use DEXA scan as the preferred method to assess bone density. This patient is at increased risk for osteoporosis, given her petite frame, family history, and smoking history. Dual-electron x-ray absorptiometry (DEXA) is currently the most widely available, accurate measure of bone density. Disadvantages to this technique include that bone density is not always equivalent to bone strength and that adjacent calcium deposits may cause an artifactual increase in the reading.

C. Learning objective: State the indications for medical treatment of osteoporosis with bone-building agents. This patient is perimenopausal, and there is no benefit to her taking ERT now, as long as she continues to have regular ovulatory menstrual cycles. She should be encouraged to ensure that she is getting adequate calcium and vitamin D, as well as regular weight-bearing and resistance exercise. Bone-building agents, such as alendronate, are not indicated unless "severe osteoporosis" (i.e., bone density is greater than 2 standard deviations below age-matched mean) or atraumatic fracture is present.

Practice Exam

1. A 50-year-old healthy man has been recently diagnosed with hypertension. Other than his BP of 160/100, he has no concerning findings on physical examination. An ECG, urinalysis, basic chemistry panel, and lipid panel are normal. Despite a 6-month course of nonpharmacologic management, his blood pressure remains elevated. Which class of antihypertensive medication would you choose for treatment based on existing evidence that it decreases morbidity and mortality from hypertension?

   A. Thiazide diuretics
   B. α-Blockers
   C. Calcium channel blockers
   D. Angiotensin-converting enzyme inhibitors
   E. Nitrates

2. A 70-year-old woman with hypertension reports shortness of breath, orthopnea, and paroxysmal nocturnal dyspnea. She denies chest pain or syncope but has a cough producing frothy sputum. On examination, HR is 104, BP 100/76, RR 26, and oxygen saturation is 92% on room air. Her JVP is 14 cm, and she has bibasilar crackles, an S_3, and pitting edema to her knees bilaterally. Which of the following studies would you order next?

   A. Exercise treadmill test
   B. Cardiac catheterization
   C. Echocardiogram
   D. Coxsackie virus titers
   E. Persantine-thallium scan

3. A 59-year-old woman with COPD has been on prednisone 10 mg PO qd for 2 years. Seven days ago, she developed a diarrheal illness that progressed to nausea and vomiting. She has not taken any medications for 3 days because of her nausea. Over the last 24 hours, she has had two syncopal episodes, as well as severe fatigue and weakness. Which of the following laboratory test results would be most consistent with adrenal insufficiency?

   A. Random cortisol of 22 μg/dl
   B. Metabolic alkalosis
   C. Hyperglycemia
   D. Hypokalemia
   E. Hyponatremia

4. A 50-year-old alcoholic person is found lying in an alley. He is brought to the ER, where his alcohol level is three times the legal limit. Additional laboratory tests show a BUN of 71 and creatinine of 4.2, up from his baseline of 1.1. A urine dipstick shows 3+ blood but is otherwise negative. Urine microscopy shows no red or white blood cells but occasional renal tubular cells and muddy brown casts. The cause of his renal failure is most likely:

   A. Hepatitis B
   B. Hypotension
   C. Interstitial nephritis
   D. Rhabdomyolysis
   E. Urinary obstruction

5. A 33-year-old man is referred for a renal artery duplex as a part of a hypertension evaluation. The test comes back positive. The renal artery duplex is highly sensitive (92%) and specific (94%) for renal artery stenosis as a cause of hypertension. The incidence of renal artery stenosis in the population is 2%. Which of the following statements is accurate in interpreting the results of the test for the patient?

   A. The test rules in the diagnosis of renal artery stenosis because of its high sensitivity
   B. The test rules out the diagnosis of renal artery stenosis because of its high specificity
   C. The high sensitivity and specificity reliably predict the accuracy of the diagnosis
   D. The low disease incidence results in a low positive predictive value for the test
   E. The low disease incidence results in a low negative predictive value for the test

6. A 42-year-old woman comes to clinic reporting that she has had three disabling headaches this month. She describes a regular pattern of unilateral throbbing with associated nausea and vomiting. The headache was so disabling that she had to lie down. She is worried that she may have a brain tumor or stroke. What is the most likely cause of this headache?

   A. Subarachnoid hemorrhage
   B. Cluster headache
   C. Tension-type headache
   D. Migraine headache
   E. Brain tumor

7. A sexually active, athletic 23-year-old man comes to clinic with an exquisitely painful right knee. The patient reports that the knee has become progressively more painful over the last day, and he notes swelling and warmth to the touch. Small amounts of knee flexion and extension cause extreme pain. What is the most appropriate initial diagnostic study?

A. Knee films
B. Arthrocentesis
C. Uric acid
D. CBC
E. MRI

8. A 20-year-old college student presents to the student health service with sore throat, low-grade fever, and fatigue. Physical examination reveals bilateral lymphadenopathy of the neck, axilla, and groin. She has previously been in excellent health and denies weight loss or night sweats. CBC and differential show many atypical lymphocytes. What is the most likely cause of this student's illness?

A. Gonorrhea
B. HIV
C. Mononucleosis
D. Hodgkin's disease
E. Herpes simplex virus

9. A 34-year-old man with a long history of alcohol abuse presents to clinic with nausea and abdominal pain. He has been drinking heavily (beer and vodka) for the past 3 weeks but stopped yesterday because of severe pain and nausea. What abnormalities would you expect to see?

A. Low phosphate, high magnesium, low bicarbonate, high amylase, high calcium
B. Low phosphate, low magnesium, low bicarbonate, high amylase, low calcium
C. High phosphate, high magnesium, high bicarbonate, high amylase, low calcium
D. Low phosphate, low magnesium, high bicarbonate, normal amylase, low calcium
E. High phosphate, low magnesium, low bicarbonate, high amylase, high calcium

10. A 72-year-old World War II veteran is hospitalized with congestive heart failure. He develops pain involving the great toe shortly after admission. The toe appears red and warm and is extremely painful to the touch. He informs you that this is probably a recurrence of his gout. Which medication would you choose in initially treating this patient?

A. Indomethacin
B. Prednisone
C. Allopurinol
D. Probenecid
E. Do not treat without arthrocentesis

11. A 45-year-old man comes to clinic for a general physical examination. You note that he was diagnosed with ulcerative colitis at age 25. He reports that he has not had much problem with the colitis over the years. He denies melena, hematochezia, or change in stool pattern. The most appropriate recommendation for colorectal cancer screening in this patient is:

A. Annual digital rectal examination
B. Annual stool occult blood testing
C. Flexible sigmoidoscopy
D. Colonoscopy
E. Delay screening until age 50

12. A 40-year-old woman has a WBC of 40,000 and a high serum leukocyte alkaline phosphatase score. What is the most appropriate next step in her workup?

A. Referral for possible bone marrow transplant
B. Infection workup
C. Begin hydroxyurea
D. Chromosome analysis
E. Bone marrow biopsy

13. A 65-year-old man presents with hemoptysis, dyspnea, and cough. He recently quit smoking. Chest x-ray demonstrates a mediastinal mass. CT scan confirms the mass, and an additional lesion is found in the liver. A biopsy is performed of the mediastinal mass confirming a diagnosis of non–small-cell lung cancer. What is the most appropriate intervention at this point?

A. Begin chemotherapy
B. Referral for surgical resection
C. Biopsy of the liver lesion
D. Further staging, including head CT and bone scan
E. Referral for hospice services

14. An unstable patient is airlifted to your medical center. The referring physician notes that the patient had a metabolic acidosis. The osmolar gap was 15, and oxalate crystals were seen in the urine. The most likely cause of this patient's acidosis is:

A. Uremia
B. Aspirin ingestion
C. Ketoacidosis
D. Sepsis
E. Ethylene glycol ingestion

15. A 43-year-old woman with a 23-year history of type 1 diabetes is seen in clinic with fatigue and postprandial nausea. Laboratory test result are as follows: Na 136, Cl 112, K 5.3, HCO_3 14, BUN 16, Cr 1.3, Glu 146, and Hb_{alc} 6.8. What is the most likely cause for the patient's low HCO_3?

    A. Diabetic ketoacidosis
    B. Renal tubular acidosis
    C. Lactic acidosis
    D. Recurrent vomiting
    E. Aspirin ingestion

16. A 23-year-old man is noted to have sudden onset of nausea, vomiting, and headache. He appears lethargic and has difficulty answering questions. You consider the diagnosis of encephalitis. What is the most appropriate intervention at this point?

    A. Begin IV acyclovir
    B. Lumbar puncture
    C. Head CT
    D. EEG
    E. MRI

17. A 49-year-old man has worsening hypertension over the past 6 months. Home blood pressure readings have been 180-200/100-110. Three years ago, he had a normal blood pressure. His physical examination is unremarkable. Laboratory test results are as follows: Na 138, K 2.9, BUN 10, Cr 1.2, and Glu 90. A renal duplex scan is negative. What would be the best next step?

    A. No testing, treat essential hypertension
    B. Aldosterone/renin ratio
    C. 24-hour urine catecholamines
    D. TSH
    E. Abdominal CT scan

18. A 29-year-old alcoholic patient presents with fever, headache, and mental status changes. His physical examination is significant for nuchal rigidity, a Kernig's sign, and disorientation on mental status examination. Laboratory tests reveal HCT 36, MCV 104, and WBC 23,000. What organism is the most likely cause of his symptoms?

    A. Streptococcus pneumonia
    B. Neisseria meningitides
    C. Haemophilus influenzae
    D. Listeria monocytogenes
    E. Coxsackie virus

19. A 65-year-old smoker has an HDL cholesterol of 30 and an LDL cholesterol of 170. You advise him that his cholesterol is too high and suggest which of the following?

    A. A goal LDL of 160
    B. Step 1 diet with the goal of lowering his cholesterol to 130
    C. Mild-to-moderate consumption of alcohol to raise his HDL cholesterol
    D. A goal LDL cholesterol of 100
    E. Repeat cholesterol screening every 5 years

20. A 72-year-old man with a history of hypertension and hyperlipidemia presents with 4 hours of substernal chest pressure radiating to his left arm. He also reports nausea and sweatiness. On examination, his BP is 100/74, HR is 98, and RR is 22. He is pale and diaphoretic and has a II/VI systolic murmur and clear lungs. An ECG shows normal sinus rhythm with 3-mm ST elevations in leads V2-V4 compared with an ECG 2 months ago that was normal. His chest x-ray shows no infiltrates or cardiomegaly. The most appropriate course of action would be:

    A. Obtain an echocardiogram to evaluate his murmur
    B. Give aspirin and thrombolytics if there are no contraindications
    C. Give aspirin, start heparin and a β-blocker, and rule out for a myocardial infarction
    D. Give aspirin, and start heparin and a calcium channel blocker for unstable angina
    E. Order a ventilation/perfusion scan to evaluate for a pulmonary embolus

21. A 70-year-old woman with a history of advanced osteoarthritis of her knees and hips presents with chest pressure, which occurs with emotional distress and exertion. The chest pressure does not radiate, and she has no associated dyspnea. ECG shows left bundle branch block. What diagnostic test would be most helpful?

    A. Exercise treadmill test
    B. Exercise treadmill with thallium
    C. Echocardiogram
    D. Dipyridamole (Persantine) thallium
    E. Exercise echocardiogram

22. A 44-year-old alcoholic man reports sharp epigastric pain radiating to his back. He has had similar pains in his epigastrium for years that are exacerbated by alcohol use. The patient's current symptoms started after a 7-day binge and have been increasing over the last 3 weeks. Initially the pain was improved by eating but it is now constant. He states that he has also been having loose stools, which are black in color. Which of the following abdominal x-ray findings would be most worrisome given his likely diagnosis?

    A.   Subdiaphragmatic "free" air
    B.   Multiple pancreatic calcifications
    C.   Dilated small bowel with air-fluid levels
    D.   Markedly dilated colon
    E.   Pneumatosis intestinalis (air in the bowel wall)

23. A 50-year-old woman with a history of heavy alcohol use presents to her primary care physician with new onset abdominal swelling. She denies any pain or fever. On physical examination her BP is 96/70, HR is 110, and she has evidence of shifting dullness in the abdomen. The most appropriate way to evaluate the cause of her ascites is:

    A.   Abdominal CT scan
    B.   Abdominal ultrasound
    C.   Pelvic ultrasound
    D.   Paracentesis
    E.   Colonoscopy

24. A 45-year-old man with long-standing cirrhosis resulting from hepatitis B comes to clinic to establish care. He denies any weight loss, abdominal swelling, or pain. Which of the following tumor markers would be the best screen for hepatocellular carcinoma?

    A.   β-HCG
    B.   CEA
    C.   α-Fetoprotein
    D.   CA 125
    E.   BrCA-1

25. A 69-year-old man with a history of COPD is hospitalized in an intensive care unit with respiratory failure. He is on a ventilator for 5 days. On the sixth day, he becomes febrile and a blood culture reveals *Pseudomonas aeruginosa*. Which antibiotic has the best pseudomonal coverage?

    A.   Trimethoprim/sulfamethoxazole
    B.   Ceftriaxone
    C.   Ampicillin/sulbactam
    D.   Ceftazidime
    E.   Vancomycin

26. A 72-year-old man presents for evaluation of his fatigue. He states that he drinks one fifth of whiskey each day and has a poor diet. Laboratory tests show a hematocrit of 28 with an MCV of 109. Which of the following would you expect to see on his peripheral blood smear?

    A.   Schistocytes
    B.   Tear drops
    C.   Döhle bodies
    D.   Hypersegmented neutrophils
    E.   Spherocytes

27. A 40-year-old woman reports a cough for the last 8 months. She does not smoke or take any medications, and she denies fever or hemoptysis. Over the last year, she has gained 20 pounds because her new job does not allow time for exercise. Her cough tends to be worse after dinner and when she is trying to go to sleep at night. She recently stopped drinking alcohol and thinks that the cough improved some after stopping. Which of the following is the most appropriate initial therapy based on her history?

    A.   Azithromycin
    B.   Diphenhydramine
    C.   Nasal steroid spray
    D.   Albuterol metered-dose inhaler
    E.   Omeprazole

28. A 33-year-old woman reports intermittent loose stools for the past year. Her symptoms are associated with crampy abdominal pain and a bloating sensation. Defecation seems to relieve the discomfort. She has not noticed any blood in her stool. When her symptoms are flaring, she sometimes needs to have five to seven bowel movements a day to control the discomfort. Between episodes, however, she is often constipated. The most likely cause of this patient's diarrhea is:

    A.   Inflammatory bowel disease
    B.   Irritable bowel syndrome
    C.   *Giardia lamblia* infection
    D.   Lactose intolerance
    E.   Celiac sprue

29. A 72-year-old woman reports 2 weeks of episodic dizziness. She describes the room "spinning in circles" when she gets in and out of bed or if she looks up towards the ceiling. The episodes typically last less than 2 minutes. She denies any hearing problems or tinnitus. On examination, a Hallpike-Dix maneuver produces rotary nystagmus. The most likely cause of this patient's symptoms is:

    A.   Benign positional vertigo
    B.   Acute labyrinthitis
    C.   Meniere's syndrome
    D.   Brainstem ischemia
    E.   Acoustic neuroma

30. A 58-year-old man with a history of a myocardial infarction presents with light-headedness and palpitations. He takes aspirin and a β-blocker and occasionally needs a sublingual nitroglycerin tablet for exertional chest pain. His rhythm strip is shown below:

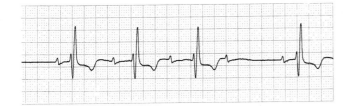

This rhythm is best described as:

A. First-degree AV nodal block
B. Second-degree AV nodal block, Mobitz type I (Wenckebach)
C. Second-degree AV nodal block, Mobitz type II
D. Third-degree nodal block
E. Junctional rhythm

31. A 30-year-old man presents with chest pain. He describes the pain as crushing substernal chest pressure radiating to his left arm. It started 1 hour after eating lunch and is associated with nausea and sweatiness. On examination, he is pale and diaphoretic but has normal vital signs and a normal heart and lung examination. An ECG during the examination is normal, but his pain improves 10 minutes after taking a sublingual nitroglycerin tablet. The most likely cause of this patient's chest pain is:

A. Myocardial infarction
B. Pulmonary embolus
C. Esophageal spasm
D. Aortic dissection
E. Pericarditis

32. A 59-year-old Peruvian woman reports nausea and achy epigastric pain for the last 2 months. She does not drink alcohol or take any medications and has not had any vomiting or diarrhea. A serum *H. pylori* serology is positive. Which of the following causes of dyspepsia will respond to *H. pylori* eradication?

A. Gastroesophageal reflux disease
B. Irritable bowel syndrome
C. Chronic pancreatitis
D. Diabetic gastroparesis
E. Peptic ulcer disease

33. A 31-year-old construction worker reports that she feels tired all the time. She has trouble getting through the workday and worries that she may have a serious illness. Her fatigue has worsened since she was recently promoted to foreman, a job that involves longer work hours and a higher stress level. Which of the following symptoms are concerning for a physical rather than a psychological cause of her fatigue?

A. Symptoms relieved by sleep
B. Symptoms increased during periods of stress
C. Symptoms better later in the day
D. Symptoms for the last 10 months
E. Symptoms that began at the time her father died

34. A 50-year-old woman with long-standing alcohol abuse and cirrhosis presents with hematemesis. Her BP is 120/80, her HR is 95, and she has spider telangiectasias, palmar erythema, and splenomegaly. Her hematocrit is 28. An EGD shows bleeding esophageal varices that are successfully banded. She improves over the next several days in the hospital and is able to be discharged home. In addition to abstinence from alcohol, what is the best prophylaxis against a repeat variceal bleed?

A. Omeprazole
B. Lisinopril
C. Perphenazine
D. Nadolol
E. Cisapride

35. A 31-year-old woman presents with pain and swelling in her wrists and hands. She also has pain in the ball of her foot. She has a history of pneumococcal pneumonia with sepsis 1 year ago and 2 prior spontaneous abortions in the past 4 years. On examination, she has spongy, tender swelling in the wrists and MCP and MTP joints. Laboratory test results are as follows: Hct 33, platelets 114,000, BUN 20, Cr 1.2, and urinalysis 2+ protein with 10-30 red cells/high power field. Which laboratory test is the most likely to confirm a diagnosis?

A. ANA
B. Rheumatoid factor
C. ESR
D. c-ANCA
E. Total complement (CH50)

36. A 40-year-old man presents to establish care. He has no chronic diseases and has had no preventive health screening. Review of systems reveals no concerning symptoms, and his physical examination is normal. Which of the following screening tests would be most appropriate to do in this patient?

A. Prostate-specific antigen
B. *H. pylori* serologies
C. Total cholesterol
D. Fecal occult blood test
E. Flexible sigmoidoscopy

37. A 50-year-old man reports pain in his lower back since lifting a heavy crate. He rested and took ibuprofen without relief. He has restricted his activity and is worried that he may not be able to ski this winter because of his pain. Which of the following would be most concerning for a dangerous cause of this patient's low back pain?

A. New onset of marked constipation
B. No improvement after 1 week of ibuprofen
C. No relief with weekly chiropractic intervention
D. Pain in the lower back with straight leg raise
E. Worsened symptoms after 7 days of bed rest

38. A 43-year-old female IV drug user presents with fever, right upper quadrant pain, and diarrhea. She has been sharing needles but has no history of hepatitis or HIV. On examination, she is jaundiced and has tenderness in her right upper quadrant. Her AST is 468, her ALT is 650, and serologies are consistent with hepatitis B infection. Which of the following statements about hepatitis B virus is most correct?

A. Approximately 80% of patients with hepatitis B develop chronic infection
B. HB_eAg indicates increased infectivity
C. HB_cIgM indicates chronic infection
D. HBV requires coinfection with hepatitis D virus to replicate
E. HBV infection does not respond to α-interferon treatment

39. A 20-year-old man with C3 HIV disease (CD4 count 29/viral load 23,000) returns to clinic for discussion of therapy options. He has previously taken AZT, then ddI monotherapy. He is interested in treatment and has not missed previous clinic visits. What therapy do you recommend?

A. Lamivudine (3TC) + zidovudine (AZT)
B. Stavudine (D4T) + lamivudine (3TC)
C. Indinavir + zidovudine (AZT) + didanosine (ddI)
D. Indinavir + stavudine (D4T) + lamivudine (3TC)
E. Zidovudine (AZT) + stavudine (D4T) + zalcitabine (ddC)

40. A 32-year-old HIV-positive patient reports difficult and painful swallowing for 3 days. Her CD4 count was 100 last month, but she has done well other than occasional oral thrush. She takes trimethoprim/sulfamethoxazole, D4T, 3TC, and nelfinavir. Her examination is remarkable for a temperature of 38.5° C and oral thrush. The most likely cause of this patient's symptoms is:

A. Hairy leukoplakia
B. CMV esophagitis
C. HSV esophagitis
D. Candidal esophagitis
E. d4T-related esophageal ulcerations

41. A 25-year-old woman presents with 4 days of dysuria and frequency. She has had no fevers or flank pain. She has one sexual partner with no new partners in the past 12 months. Physical examination is unremarkable. What test(s) should be ordered?

A. Urinalysis
B. Urinalysis and urine culture
C. Urinalysis, urine culture, and chlamydia culture
D. Urinalysis, urine culture, gonorrhea culture, and chlamydia culture
E. Urine culture

42. A 37-year-old man with C3 HIV disease and a history of IV drug use presents with fever, weight loss, and nonproductive cough. He has adenopathy in the axilla and neck. His chest x-ray shows bilateral hilar and paratracheal adenopathy. No infiltrates are present. What is the most likely cause?

A. *Pneumocystis carinii*
B. Sarcoidosis
C. *Mycobacterium* tuberculosis
D. Endocarditis
E. Persistent generalized lymphadenopathy

43. A 41-year-old man with a long history of recurrent sinusitis reports a new episode of nasal discharge, cough, and fatigue. On physical examination, he has crusted blood in the nares and a tender right maxillary sinus with opacification on transillumination. Chest x-ray reveals bilateral nodules. Laboratory test results are as follows: HCT 33, WBC 10,000, BUN 33, Cr 2.6, and urinalysis shows 2+ protein, 0-3 WBCs, and 30-50 RBCs. What test is the most likely to explain his sinus disease and laboratory findings?

A. ANA
B. Anticardiolipin antibody
C. ESR
D. c-ANCA
E. CEA

44. A 27-year-old elementary school teacher is seen for evaluation of fever and cough. She has had a nonproductive cough for the past 5 days, myalgias, sore throat, and fevers (T_{max} 101.8° F). On examination, she has rhonchi and wheezes in the right lower lobe. Laboratory test results are as follows: WBC 10.8, HCT 37, and chest x-ray shows a subsegmental right lower lobe infiltrate. What is the most likely organism?

A. *Haemophilus influenzae*
B. Influenza A
C. Mixed anaerobes
D. *Mycoplasma pneumoniae*
E. *Streptococcus pneumoniae*

45. A 79-year-old woman presents with fever, nausea, vomiting, jaundice, and right upper quadrant pain. Laboratory test results are as follows: bilirubin 2.5, alkaline phosphatase 360, and WBC 23,000. Ultrasound shows gallstones and dilated common bile duct. What is the most appropriate course of action?

A. Consult surgery for urgent cholecystectomy
B. Treat with IV azithromycin
C. Treat with IV cefazolin
D. Treat with IV ampicillin
E. Consult a gastroenterologist for emergent ERCP

46. A 33-year-old IV drug user presents with 3-day history of cough, fever, and pleuritic chest pain. Cardiac examination reveals a grade II/VI systolic murmur at the sternum, normal skin examination, and bilateral rhonchi on chest auscultation. Chest x-ray shows bilateral, patchy peripheral infiltrates. What test is most important for making a diagnosis?

A. Three sets of blood cultures
B. Chest CT scan
C. Sputum Gram stain
D. Echocardiogram
E. Sputum culture

47. A 33-year-old woman presents with fatigue and weight gain. She reports a family history of hypothyroidism. Which set of clinical features would be most consistent with hypothyroidism?

A. Macroglossia, tachypnea, increased CPK, amenorrhea
B. Amenorrhea, bradycardia, increased cholesterol, cool skin
C. Macroglossia, tachycardia, increased cholesterol, menorrhagia
D. Menorrhagia, increased CPK, increased cholesterol, carpal tunnel syndrome
E. Amenorrhea, decreased cholesterol, bradycardia, macroglossia

48. A 47-year-old obese man presents for annual examination. He reports a family history of type 2 diabetes. A screening fasting blood glucose is 200. He begins a diet, loses 10 pounds over 3 months, and a repeat fasting blood glucose is 160 with a Hb_{alc} of 7.8. Cholesterol is 220 with triglycerides of 400 and HDL 30. What is the best initial therapy for this patient?

A. Insulin
B. Metformin
C. Metformin + sulfonylurea
D. Troglitazone
E. Sulfonylurea + troglitazone

49. A 45-year-old woman with type 1 diabetes for 18 years presents as a new patient for evaluation. Her physical examination is remarkable for nonproliferative diabetic retinopathy and a BP of 146/92. Laboratory test results are as follows: Hgb_{alc} 7.0, BUN 12, Cr 0.8, and urinalysis shows trace protein. What would you recommend for this patient?

A. Follow blood pressure, no treatment at this time
B. Begin hydrochlorothiazide
C. Begin ACE inhibitor
D. Begin calcium channel blocker
E. Begin β-blocker

50. A 34-year-old pregnant woman from Cambodia who is in her second trimester presents with increasing dyspnea on exertion. She has also coughed up occasional bloody sputum. On examination, she has a low-pitched diastolic murmur heard best at the apex. What is the most likely diagnosis?

A. Bacterial pneumonia
B. Primary pulmonary hypertension
C. Aortic regurgitation
D. Aortic stenosis
E. Mitral stenosis

51. A 25-year-old man with HIV infection and a CD4 count of 100 presents with fever, headache, and mild photophobia. Funduscopic examination reveals normal optic disks, and the patient has a nonfocal neurologic examination. Diagnostic evaluation should begin with which of the following?

A. Lumbar puncture
B. Head CT scan
C. Monitor clinical symptoms
D. Begin IV acyclovir
E. Begin IV amphotericin

52. A 54-year-old man presents to the hospital with a 6-month history of fever, night sweats, and weight loss. CT scan reveals evidence of multiple tumors confined above the diaphragm. Biopsy reveals low-grade lymphoma. What is the correct stage of this patient's non-Hodgkin's lymphoma?

A. I
B. IB
C. II
D. IIB
E. IIIB

53. A 55-year-old man with type 2 diabetes reports progressive lower-extremity pain over the last 3 months. The pain is bilateral and varies from a burning pain to an uncomfortable tingling sensation. It started in his feet and has progressed to involve both ankles, as well. The pain is most bothersome at night. On examination, an ankle/brachial index is 1.1 and he has decreased vibration and proprioception in his feet. What is the most likely cause of this patient's leg pain?

A. Peripheral vascular disease
B. Venous obstruction
C. Nocturnal cramps
D. Multiple myeloma
E. Diabetic peripheral neuropathy

54. A 30-year-old female smoker reports 3 days of left lower extremity swelling. She denies any trauma to the leg and states that in the last day it has started aching, as well. She has also developed a low-grade temperature but denies chills, sweats, or rash. Which of the following would increase her risk of deep venous thrombosis the most?

A. Corticosteroid therapy
B. History of asthma
C. History of myocardial infarction
D. History of nephrotic syndrome
E. Laparoscopic cholecystectomy

55. A 31-year-old man undergoes HIV testing because his partner is newly HIV positive; he is found to be HIV positive by ELISA and by Western blot. He has no symptoms, and his examination is normal. Which of the following statements is correct regarding the initial management of this patient?

A. Start azithromycin prophylaxis against *Mycobacterium avium* if his CD count is less than 75
B. Start trimethoprim/sulfamethoxazole prophylaxis against *Pneumocystis* if his CD4 count is less than 500
C. Check an HIV viral load only when the patient becomes symptomatic
D. Start AZT monotherapy if his CD4 count is less than 200
E. Check a p24 antigen to verify the ELISA and Western blot results

Exam Answers

1. A (30, Hypertension)
2. C (23, Congestive Heart Failure)
3. E (25, Adrenal Disorders)
4. D (30, Acute Renal Failure)
5. D (6, How to Interpret Sensitivity and Specificity)
6. D (17, Headache)
7. B (19, Joint Pain)
8. C (22, Lymphadenopathy)
9. B (35, Alcohol)
10. B (34, Gout)
11. D (28, Colon Cancer)
12. B (28, Leukemia)
13. D (28, Lung Cancer)
14. E (30, Acid-Base Disturbances)
15. B (30, Acid-Base Disturbances)
16. A (29, Encephalitis)
17. B (30, Hypertension)
18. A (29, Meningitis)
19. B (25, Hyperlipidemia)
20. B (23, Ischemic Heart Disease)
21. D (23, Ischemic Heart Disease)
22. A (6, How to Read an Abdominal Film)
23. D (6, How to Perform Basic Procedures and Body Fluid Analysis)
24. C (6, How to Interpret Abnormal Laboratory Results)
25. D (6, How to Use Antibiotics)
26. D (8, Anemia)
27. E (10, Cough)
28. B (11, Diarrhea)
29. A (12, Dizziness and Syncope)
30. B (23, Common Cardiac Arrhythmias)
31. C (9, Chest Pain)
32. E (13, Dyspepsia)
33. A (15, Fatigue)
34. D (16, Gastrointestinal Bleeding)
35. A (34, Systemic Lupus Erythematosus)
36. C (18, Healthy Patients)
37. A (20, Low Back Pain)
38. B (26, Liver Disease)
39. D (29, HIV Infection Primary Care)
40. D (29, HIV Infection Complications)
41. A (29, Urinary Tract Infections)
42. C (29, Tuberculosis)
43. D (34, Vasculitis)
44. D (29, Pneumonia)
45. E (26, Biliary Tract Disease)
46. A (29, Endocarditis)
47. D (25, Thyroid Disease)
48. B (25, Diabetes Mellitus)
49. C (25, Diabetes Mellitus)
50. E (23, Valvular Heart Disease)
51. B (29, Meningitis)
52. D (28, Non-Hodgkin's Lymphoma)
53. E (21, Lower Extremity Problems)
54. D (21, Lower Extremity Problems)
55. A (29, HIV Infection Primary Care)

Index

Page numbers in italics indicate illustrations; *t* indicates tables.

Abbreviation	Term
ABCs	airway, breathing, circulation
ABG	arterial blood gas
ABPA	allergic bronchopulmonary aspergillosis
ACEI	angiotensin-converting enzyme inhibitor
ACTH	adrenocorticotropic hormone
ADH	antidiuretic hormone
AFB	acid-fast bacilli, usually a mycobacterium species
AFP	alpha-fetoprotein
AI	aortic insufficiency, also called aortic regurgitation
AICD	automatic implantable cardiac defibrillating device
AIDS	acquired immunodeficiency syndrome
AIN	acute interstitial nephritis
ALL	acute lymphocytic leukemia
ALT	alanine aminotransaminase, same as SGPT
AML	acute myelogenous leukemia, exists as types 1-7
ANA	antinuclear antibody
ANCA	antineutrophil cytoplasmic antibody, may be "c" for cytoplasmic or "p" for perinuclear pattern
AP	anterior-posterior, usually in reference to direction x-ray beam travels through body
APAS	antiphospholipid antibody syndrome
ARF	acute renal failure
AS	aortic stenosis
ASA	acetylsalicylic acid (aspirin)
AST	aspartate aminotransaminase, same as SGOT
ATN	acute tubular necrosis
AV	atrioventricular
AVNRT	AV node reentrant tachycardia
BCC	basal cell carcinoma
β-HCG	human chorionic gonadotropin, beta subunit
bid	twice a day
BMD	bone mineral density
BPH	benign prostatic hyperplasia
BPV	benign positional vertigo
BRCA	gene mutation that increases risk of breast and other cancers
BUN	blood urea nitrogen
Ca	calcium
CABG	coronary artery bypass graft (pronounced "cabbage")
CAD	coronary artery disease
CBC	complete blood count
CEA	carcinoembryonic antigen
chemistry panel	sodium, potassium, chloride, bicarbonate, BUN, creatinine, glucose
CHF	congestive heart failure
CLL	chronic lymphocytic leukemia
CML	chronic myelogenous leukemia
CMV	cytomegalovirus
CNS	central nervous system
COPD	chronic obstructive pulmonary disease
CPK	creatine phosphokinase
CPR	cardiopulmonary resuscitation
CSF	cerebrospinal fluid
CT	*Chlamydia trachomatis*
CT	computed tomography, "cat" scan
CVA	cerebrovascular accident, also called stroke
CXR	chest x-ray
D5½NS	IV solution with 5% glucose in ½ normal saline
D5NS	IV solution with 5% glucose in normal saline
D5W	IV solution with 5% glucose in water
DEXA scan	dual electron x-ray absorptiometry, bone density test
DHT	dihydrotestosterone
DIC	disseminated intravascular coagulopathy
DM	diabetes mellitus (type 1 or 2)
DMARD	disease-modifying antirheumatic drug
DNR	do not resuscitate
DUB	dysfunctional uterine bleeding
DVT	deep venous thrombosis
ECG	eletrocardiogram
echo	echocardiogram
EEG	electroencephalogram
EF	ejection fraction
EGD	esophagogastroduodenoscopy
EMG	electromyogram
ER	emergency room
ER	estrogen receptors, present on some breast cancer cells
ERCP	endoscopic retrograde cholangiopancreatogram
ERT	estrogen replacement therapy
ESLD	end stage liver disease
ESR	erythrocyte sedimentation rate
ESRD	end stage renal disease
ETT	exercise treadmill test
FeNa	fractional excretion of sodium
FEV$_1$	forced expiratory volume in one second
FFP	fresh frozen plasma
FMP	final menstrual period
FNA	fine-needle aspirate
FOBT	fecal occult blood testing
FSH	follicle-stimulating hormone
FVC	forced vital capacity
GC	gonorrhea
GERD	gastroesophageal reflux disease
GGT	serum gamma-glutamyltransferase
GI	gastrointestinal
GU	genitourinary tract or system
HBV	hepatitis B virus
HCV	hepatitis C virus
HDL	high-density lipoprotein, "good" cholesterol
HgbA$_{1c}$	hemoglobin AIC, or glycohemoglobin, reflects average blood glucose over past 3 months
HIT	heparin-induced thrombocytopenia
HITT	HIT-associated thrombosis
HIV	human immunodeficiency virus
HL	hairy leukoplakia
HMG CoA reductase inhibitor	3-hydroxy-3-methylglutaryl coenzyme A reductase inhibitor, also called "statins," used to reduce cholesterol
HPV	human papilloma virus
HRT	hormone replacement therapy
HSP	Henoch-Schönlein purpura
HSV	herpes simplex virus
HTN	hypertension
HZV	herpes zoster virus
IBD	inflammatory bowel disease
IBS	irritable bowel syndrome
ICU	intensive care unit
INH	isoniazid
INR	international normalized ratio, a standardized prothrombin time
ITP	immune thrombocytopenic purpura
IUD	intrauterine device
IV	intravenous
IVIG	intravenous immunoglobulin
JVD	jugular venous distension
JVP	jugular venous pressure
K	potassium
KOH	potassium hydroxide
KS	Kaposi's sarcoma
LCR	ligase chain reaction
LDH	lactate dehydrogenase
LDL	low-density lipoprotein, "bad" cholesterol
LFTs	liver function tests
LH	luteinizing hormone
LLQ	left lower quadrant
LMWH	low-molecular-weight heparin
LP	lumbar puncture
LS-spine	lumbosacral spine radiograph
LUQ	left upper quadrant
LV	left ventricle
MAC	*Mycobacterium avium* complex
MAT	multifocal atrial tachycardia
MCP	metacarpophalangeal joint
MCV	mean corpuscular volume
MDI	metered-dose inhaler
MEN	multiple endocrine neoplasia
Mg	magnesium
MI	myocardial infarction
MMSE	mini-mental status exam
MR	mitral regurgitation
MRI	magnetic resonance imaging
MS	mitral stenosis
MTP	metatarsophalangeal joint
Na	sodium
NG	nasogastric tube
NHL	non-Hodgkin's lymphoma
NPV	negative predictive value
NSAID	nonsteroidal antiinflammatory drug
NSCLC	non–small-cell lung cancer
OA	osteoarthritis
OHL	oral hairy leukoplakia
OR	operating room
PA	pulmonary artery
PA	posterior-anterior, usually in reference to direction x-ray beam travels through body
PAC	premature atrial contraction
PA-gram	pulmonary arteriogram
PAN	polyarteritis nodosa
PCN	penicillin
PCOS	polycystic ovary syndrome
PCP	*Pneumocystis carinii* pneumonia
PCR	polymerase chain reaction
PE	pulmonary embolism
PEEP	positive end expiratory pressure
PEFR	peak expiratory flow rate
PFT	pulmonary function test
PHN	postherpetic neuralgia
Phos	phosphorous
PID	pelvic inflammatory disease
PMI	point of maximal impulse (of the heart against the chest wall)
PML	progressive multifocal leukoencephalopathy
PMN	polymorphonuclear cell, neutrophil
PMR	polymyalgia rheumatica
PN	peripheral neuropathy
PND	postnasal drip or paroxysmal nocturnal dyspnea
PO	to take by mouth
PPV	positive predictive value

Abbreviation	Term	Abbreviation	Term	Abbreviation	Term
PR	to take by rectum	SA node	sinoatrial node	Td	tetanus booster
PSA	prostate-specific antigen	SAAG	serum to ascites albumin gradient, diagnoses portal hypertension when >1.1	TG	triglycerides
PSC	primary sclerosing cholangitis			TIA	transient ischemic attack
PT	protime			TIBC	total iron-binding capacity
PTCA	percutaneous transluminal coronary angioplasty (pronounced "pizza")	SAH	subarachnoid hemorrhage	tid	three times a day
		SBE	subacute bacterial endocarditis	TIPS	transjugular intrahepatic portocaval shunt
PTH	parathyroid hormone	SBP	spontaneous bacterial peritonitis	tPA	tissue plasminogen activator, used as a thrombolytic
PTT	prothombin time	SCC	squamous cell carcinoma		
PUD	peptic ulcer disease	SCLC	small-cell lung cancer		
PVC	premature ventricular contraction	SERM	selective estrogen receptor modulator	TSH	thyroid-stimulating hormone
PVD	peripheral vascular disease			TURP	transurethral resection of the prostate
PVR	postvoid residual	SGOT	serum glutamic-oxaloacetic transaminase, same as AST		
qd	once a day			UA	urinalysis
qid	four times a day	SGPT	serum glutamic-pyruvic transaminase, same as ALT	UGIB	upper GI bleed
RA	rheumatoid arthritis			URI	upper respiratory infection
RBC	red blood cells	SIADH	syndrome of inappropriate ADH secretion	US	ultrasound
RES	reticuloendothelial system			USPSTF	U.S. Preventive Services Task Force
RF	rheumatoid factor, serum test for rheumatoid arthritis	SIL	squamous intraepithelial lesion (of the cervix)	UTI	urinary tract infection (cystitis or pyelonephritis)
RLQ	right lower quadrant	SLE	systemic lupus erythematosus	V/Q	ventilation perfusion lung scan (looking for PE)
ROM	range of motion	SPEP	serum protein electrophoresis		
RPR	rapid plasma reagin, test for syphilis	SSRI	selective serotonin reuptake inhibitor antidepressant	VDRL	Venereal Disease Research Laboratory, a test for syphilis
RR	respiratory rate				
RTA	renal tubular acidosis	STD	sexually transmitted disease	VF	ventricular fibrillation
RUQ	right upper quadrant	SVT	supraventricular tachycardia	VSD	ventricular septal defect
RV	right ventricle	TA	temporal arteritis	VT	ventricular tachycardia
S1, S2, S3, S4	heart sounds 1 through 4	TB	tuberculosis	vWD	von Willebrand's disease
		TCA	tricyclic antidepressant	WBC	white blood cells

Formulas

Fractional excretion of sodium:

$$\text{FeNa} = \frac{Cr^s \times Na^u}{Cr^u \times Na^s} \times 100$$

Creatinine clearance:

$$\text{CrCl} = \frac{(140 - \text{age}) \times \text{ideal weight (kg)}}{72 \times (\text{serum creatinine})}$$

Osmolal gap:

$$\text{Osm gap} = (\text{measured serum Osms}) - (\text{calculated Osms})$$

Osmolality:

$$\text{Osm} = 2(\text{sodium}) + \text{BUN}/2.8 + \text{glucose}/18$$

Free water deficit:

$$\text{Free water deficit} = [(\text{serum sodium}/140) - 1] \times 0.6 \times \text{weight (kg)}$$

Alveolar oxygen concentration, P_{AO_2}:

$$P_{AO_2} = F_{IO_2}(P_B - 47) - P_{CO_2}/0.8$$
$$= \text{approximately 100 at sea level with normal } P_{CO_2}$$

Where: P_B = atmospheric pressure = 760 mm Hg at sea level
F_{IO_2} = fraction of oxygen in inspired = 0.21 at sea level
P_{AO_2} = arterial oxygen concentration = blood gas P_{O_2}
P_{CO_2} = arterial carbon dioxide concentration

Alveolar-arterial oxygen gradient, A-a gradient:

$$\text{A-a gradient} = P_{AO_2} - P_{aO_2}$$

Laboratory Test	Normal Value*	Laboratory Test	Normal Value*
albumin	3.5-5.2 g/dl	erythrocyte sedimentation rate (ESR)	0-15 mm/hr
alkaline phosphatase	38-172 U/L	glucose (Glu)	62-125 mg/dl
amylase	27-144 U/L	hematocrit (HCT)	36-45% female, 38-50% male
arterial P_{CO_2}	33-48 mm Hg	lactate dehydrogenase (LDH)	0-190 U/L
arterial pH	7.35-7.45	lipase	7-51 U/L
arterial P_{O_2}	70-100 mm Hg	mean corpuscular volume (MCV)	81-98 fl
bicarbonate (HCO₃)	24-31 mEq/L	osmolality (Osms)	280-300 mOsm/kg
bilirubin, direct (conjugated)	0.0-0.3 mg/dl	platelets (PLT)	150,000-400,000/μl
bilirubin, indirect (unconjugated)	0.1-0.7 mg/dl	potassium (K)	3.7-5.2 mEq/L
bilirubin, total	0.1-1.0 mg/dl	SGOT = AST	10-44 U/L
blood urea nitrogen (BUN)	8-21 mg/dl	SGPT = ALT	11-39 U/L
calcium (Ca)	8.9-10.2 mg/dl	sodium (Na)	136-145 mEq/L
chloride (Cl)	98-108 mEq/L	uric acid	2.4-5.7 mg/dl female, 3.4-7.0 mg/dl male
creatine phosphokinase (CPK)	30-285 U/L		
creatinine (Cr)	0.3-1.2 mg/dl	white blood cell count (WBC)	4300-10,000/μl

*Normal values for the University of Washington Medical Center Laboratory.